This book provides the practitioner with ways to measure progress. The author has provided clear user-friendly forms, which delineate the process of progress from dependency to independence. Additionally, the book provides examples of goals and objectives for clients with specific problems. The problem areas are organized around the domains: the cognitive domain, the physical domain and the psychosocial domain. Within each one of these sections, examples of problems, goals, and objectives are provided. Specific activities are analyzed in the book to illustrate how to utilize the measurements towards progress. This method of measurement of progress is what makes this book unique. The tools provided can potentially help recreation providers develop programming, which will address the needs of their clients. The tools and charts in this book will help the practitioner assess individual clients, observe the client's strengths, and plot a course towards independence.

Jeremy Cash, MS in Education, CTRS, Adjunct Professor Lehman College, City University of New York, Adjunct Professor Kean University

This book embraces the concept of successful aging in terms of strategies for coping. Gibson (1995), stated that successful aging "refers to reaching one's potential and arriving at a level of physical, social, and psychological well-being in old age that is pleasing to both self and others." We now embrace a shift from medically not just prolonging life to ensuring that a prolonged life is worth living. Susan Brhel's helpful book gives us a recipe that demonstrates why decline is not inevitable. She carefully compiles components of successful aging. These are outlined as good health, how to avoid risk of disease and disability, high mental and physical functioning and ultimately how to actively engage with life. The book is important as it dispels the aging myths by promoting function.

Susan Henderson, R.P., LCSW/SAP, Clinical Coordinator, Counselor

Six years ago my father-in-law was diagnosed with Alzheimer's. I discovered a great need to improve the quality of life for these patients. Fulfilling their individual needs on a daily basis, Susan has scored a victory for these and all nursing home patients. This book is a must need for every nursing home facility.

Phyllis L. Callaghan, RN, former health consultant for Liberty Mutual Insurance

A caregiver can access information on all aspects of the many-faceted issues of patient-based care in one volume, rather then having to research "a dozen" separate texts.

Carol Potts, L.M.T.

User-friendly, easy-to-follow the step-by-step process of evaluating clients; definitions are easy to understand. Implementation of programs in the health and fitness field would be very beneficial in many areas of care.

Jen Sweeney, Aerobics Coordinator at West Family Y. W. C.A., Johnson City, N.Y.

Susan Brhel

The Bio-Psychosocial Approach to Therapeutic Activities & Successful Aging

A Guide for Professionals
Working with the Geriatric Population

Edited by John Brhel

*G*oals *S*eminars & *C*onsultants
Binghamton, New York

The Bio-Psychosocial Approach to Therapeutic Activities & Successful Aging

A Guide for Professionals Working with the Geriatric Population

by Susan Brhel

Published by Goals Seminars and Consultants
1647 Airport Road
Binghamton, NY 13905
USA

Jacket designed by Christine McCord

ISBN 10: 0-9779214-0-9
ISBN 13: 978-0-9779214-0-9

Printed in the United States of America

This book is dedicated to all people who promote the quality of living
of older adults through research, education, and all aspects of quality care.

BRIEF TABLE OF CONTENTS

EXTENDED TABLE OF CONTENTS

Figures

Activities Charts and Tables

FOREWORD

Ongoing research continues to validate the necessary intricate balance for both quality of life and longevity goals found in elders who stay active through the use of physical, cognitive, and psychosocial activities.

Medical researchers mindful of the surge in baby boomers are actively pursuing the need for understanding the aging process and addressing health concerns for today's aging population.

Advancements in medical technology, such as the use of PET scans and Magnetic Resonance Imaging, offer a wealth of information on how the body ages, attempts to compensate, and ada-pts, from physical, cognitive and psychosocial standpoints.

The promotion of activities for the older adult's physical health has contributed to better physical health and longevity.

Research and the promotion of activities particularly in the areas of cognitive health continue to show promise to combat cognitive deficits and enhance cognitive well-being.

The promotion of active living and use of activities in support of socio-emotional well being continues to show promise towards physical, psychological, and spiritual welfare.

Those involved in the study of psychology, social sciences and various fields within social agencies are promoting and advocating social policy changes and a higher emphasis on "inclusive services" to continue to seek ways to fully address aging issues.

Psychological studies identify activities and active living as an important factor when addressing various domains within the bio-psychosocial framework and aging issues.

With heightened focus on the bio-psychosocial aspects of aging and quality living in the home or in the nursing home setting, these specialists are looking more closely at the use of therapeutic activities, rehabilitative, and recreational therapy regarding the full spectrum of elder needs and issues.

As a result of research and heightened awareness of a proactive bio-psychosocial approach, higher government standards have been initiated to implement effective therapeutic and activity programs for elders in facility settings.

As medical researchers continue to look at the benefits of activities for their scientific qualities, social agencies address the bio-psychosocial framework and inclusion of therapeutic recreational/activity programs, and government agencies institute therapeutic activities as a quality of life concern, we will continue to recognize the opportunities that can be found in promoting activities/active living.

DISCLAIMER

Every older adult must have an assessment and diagnosis from a physician before engaging in any activity that requires physical exertion; this is imperative to ensure the older adult is indeed capable of such activity. It is also important to use good judgment and monitor the older adults throughout all activities. The author of this book has suggested therapeutic activities for older adults. However, each adult must be assessed and diagnosed by a competent medical professional prior to engaging in any of these activities. Furthermore, all activities must be undertaken with appropriate supervision and safety requirements in place. No activities in this book can substitute the needs of safety protocol for a particular setting, and there is an absolute requirement to follow the state and federal regulations pertaining to safety.

ACKNOWLEDGEMENTS

I would like to thank the following professionals:

Lynn Crummy, for reading a second book and offering valuable recommendations and critical details.

J Crosby, MD, for reading through the medical information and offering critical suggestions.

Liz Carter and Susan Henderson, for their support and help with valuable activities needed for successful aging and its importance in the quality of life and lifespan issues.

Jeremy Cash and Arnie Idelson, for their helpful suggestions and support. I hope that their commitment to the care of older adults and the belief in the power of joyful living, including recreational activities, are reflected in this book.

Dayo Adekoya, for taking the time to read and point out important details the book should cover to be both practical and supportive to those working in the field of occupational therapy.

The staff and residents of HillTop Retirement Center, for allowing me to do research in your facility. Your generosity of time and support allowed me to implement practical use of this program in a nursing facility setting.

John R.Brhel, for editing this book (including the charts) and for helping me to bring this book to completion.

CONSULTANTS

James Crosby, MD – Director of United Health Services Geriatric Fellowship, Assistant Director of Family Practice Residency, Johnson City, NY, Medical Director at Ideal Senior Living Center in Endicott, NY.

Elizabeth Carter – Ph.D. Child and Family Studies, Johnson City, NY.

Lynn Crummy – MS, Physical Therapy, Endicott, NY.

Dayo Adekoya – MS, Occupational Therapist, Johnson City, NY.

Susan Henderson – R. P. LCSW/S.A.P, MSW, Clinical Social Worker.

Jeremy Cash – MS in Education, Adjunct Professor at Lehman College, City University of New York, Adjunct Professor Kean University, Bachelors of Fine Arts, CTRS.

Arnie Idelson – MS in Therapeutic Recreation, BS in Music Therapy, CTRS/ C.M.T, Director of Therapeutic Recreation, Hamilton Park Health Care Center, Jersey City, NJ.

Donna Zajac – MS, Physical Education Teacher, Binghamton, NY.

Peter Balzani – MS, Nutrition Dietitian, Binghamton, NY.

Carol Potts – Licensed Massage Therapist, Therapeutic Massage Center, Vestal, NY.

Paul Bendert – New York State Licensed Massage Therapist, Vestal, NY.

Phyllis Callaghan – RN, Former Health Consultant, Loss Prevention at Liberty Mutual Insurance Co.

Shelley Kinney – BS, Human Services, Addictions Counselor, Whitney Point, NY.

Faye Clark– Director of Activities for Hilltop Retirement Center, Johnson City, NY.

Sue Baron – Computer consultant.

Sheila Dzuba – Aquatic Director for West Family Y.W.C.A. Johnson City, NY.

Jen Sweeney – Aerobics Coordinator for West Family YWCA, Johnson City, NY.

Rosie Roe – PT Assistant, Endicott, NY.

INTRODUCTION

AGING TODAY

By the year 2011, the first set of baby boomers will reach old age. The changes and dynamics of aging today are much different then the experiences of those aging even 40 years ago.

The aging population today and the upcoming baby boomers were part of an era that saw dramatic changes in healthcare systems, a heightened awareness of environmental concerns, and the institution of more civil rights.

This is a generation exposed to books and media advocating awareness and promotion of self-help concepts, an influx of interest-specific support groups, and the introduction of educational and wellness programs. So, it is no surprise that older adults today are more apt to be active in their health, well-being, and rights.

As a result of medical advancements and quality of life initiatives, older adults are living much longer. In fact, the number of older adults celebrating the age of 100 is becoming more and more commonplace. Today's "young old" are considered to be between the ages of 65 and 74. Today's "middle old" as they are known, are between the ages of 75 and 84. Today's "old-old" are 85 years and older.

If people can reasonably expect to live to 90, it is important that we support them to ensure the last decades of their lives are ones that stimulate them mentally, physically, and socially.

Two emerging elements and advancements in older adult care involve the validated research recognizing the significance of activities for their medical, cognitive, and psychosocial attributes and the relevance of activities within the bio-psychosocial framework of elder care issues.

MEDICAL RESEARCH FINDINGS ON THE VALUE OF ACTIVITIES

For many years, the value of activities was considered as mere fun, just to fill in time for older adults. Today it is more deeply understood that when we talk about offering activities for the elderly, we are referring to the benefits to physical health, cognitive boosters and successful aging. Looking even more closely, we are referring to enhancing daily living and experiences that are the very essence of fulfillment, existence and living.

Some ways to fully appraise and respect the opportunities and goals found in the inclusion of activities in all aspects of adult care is by continuing to recognize and tap into research findings and validated studies on activities.

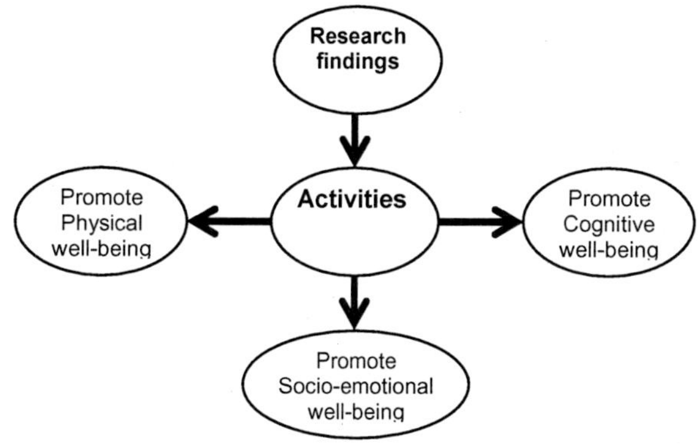

Figure 1.0 -Cognitive, physical socio-emotional aspects of aging
A high amount of data points to the correlation of exercise and the positive effects on reduced depression, benefits to cognitive, socio-emotional, physical well-being and longevity. For example, in one study, weight lifting was shown to preserve and possibly increase muscle mass in older adults. In another, it reduced depression in the elderly (Singh, Clements & Fiatarone, 1997).

Five particular forms of activities have been linked with lowering the risks of dementia and cognitive decline. These five activities include: dancing, the use of board games, the playing of musical instruments, doing crossword puzzles and reading. Researchers have found that aerobic exercise is related to improved memory reasoning (Clarkson-Smith & Harley, 1989).

These issues are not minor. Research points to findings noting what has been termed the "terminal drop hypothesis," which states that a decline in cognition has been associated with a five year span and an associated death ratio. (Riegel & Riegel, 1972).

An article in The Journal of the American Medical Association (2003) states that "the health benefits of regular walking may include helping prevent mental decline and Alzheimer's."

Alzheimer's disease and dementia are of concern and pertinent in all areas of healthcare and professionals working with the elderly.

When working with Alzheimer's/dementia patients, if we know activities possibly slow down the progress of cognitive declines or disease, we can promote these activities in whatever discipline we are focused in. We can also find similar activities that promote the same outcome. This is true whether we are looking to enhance cognitive, physical, or socio-emotional well-being. (Fig. 1.0)

Activities are not just advantageous. When they take place within a clinical setting, they also present a critical time within the day to observe the residents' level of function.

When the therapeutic team/ staff have the ability to document and take part in enhancing wellness, two benefits are gained. The entire staff can be made aware of residents' skills observed during recreational activities and the therapeutic team/activity staff can promote activities that effectively enhance individual patient skills and needs.

ADDRESSING THE BIO-PSYCHO-SOCIAL ASPECTS OF AGING

All of these issues will require us to explore factors that contribute to aging today: current medical research, support services, and the resources needed to enhance quality activity programs.

The overall well-being of the aging adult, the health care benefits, and ultimately the fiscal savings regarding wellness, health care and the possibility of reduced long-term care costs, are key factors for advocating and respect for "the activity/active living factor."

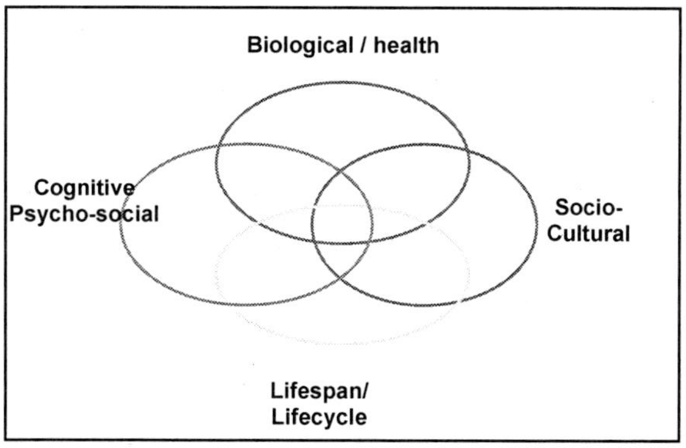

Figure 1.1 Multi-faceted forces that impact human development

Addressing successful aging and activities within the bio-psychosocial framework involves the examination of multi-faceted forces that impact human development as we age.

We must be able to take into consideration the biological, genetic, and health-related factors for the elderly. We must look at psychological forces of cognition, perception, emotional and personality factors. We must look at socio-cultural forces: inter-personal, societal, cultural, and ethnic factors. And we must look at life cycle forces and how events affect the aging population.

Educating medical professionals, legislators, researchers, and anyone involved in decision-making regarding elders on the valuable impact of activities on all outcomes of health and well-being are paramount.

Having funds available for supplies, resources, research, and education are all important measures to make certain older adults receive these valuable services and that research and programs can continue to grow.

In truth, no matter what field of study we are in, every discipline can tap into activities as a resource. When we can incorporate activities into various clinical settings as an additional tool to fully impact and correlate scientific and therapeutic value, we can then continue to promote physical, cognitive, and socio-emotional activities for their positive outcome findings.

Cognitive, Physical, Socio-Emotional Aspects of Aging

As clinicians, before we can begin to understand and evaluate how to include therapeutic activities/ promote active living as pertinent to our field of study, we need to be able to explore all three domains of cognitive, physical, and socio-emotional aspects in aging. We can start by looking at the changes that take place as a natural biological condition of aging, environmental factors that affect aging, and what we can do to influence and enhance the quality of life.

COGNITIVE ASPECTS OF AGING

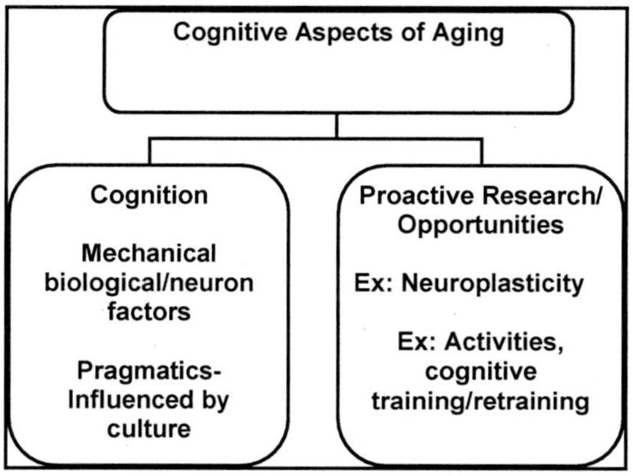

Figure 2.1 -Promoting Cognitive Opportunities
Deeper understanding of cognition and the role of neuron-plasticity have sparked greater interest in offering cognitive boosting programs.

Research has been conducted by Paul Baltes that explores what is called mechanical cognition and pragmatics cognition.

Mechanical cognition is what takes place in cognition as we age, including changes in sensory input, visual and motor memory, categorizing, discrimination, and comparison. It is more related to structural/ neuro-physiologic "hardware" changes due to evolution, hereditary factors and biological changes of wear and tear. Baltes believes that cognitive mechanics will decline as part of the natural progression of aging.

Pragmatics cognition involves skills such as reading and writing, language, and communication comprehension. It also includes knowledge and skills acquired through work, education, life experiences, and wisdom and coping strategies. Baltes believes pragmatics cognition is more affected by cultural influences, and therefore it can be affected by exposure/stimulus. Baltes also believes that we have the opportunity to retain pragmatics cognition and even improve it.

Research findings related to neuron-plasticity

While cognitive mechanics may decline, the older adult brain has shown the potential to compensate for these changes.

Scientists continue to research neuron-plasticity as a promising possibility for cognitive well-being. Plasticity shows the brains ability to redirect "learning" to other areas to compensate for loss of abilities.

Merzenich (2005) a neuroscientist studying neuro-plasticity and the developer of games/ therapies to enhance brain function defines neuron-plasticity as, "the capacity of the brain to change itself." "It actually changes physically, functionally, in ways that you can measure." Merzenich is the developer of a promising new program called Brain Gym computer program.

This program is currently being tested by Stanford University to study the effects of the program as a tool for memory enhancement.

PET scans and Magnetic Resonance Imaging have also shown that in addition to redirection to compensate for losses, injury or wear and tear, the brain wiring between the left and right hemsphere function intertwines as we age. This phenomenon has been termed Hemispheric Asymmetry Reduction in Older Adults by Robert Cabeza, a neuroscientist at Duke University.

Generally, the left hemisphere of the brain is responsible for speech, language and reasoning and the right hemisphere is responsible for emotional perceptions, inklings, cues and facial recognition.

These findings may have implications for how older adults, when given optimum conditions for cognitive boosters, may continue to obtain cognitive skills and well-being. (fig.2.1) The possibilities of these findings and the possibilities of enhancements through the use of cognitive training, memory enhancement programs, and activities are all promising opportunities for cognitive enhancement and function.

Cognition Changes Related to Aging

Cognitive changes affect sensory/motor skills, speed of processing information, and memory. Cognitive changes in aging are different for every older adult. However, some general findings are known that affect older adults as they age.

Changes in the nervous system include reduced efficiency of neural transmission, sensory/motor deficits with a decline in reaction time, the slowed speed of processing information, and memory function changes.

Memory changes are more related to the ability to store information while performing a task and a slower ability to remember information. Some effects and concerns include the fact that older adults may need more time to think and to problem-solve, and the second feature, a decline in sensory input/response time and coordination of actions.

Older adults may have trouble with short-term memory and will show a decline in the ability of storage and organization needed within the moment to do a task. This is called working memory. Not all adults have problems with short-term or working memory. Some older adults continue to have sharp and quick memory. The more active an older adult remains by doing activities, the less effect there is on memory. Effects and concerns include forgetting to take medications on time or forgetting to turn off appliances. We can all be forgetful, and the elderly struggle a bit more sometimes. However, extreme memory loss, disorientation to time frames, surroundings, or events, and misplacing items are usually more related to diseases like Alzheimer's/dementia.

Generally, older adults retain long-term memory. **Long-term memory** is information permanently embedded within the memory banks of the brain over long periods of time. Older adults may believe that their memory has declined due to aging. However, although it may take an older adult a longer time to recall information, in most cases, when they are given enough time to recall the information, they are actually quite good at recollecting the event.

Prospective memory is an area of memory function currently being highly researched. An example of a concern regarding prospective memory involves being distracted and forgetting to take medications on time. This is generally a problem with short-term memory and working memory problems seen in older adults.

Explicit memory is another example of mild memory loss or the need to have enough time for the older adult to remember what they were doing. An example of explicit memory is remembering things you went to buy or details of a television show you watched.

A complete inability to remember the event even with a fair amount of time is usually a sign of Alzheimer's disease/dementia.

Semantic memory is a memory process involving knowledge and what we have learned through books, our jobs, schooling, or personal experiences.

Episodic memory is a long-term memory process and involves the ability to recall long-term events. The type of information stored includes memories of one's past, one's high-school years, or remembering important historical events.

Implicit memory is the unconscious ability to perform a task without deep thought or instruction. Some examples include driving a car or some other rote activity.

We have the opportunity to promote cognitive function by finding creative activities that offer cognitive challenges and stimulation. Some examples include the use and availability of books, the arts and music, science, games, educative opportunities, sensory simulation equipment, and exercise programs.

Research has also shown additional activities that help cognition of sensory/motor and speed processing will be geared towards help in visual and motor memory, discrimination, comparison, and categorizing areas. Activities that help with memory include reminiscing, storytelling, games like memory and concentration, and aroma-therapy.

Long-term studies (Arbuckle and others, 1998) have consistently showed that stimulating the brain with activities helps cognitive function in a similar way exercise helps muscle function.

PHYSICAL ASPECTS OF AGING

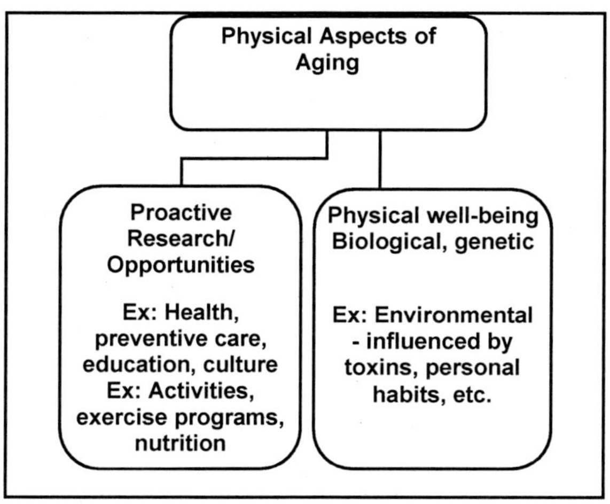

Figure 2.2 -Promoting Physical Opportunities
Research findings on the benefits of physical activities have promoted exercise programs as an important component in proactive healthcare

When considering physical changes related to aging, we can explore questions such as "What is a natural biological process of aging?" "What is genetic?" "How much of aging is influenced by the environment, and therefore a result of pollution, our food choices, and other factors?," or "Do things such as stress, pleasure, and fulfillment affect not just the quality of life, but extension of life?" Let's start out by talking about physiological changes and the theories of aging.

The Theories of Aging

There are many hypotheses, as well as ongoing research, regarding theories on aging. Theories considered include: a simple process of wear and tear, a biological clock, changes in hormones, genetic control, a limited number of cell divisions, the free radicals theory, and many more. Let's talk about a few of these examples.

The **Wear and Tear Theory** (August Weisman) states that: (a) aging is a response to care of the body; and (b) aging is also an inevitable physiological process.

While we know this to be true today, the question of what affects the body and what we can do to prevent or stall these processes has become the focus. For example, we know strategies such as good nutrition, proper hydration, proper rest, exercise, avoiding smoking and drinking, and proper hygiene are all preventive measures to health. But, we also know aging is inevitable.

The **Free Radical Theory** (R. Gerschman & D. Harman) argues that aging is influenced by consequences of free radicals. Free radicals are the result of natural changes that occur as cells metabolize energy. As this metabolism process takes place, it produces unstable oxygen molecules (free radicals.) These molecules multiply and damage cells, which leads to an advancement in the aging process.

Scientists have been studying the large amount of free radicals (which attack proteins) that have been found deep in the heart muscle. Some believe that if they can understand this process, it could be a key to understanding how we age.

This research may also help us to understand how the heart is affected by aging, and may help us to prevent damage to the heart. Heart disease is the leading cause of death in older adults. This is just one example of the search to improve healthcare issues and aging.

The **Hormonal Stress Theory** states that, as we age, the HPA axis relating to the hypothalamus, pituitary, and adrenal glands is affected. The HPA helps to regulate the body's internal regulatory functions and external stresses. It is thought that, as we age, the hormones that react to stress can not slow down properly, and stay elevated. These higher levels of stress induced hormones lead to risk of disease.

Physical Changes Related to Aging

Many factors will determine an individual's physical changes related to aging including genetics, nutritional choices, exposure to toxins, exercise levels, stress factors, smoking, and an array of personal habits. The changes listed vary per person and even in degree.

As older adults age, there is a decline in cell activity leading to deterioration and slowing down of all body systems.

Changes in physical function include: muscle atrophy/ weight loss, skin/ hair changes, sensory/ neuron changes, heart/ cardiovascular changes, kidney/liver function changes, respiratory/ lung capacity changes, bone loss/height loss, endocrine and metabolic system changes, sexual changes, and gastrointestinal changes.

Both visual and auditory perception change with age (Helfer, 1998).

Changes in vision include: near-sightedness and possible deterioration to retina, blood vessels, and lens. Many older adults suffer from diseases such as glaucoma and cataracts, and those with Degenerative Macular disease continue to regress in vision. Night blindness and colorblindness can also be concerns for older adults. Per-ceptual changes may include problems with depth perception and visual acuity.

Effects and concerns include isolation and the inability to drive or even walk down a hall safely.

Dangers of falling, walking into something, or not clearly being able to see what is in front of the older adult may leave them very vulnerable to injury.

Hearing loss can occur as a result of damage to the hearing organ, the peripheral nervous system, and/or the central nervous system.

Effects and concerns include difficulty understanding or distinguishing words. Hearing loss can affect the communication skills of the person, not only in receiving information, but also in giving the correct response (Amber Stary, 2002). It can lead to incorrect assumptions, such as an older adult being mislabeled or misconstrued as having a cognitive defect related to intelligence level or dementia.

Hearing loss can be incapacitating. The older adult may become isolated or not be able to engage in a conversation, including those with family and friends, or much-needed communication, such as a conversation with the pharmacist.

Hearing loss can leave the older adult vulnerable to injury. They may be unable to hear high pitch sounds like the sound of a smoke alarm or warning system. They may not hear cars coming or be able to respond to other dangerous situations.

Changes in smell and taste include a reduction in taste buds and smell diminished by changes in the olfactory senses.

Effects and concerns include: the inability to smell bad food or smoke and an increased desire to choose salty or spicy foods, which may lead to problems in an already sensitive digestive system. This can also be dangerous for those who require low-salt diets. Because food tastes blander, and the older adult possibly having a decreased desire to eat, nutrition can become a concern. Smell and taste are some of the last senses to leave the elderly, so preparing food that looks tempting is important (Helen Battisti, 2006).

Touch is also affected by neural/sensory changes.

Effects and concerns include failure to be aware of an injury. This, and the fact that they do not heal well, can lead to very serious consequences. They may not be aware of temperature changes, and therefore are susceptible to hypothermia and hyperthermia.

Stimulation and sensation are diminished, and therefore older adults have a harder time being stimulated by external events or nurturing experiences, such as therapeutic or human touch. Sexual stimulation is also diminished.

Changes in skin and appearances include changes in oil/sweat gland production, less elasticity of skin, and pigment/melanin changes. Effects and concerns include: wrinkles, age spots, hair turning gray, blood flow problems which create thickening of nails, easy bruising, and bedsores.

As stated earlier, sensory perception may be altered, leading to dangers regarding recognition of hot or cold, or leading to an inability to recognize an injury.

Changes in muscles include the muscle tissue being replaced by fat deposits. Muscle tone and strength may be affected in all organs. Effects and concerns include the slowing down of blood pumping and circulation problems and the ability to transport nutrients for optimum system function. Older adults will have trouble with the ability to breathe deeply and with exchange of oxygen and ridding the body of carbon dioxide. Muscle weakness will also affect gastrointestinal activity/acids, hormonal exchanges, and other systems functions throughout the body.

Changes in the cardio-vascular system include atrophy of the heart muscle and the loss of elasticity in artery walls. There will be slower blood pumping/less oxygen being exchanged. It should be noted that if the older adult does not have heart disease, their heart/circulatory system may function at a normal level.

Effects and concerns include: kidney and liver function becoming less effective, hardening of the arteries and clogging of the artery which may lead to hypertension, stroke, heart attack, and/or congestive heart failure. They may be susceptible to drug toxicity, have a harder time healing, as well as less tolerance to stress.

Changes in the respiratory system include loss of elasticity to the lung tissue and the airways. There may be problems in breathing adequately due to muscle atrophy/weakening of the diaphragm. The chest also becomes smaller. There will be a reduction in cilia activity and a decreased oxygen uptake and exchange.

Effects and concerns include weakness in ability to breathe deeply, cough, and get rid of carbon dioxide, a decreased stamina/shortness of breath, and fatigue. All of these respiratory concerns may lead to pulmonary diseases, which cause deterioration to lung capacities and muscle, and blockages to breathing passages.

As we age, lung function capacity decreases. Older adults can improve lung function capacity by doing exercises that strengthen the diaphragm muscles.

Changes in the gastrointestinal system /endocrine system include slowed digestion of food and slow movement of food emptying from the stomach. For these reasons, older adults may have trouble enjoying mealtime.

There may be a reduced production of hydrochloric acid, digestive enzymes and a decrease in saliva and taste buds.

Effects and concerns include impaired swallowing, gastrointestinal upset, slow digestion of foods, emptying of the stomach, and malnutrition. Some concerns and effects include: impaired swallowing due to problems associated with a lack of saliva, slowed swallowing abilities, inadequate swallowing ability.

As mentioned earlier, changes in the endocrine system may alter the hypothalamic-pituitary-adrenal axis. Increased stress-related hormone levels can lead to vulnerability to diseases, such as cardio-vascular disease, diabetes, cancer, and hypertension.

The **metabolic system** also slows down. The metabolic system is responsible for changing food into energy. Problems of malnutrition may be associated with a lack of desire to eat or inability to metabolize and transport important nutrients.

Changes in the **skeletal system** may include calcium loss or other types of absorption problems. There may be a thinning of the vertebrae or calcium deposit build-ups and vertebrae calcification.

Effects and concerns include a reduction in height and postural changes. Changes may lead to bones becoming less dense (which is known as osteoporosis); inflammation of the joints/ arthritis, a wearing away of the joint cartilage called osteoarthritis, or rheumatoid arthritis, a disease of the connective tissue.

We can promote physical well-being by encouraging and finding activities that promote wellness and exercise programs. Some examples of physical activities include walking, swimming, golfing, bowling, yoga exercises, and any strength-training activities.

Older adults who exercise and have better balance as a result of posture and strength training are less likely to be susceptible to falls. This is a critical issue because falls account for not only injuries and fractures that decrease mobility, but have been associated with a high likeliness of needing care in a long-term care facility.

Studies have also shown correlation to deaths not just attributed to the fall, but as a secondary cause, such as the exposure to disease, infections, and pneumonia, while inpatient or immobilized.

Researchers continue to look at the possibilities of altering the aging process. Futhermore, proactive healthcare involving education, prevention, and intervention are all factors that have greatly improved the well-being of the aging population.

Dr. David Buchner, Chief of CDC's Physical Activity and Health Branch states " Health clubs also provide older adults with a variety of opportunities to improve their aerobic fitness, muscular strength, and flexibility. Dr. Buchner adds, "Traditionally health and fitness facilities have marketed mainly to body-conscious younger adults, who focus on the cosmetic effects. It's great to see that health clubs have developed more programs for older adults, and we hope this trend continues." (Special focus: healthy aging. Chronic Disease Notes and Reports 1999;12(3): 10-11).

Along with physical benefits, studies have shown that physical well-being helps older adults maintain their self-sufficiency, dignity, and well-being (Burke et al, 2001: Evan, 2000: Kabitsis et al., 1999: Prohaska & Peters, 1999: Wang, Bashore & Friedman, (1995)

SOCIO-EMOTIONAL ASPECTS OF AGING

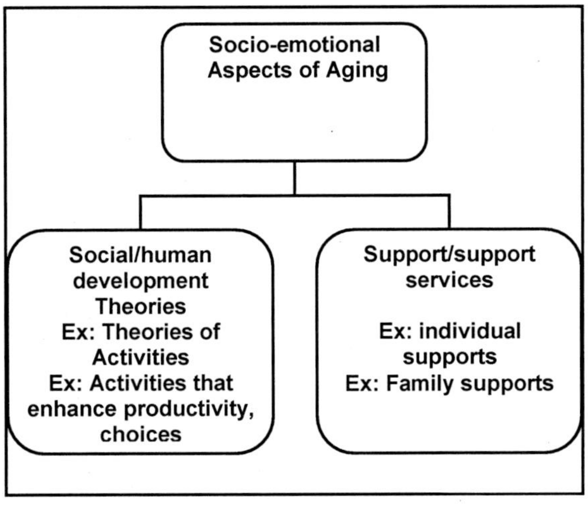

Figure 2.3 **-Promoting Socio- emotional Opportunities**
Activities have been found to be a valuable tool to support quality of life and psychosocial needs for older adults

SOCIO-EMOTIONAL CHANGES RELATED TO AGING

Social-emotional/psychosocial aspects of aging can be broken down into three areas of concentration.

The first area of concentration involves looking at social and human development related to research, lifespan issues, and theories on the aging process. Some theories of consideration regarding social and human development and the aging process include Maslow's Theory on Basic Human Needs and Motivation, Successful Aging, Theories of Activities, and the Psychosocial Reactions to Aging.

Maslow believed that humans have basic needs, and that the focus and motivation of the individual will stay geared at that need until it is met. Once that need is met, they will then aspire towards the next level of need.

The first basic need is physiological and includes things like oxygen, food, and drink. The second step is safety, and has to do with psychological aspects related to our environment. The third step is love and the need to belong, be loved, or accepted by others. The fourth step is self-esteem. Self-esteem is gained by mastering a task or receiving acknowledgement of your skill/worth from others. Once all of these needs are met, the individual can then look to obtain self-actualization. This is the process of self-discovery and finding out who we are, and the ability to aspire and accomplish all we are capable of.

Once we have met the older adult's physiological and safety needs, we can promote social-emotional support and well-being by encouraging social activities.

Some ways we can do this is helping older adults to stay productive and have choices and control of their life decisions, as well as remaining involved in social interaction, community integration, and volunteer work. Actively listening to what older adults say is critical to offering constructive, dignified, and fulfilling experiences.

For example, in a large-scale study commissioned by CMS, 160 residents in 40 nursing homes were interviewed in 1992 and asked about what the quality of life meant to them. The residents overwhelmingly listed meaningful activities (not just availability) as a key factor that contributed to their positive self-image, and reported that they feel no sense of purpose without them. Residents also said they like to take part in activities that "amount to something," not just a way to "keep busy." For example, religious activities and activities that allow the resident to contribute to the nursing home in some manner (delivering the mail or helping set up activities).

Another example might be to offer residents activity experiences, which allow them to use the skills and talents they learned in a lifetime of work. All of these activities can enhance socio-emotional well-being.

THEORIES OF ACTIVITIES/ SUCCESSFUL AGING

For a long time, the goal of helping older ad-ults was centered on taking care of health and attempting to prolong life.

As older adults began to live longer as a result of better medical care, quantity vs. quality of life became a larger question.

Successful Aging is a term that was used by R. J. Havighurst in 1961. The term caught on as a way to talk about the goal for quote "Successful Aging". There are countless attempts to understand what "successful aging" means and "having lived a quality life." The theories of activities are based on the psychosocial processes that take place as we age.

"When we talk about activities we are referring to daily living experiences. We are referring to everyday living activities such as working, education, hobbies, how we relate to these everyday occurrences and further the inclusion (in this case) of aging factors.

There are various theories on the psychosocial meaning of activities pertaining to the older adult and how they respond to aging and "going about living" activities.

To understand and support quality living or successful aging, we need to be able to understand the psychosocial effects of aging on the older adult.

Once we can understand what matters to them and how they relate to aging, we can then help them to successfully age. These theories can also help us to understand the older adults' feelings about being involved in activities.

THEORIES OF ACTIVITIES AND PSYCHOSOCIAL REACTIONS TO AGING

The Model of Human Occupation theory (Kielhofner) is based on the idea that aging itself is just another natural progression in the mastery of life, and that seniors will just have new sources of "learning" to master.

The **Lifespan theory** (Negarten & Levinson) is a hypothesis that considers aging issues and the receptiveness to activities as being unique needs and developmental steps/stages for this time of life.

Erickson's eighth and final stage of human development centers on what he called Integrity vs. Despair. Erickson's theory of aging revolves around the idea that, as older adults reflect on the life that they have led, it effects how they view themselves. If they feel they have lived well and accomplished a well life, they will have integrity. If they feel they failed in how they lived or succeeded in life, they will have despair.

The **Selective optimization with compensation theory** (Baltes & Baltes, 1990: Mariske et al, 1995) states that, as older adults' age, they use a process of selection, optimization, and compensation. They become more selective of the activities they do in order to make up for reduced capacity and function level. They take the abilities they do have and maintain, optimize, and enhance these areas as much as they can. They compensate and find ways to cope, function, and adapt within, around the aging process and limitations.

Dr. Gene Cohen, founding director of the Center on Aging, Health and Humanities at George Washington University Medical Center, has identified four distinct developmental phases of aging. These developmental phases unfold in overlapping 20-year periods. They begin in a person's early 40's: with **a midlife-re-evaluation** (typically encountered between 40 and 65) during which we set new goals and priorities. We then begin a **liberation phase** (55-75) that involves shedding past inhibitions to express ourselves more freely. This is followed by **a summing up phase** (65-85) when we begin to review our lives and concentrate on giving back. The final developmental phase is called **an**

encore phase (75 and beyond) which involves finding affirmation and fellowship in the face of adversity and loss. (Cohen, 2005)

The **Activities theory** by Lemon, Bengtson and Peterson points to the idea that seniors would readapt from the change of raising a family and working, and as they aged, replace this with a healthy balance of activities, such as volun-teering, joining clubs, etc.

When initiating activities, the older adults may need support and encouragement. It is important to be sure to honor the older adult's own feelings and thoughts regarding participation. Once you know the older adult better you can get a clearer picture of how to help them benefit from engaging in the activities.

SOCIAL FACTORS RELATED TO AGING

Individual background

Socio-emotional aspects of aging for the older adult can include issues related to loss of partner, home, financial concerns, isolation from cultural and ethnic customs and/or groups, and loss of independence, privacy, and productivity.

Exploring socio-emotional/ psychosocial issues involves looking at an individual's background. This usually includes what the older adult's life was like before they reached old age, where they lived, what hobbies they had, what type of work they did for a living, religious/ cultural background, the time-era they grew up in, and their personal experiences and personality.

It is crucial to remember the individual older adult. Every older adult has his or her own history, life choices they have made, and lifestyle.

Some concerns regarding aging issues include depression and isolation. Findings from reviews of outcome studies indicate that therapy is effective with older adults (B. G. Knight, 1999). Helping older adults to adjust to the changes they face, such as dealing with issues of grief, death, and dying, changed roles in the family dynamics, and many other issues they face can be of great support and comfort to the elderly.

On a positive note, Dr. G Cohen, who identified the four developmental phases of aging listed earlier in this text, and author of the book *The Mature Mind: The Positive Power of the Brain.* (2005) has been doing research showing correlation and further hypothesizing on the information gained by the use of PET scans and Magnetic Resonance Imaging.

Noting the older adult's use of both right and left hemisphere brain functions, Cohen has been using this information to study the impact of brain changes and psychological well-being during aging. Older adults may have the gained ability of using both the analytical (primary left hemisphere ability) brain and the creative, intuitive brain function (primary right hemisphere function) to explore/ channel cognitive boosting ventures and experiences. G. Cohen, The Myth of the Midlife Crisis (2005) Newsweek, p 82-86 article adapted from The Mature Mind: The Positive Power of the Brain: New York, Basic Books, (2005)

Studies have also shown that as we age the limbic system (in the middle of the brain) goes through changes. As a result, the older adult's reactions to emotions (particularly negative emotions) and impulsive behavior soften. Older adults are less apt to be ruled by impulsive or high emotional states and reactions.

Cohen hypothesizes that older adult are therefore better able to seek out goals in a more organized or thought-out process, with less influence of negative emotions and more thought-out decisions. This may lead to better satisfaction and self-gratifying direction.

Additionally, studies validate how important these issues are to the older adult and their quality of life. Studies have shown having a sense of control over decision-making and other choices (Rodin & Langer, 1977) can increase the older adult's quality of living and satisfaction.

Family Involvement

Due to various changes, older adults may feel or actually experience a loss of connection to their family, friends, and community. In a nursing home setting they may even lose their privacy, freedom of roommate choice, freedom to cook, or even choice of their own meals. These changes have a major impact on their socio-emotional/ psychosocial well-being.

Whether in a nursing home setting or at home, maintaining support from family and friends can help them to stay connected to their life as much as possible. Encouraging and supporting family involvement has positive effects for the older adult's physical, cognitive, and socio-emotional well-being. Family input on the older adult's background, preferences, personality, etc. can also help the staff/homecare personnel to understand the individual better.

Cultural, Ethnic and Social Factors

It is important to include activities specific to ethnic and cultural awareness and sensitivity. This is especially needed for residents who come from another country or a setting in which the ethnic and cultural practices are strong and definitory to their identity, beliefs, and pride.

Culture is described as the shared values, traditions, norms, customs, arts, history, folklore, and institution of a group of people. Understanding culture helps us to understand how others interpret, perceive, and function.

Culture shapes the individual's as well as the group's attitudes, ideals, goals, and values.

Understanding culture can help us avoid prejudices, stereotypes, and biases. Understanding why a group of older adults react in relation to certain activities or circumstances can dispel assumptions and allow us to respect, appreciate, and support the older adult.

Cultural factors may be related to educational backgrounds, financial issues, geographic residence, and identification with community groups, religious affiliations, political beliefs, individual experiences, and place of birth.

It is important to make the environment culturally welcome, get the community's input when planning activities, and have staff with varied backgrounds to enhance understanding of every culture, or offer as many as cultural experiences as possible. Invite those in the community to join or share cultural experiences with the group.

Differences can be valued through learning as much as possible about the older adult's present or past environment, values, norms, and customs. Learning to understand how others perceive the world it is both challenging and rewarding.

Offering quality programs inclusive of cultural considerations is crucial to recognition of the older adult's self-identity, self-esteem, rights, dignity, spiritual wellness, and care.

All programs should include cultural appropriateness, cultural accessibility, and cultural acceptability.

Lifecycle and Socio-environmental Factors

Lifecycle and socio-environmental factors that can impact an older adult's well-being may include: changes and consequences associated with the loss of spouse, the loss of their own home, having to move away from their own home to live with family, loss of contact, experiences or access to cultural and ethnic customs and/or groups, lack of financial resources, loss of job, etc.

As a result of these changes in their life, they may ultimately lose the freedom or access to go and do things as they wish, leading to loss of independence, privacy, and productivity.

Awareness of support services can help enhance any services offered to the older adult.

Some ways we can help is to offer additional support services to older adults, family members, and caregivers.

This includes issues regarding: housing, financial assistance, prescription drug programs, therapeutic services, mental health and addiction services (if applicable), and additional counseling services.

It is important to not only be aware of additional services available, but also to support the older adult in receiving all the benefits available to them, and to gain maximum benefits within the bio-psychosocial perspective.

When we are looking at assessments or the inclusion of activities, understanding human nature, the individual's background, circumstances of the individual's environment, and needs of services will help us to determine how to offer activities that address the older adult's needs and fulfillment. (Fig.2.3)

Caregiver Support

The impact on caregivers is a critical concern. The caregiver plays an important role in the well-being of the older adult. Caregivers provide care for disabled or frail family members with the average timeframe being up to five years. This helps the older adult to remain at home and in their community, rather than in a long-term care facility. Not only does the older adult thrive in the comfort of home and family and friends, the benefits of homecare also play a major factor in cost reduction to states and federal spending.

Families and other "informal" caregivers provide care for almost 80 percent of those requiring long-term care.

If the services provided by informal caregivers had to be replaced with paid services, it would cost an estimated $196 billion dollars per year. All of these factors make the caregiver a valuable resource for the older adult.

Many caregivers that provide care for the elderly also continue to be employed. The sandwich generation has the added factor of caring for aging parents and raising their own children at the same time.

The combination of stress factors is incredibly challenging. Caring for the older adult, may include: managing doctor appointments, the elder's personal care needs, homecare or making sure the older adult's home is maintained and bills paid; obtaining medications, filing papers for drug prescription programs, and additional paperwork and decision-making.

These issues may be coupled with the possibility of additional care for their own young children, financial concerns, and emotional/interpersonal stresses.

All of these factors can lead to physical and emotional exhaustion, heightened anxiety levels, and depression.

A study of older spousal caregivers found that caregivers that experience mental or emotional strain have a 63% higher risk of dying than non-caregivers. Studies show that an estimated 46%-59% of caregivers are clinically depressed. Research has shown that caregiver stress, alcohol or substance abuse, and emotional and/or financial problems are factors in many instances of elder abuse.

The need for supportive services is critical for the older adult and their caregivers. Making sure families are aware of services is the first step. Studies show that many families may not be aware of all the services available to them. Even when families are aware of services, many families do not reach out for the services. Therefore, it is important to make them aware of the services and encourage them to use them.

Support services such as respite, support for Alzheimer's disease patients and their families, supplemental services, and resources can reduce stress. Respite care is gaining importance and this is one positive step towards addressing family's socio-emotional needs.

Support services can help the older adult to stay at home, can be a preventive measure for elder abuse, reduce state and federal long-term care costs, and contribute to wellness and promotion of an optimum environment for the older adult and those who care for them.

Funding to support activities and wellness

Considerations for the inclusion of activity programs and their value to the quality of life for older adults and families can also be of tremendous worth. These are important factors, whether we are talking about home care, assisted living or the quality of living that takes place in a long-term care facility.

In the book *CHECCHINO A Father & Son Journey towards Dusk*, author Francis Battisti speaks both about homecare and his personal journey as a caregiver for his father.

Fransis' book is an excellent resource for those looking to understand and empathize with the everyday experiences that take place for families as they care for their loved ones. It is also a valuable resource for those working in the gerontology social workers capacity or gerontology health fields.

In his book, Francis states "The new reality of life means being part of the sandwich generation… caring for both children and elderly family at the same time." Interpreted as…your emotions are being squeezed from many directions. (p.91).

He goes on to share his personal experiences and the journey that he, his family and his father travel through during the late stages of his father's life and eventual passing.

Francis's book provides insight into his journey as a caregiver for his father as well as his expertise as a social worker and educator.

"Home care with assistance, home of caregiver, or assisted living in a long-term care facility...all are acceptable methods of dealing appropriately with the needs of the elder or infirm. (P.93)

While trying to find fair equitable care, the costs and the need for medical services must be considered. The amounts have increased dramatically and the issue of adequate health care has become center stage in our society. (P.93)

Long-term care is evolving in the most enlightened facilities. The environment is being designed with a home atmosphere with the focus on the individual and not facilities-centered care. We are transforming institutions into homes. (p.94)

Treatment patterns are adaptable to the residents, with the resident participating in all facets of a well-rounded lifestyle.

Residents should be able to look forward to each day and to enjoying a stimulating atmosphere, interacting with the other residents, staff, visitors, and family. Ideally, residents should thrive in the home, not vegetate as often occurred in the past.

Care must be a sharing process, taking into consideration the wishes of the resident, relatives and the facility. The goal is to build a residential family, or community of care, involving interaction with outside schools, clubs, and other groups. Also pets and plants could be introduced into the facility... all creating a more relaxed setting. "a welcoming, wellness environment.". (p.94) (Battisti, 2005).

Along with addressing the most crucial factors of basic needs, medical needs, social support services related to safety, etc., we must remember the realism, the "everyday happenings" and critical value of fostering positive daily living experiences, which take place within the family home environment, assisted living and long-term care settings.

When taking into consideration the importance of creating a wellness environment, family involvement, and caregiver services, we must provide resources to obtain the supplies or monies for these services. The inclusion of support services for activity and "wellness environments" can only enhance quality care and daily living experiences for older adults and their families.

OAA Resources and Support Services

The following list (adapted from the OAA website: (aoa.hhs.gov) provides an overview of the range of supporting services available to older residents in their communities. These services are offered through the Access Services, which help assure that elderly Americans are linked with appropriate services in the community as needed.

- **Transportation**. Transportation is one of the most common needs expressed by older people. Senior transportation programs make it possible for individuals who do not drive or whose physical condition prohibits them from using public transportation to obtain rides for essential trips, such as medical appointments, business errands, shopping and senior activities. Door-to-door transportation is available in many places.
- **Outreach,** through door-to-door canvassing, extensive public announcements or other means, is an effort to familiarize people to services and benefits available to them. Outreach identifies homebound or isolated people in need of services. Once they are identified they are assisted in receiving app-ropriate services.
- **Information and Referral**. Information and referral/assistance programs assist older persons, their families and community agencies who need information but don't know where to turn. Many State Agencies on Aging have toll free statewide 800 numbers that assist with linking older persons with appropriate services. Anyone, regardless of age, may telephone the Area Agency on aging for information on services and resources available in the community to individuals 60 and over.
- **Escort**. Escort service provides support for older people with limited mobility to obtain needed services.
- Escort service is often provided by volunteers. It might mean picking up an individual at their home, accompanying them to a doctor's appointment or spending the afternoon together running errands.
- **Case Management**. Case management services are aimed at providing a single access point in the community to reduce the distance an individual must go to initiate entry into the service system. Drawing upon a variety of

resources, the case manager meets with the individual, assesses his or her needs, and develops a service plan to meet those needs. Once services are initiated, a case manager can provide follow-up to assure that needed services are being provided.

- **In-Home Services** encompass a wide range of supporting services offered to individuals who are homebound due to illness, functional limitations in activities of daily living, or disability. Their availability often is credited for allowing people to remain in the community.
- **Home Health**. Home health care is recognized as an increasingly important alternative to hospitalization or care in a nursing home for patients who do not need 24-hour day professional supervision. Many people find it possible to remain at home for the entire duration of their illness or at least to shorten their hospital stay. In many cases readmission to the hospital can be prevented or delayed. A variety of health services are provided in a home health care program in the patient's home, under the directions of a physician.
- **Homemaker**. Homemaker service is extended to individuals who are unable to perform day-to-day household duties and have no one available to assist them.
  Services include light housekeeping, laundry, limited personal care, grocery shopping, meal preparation, and shopping assistance.
- **Chore Service**. Chore service is available to persons who are physically unable to perform tasks, such as heavy cleaning, minor repair or yard work, and unable to neither secure assistance from family or friends nor have the means to pay privately.
- **Home Delivered Meals**. A hot, nutritionally balanced meal is delivered five days a week to individuals who are physically unable to prepare their own meals and do not have anyone else to prepare meals for them.
- **Friendly Visitors and Telephone Reassurance**. These programs, which have different titles in different communities, provide regular personal or telephone contact for older persons who are homebound or live alone. Usually a volunteer provides the service. Besides developing friendships, perhaps a more important aspect of these programs is the volunteer's ability to identify needs of the individual as they occur and notify those who can help.

Services in the community enable many hundreds of thousands of older persons maintain dignity and independence within their homes and communities. Community resources available for the elderly include:

- **Adult Day Care**. Adult day care programs offer a lower cost alternative to institutionalization for newly or chronically disabled adults who cannot stay alone during the day, but who do not need 24-hour a day inpatient care. Designed to promote maximum independence, participants usually attend on a scheduled basis. Services may include nursing, counseling, social services, restorative services, medical and healthcare monitoring, exercise sessions, field trips, recreational activities, physical, occupational and speech therapy, medication administration, well-balanced meals, and transportation to and from the facility.
- **Adult day care** can provide the respite family members require to sustain healthy relationships while caring for their elderly loved one at home.
- **Senior Centers**. Literally thousands of senior centers are operating in the United States. A vital link in the service delivery network which older persons may avail themselves of, senior centers are functioning as meal sites, screening clinics, recreational centers, social service agency branch offices, mental health counseling clinics, older worker employment agencies, volunteer coordinating centers, and community meeting halls. The significance of senior centers cannot be underestimated for they provide a sense of belonging, offer the opportunity to meet old acquaintances and make new friends, and encourage individuals to pursue activities of personal interest and involvement in the community.
- **Legal Assistance**. Legal services help older persons experiencing problems in civil matters to obtain advice, counseling, information or representation.

Services are provided either by a licensed attorney or trained paralegal. Types of matters for which help is typically sought include health care, income, public benefits (Social Security, Medicare, Medicaid, SSI, and food stamps), employment, consumer complaints, nursing home resident rights, utilities, guardianship/ conservatorship, wills and estates.

- **Housing**. Housing services are aimed at providing older persons with a wide variety of assistance related to financing, building, maintaining and locating housing. Services include housing counseling, information and referral, landlord-tenant dispute resolution, tenant group supports, home equity conversion, carpentry, minor electric and plumbing repairs, low cost weatherization material. In some areas short term shelter is provided to elders who are in need of emergency housing due to fire, theft, physical or mental abuse or other similar situations beyond their immediate control.
- **Self-Help/Support Groups**. Mutual support groups lend peer support and help for those who have encountered life-threatening illness or chronic disability, either personally or as a family member.
- **Respite Care**. The provision of short-term relief (respite) to families caring for their frail elders offers tremendous potential for maintaining dependent persons in the least restrictive environment. Respite services encompass traditional home-based care, as well as adult day health, skilled nursing, home health aide and short-term institutional care. Respite can vary in time from part of a day to several weeks.
- **Protective Services**. Adult protective services are designed to meet the needs of individuals who are severely or functionally incapacitated to the point where they can no longer manage their personal and financial affairs and who have no relative or friend to provide the necessary assistance. Services include investigations and interv-ention of elder abuse, including physical and emotional abuse and neglect by a caretaker. Protective service workers provide crisis intervention, counseling, information and referral to clients and liaison with the court system.
- **Residential Repair and Renovation**.

  These programs help older people keep the condition of their housing in good repair before problems become major. Volunteers might come to an individual's home and patch a leaky roof for instance, repair faulty plumbing or insulate drafty walls. These programs could help seniors who are temporarily in a long-term care facility and who expect to return home to secure their home environment while they are away.
- **Employment**. Employment services are designed to increase older workers' employment opportunities in the general labor market as well as in community service. Income eligible persons 55 and over are recruited, trained, and referred to job openings with local employers. The ultimate goal is to place the older worker in non-subsidized employment.
- **Crime Prevention/Victim Assistance**. Many communities have active crime prevention programs to reduce elders' vulnerability to crime. In some areas police refer senior crime victims to the local Area Agency on Aging for counseling, help in obtaining lost identification or emergency financial assistance.
- **Volunteer Program**. Volunteers have always played an integral role in the OAA system. This partnership is built on the dedication of volunteers giving time to serve in a broad range of capacities such as providing escort services, delivering home bound meals, serving meals at nutrition sites, providing I&R and outreach assistance, serving as friendly visitors, offering telephone reassurance, etc. A resource for elderly Americans in need of assistance, volunteer programs also offer meaningful opportunities for older people to participate more fully in community life through volunteer service. Among the many volunteer programs established specifically for the elderly are the Retired Senior Volunteer Program (RSVP), Foster Grandparents and Senior Companion Programs.
- **Nutrition Education**. These programs help older people to identify and understand their nutrition and health needs emphasizing prevention, programs are designed to improve participants' health through improved food purchasing, diet food preparation, etc.
- **Physical Fitness/Exercise**. Programs are designed to assist older people stay physically active and healthy. An exercise expert, for example, might come to a senior center, nursing home, hospital or other facility in the community to lead exercises geared especially to older people. Or transportation might be provided to the local YMCA/ YWCA or other

community venue for older persons to attend special exercise classes.

- ❖ **Services Provided to Support Caregivers** under the National Family Caregiver Support Program include:
- • Information to caregivers about available services.
- • Assistance to caregivers in gaining access to services.
- • Individual counseling, organization of support groups, and caregiver training to caregivers to assist the caregivers in making decisions and solving problems relating to their caregiving roles.
- ❖ **Respite care** to enable caregivers to be temporarily relieved from their care giving responsibilities. In-home respite, adult day services, and institutional respite on an intermittent, occasional or emergency basis.
- ❖ **Supplemental services**, on a limited basis, to complement the care provided by caregivers. Services such as home-modifications, assistive technology, emergency response systems, equipment/supplies, and transportation.
- ❖ **Services to Residents of Care Providing Fac-ilities** are designed to protect and improve the quality of life of elderly persons living in institutions and to support relatives and other caregivers.
- ❖ **Senior Medicare Patrol**

Senior Medicare Patrols is an AoA-led effort which uses innovative, proactive partnerships across the federal, state, and community levels to identify and report healthcare waste, fraud, and abuse.

Senior Medicare Patrol projects teach volunteer retired professionals, such as doctors, nurses, accountants, investigators, law enforcement, personnel, attorneys and teachers, to help Medicare and Medicaid beneficiaries to be better health-care consumers.

- ❖ **Pension Counseling**

AoA pension counseling projects are designed to reach out, educate, and promote pension aware-ness and protection among older individuals, as well as to encourage better financial planning.

(To obtain further information please visit aoa.hhs.gov 2005.)

FUNCTIONAL SKILLS

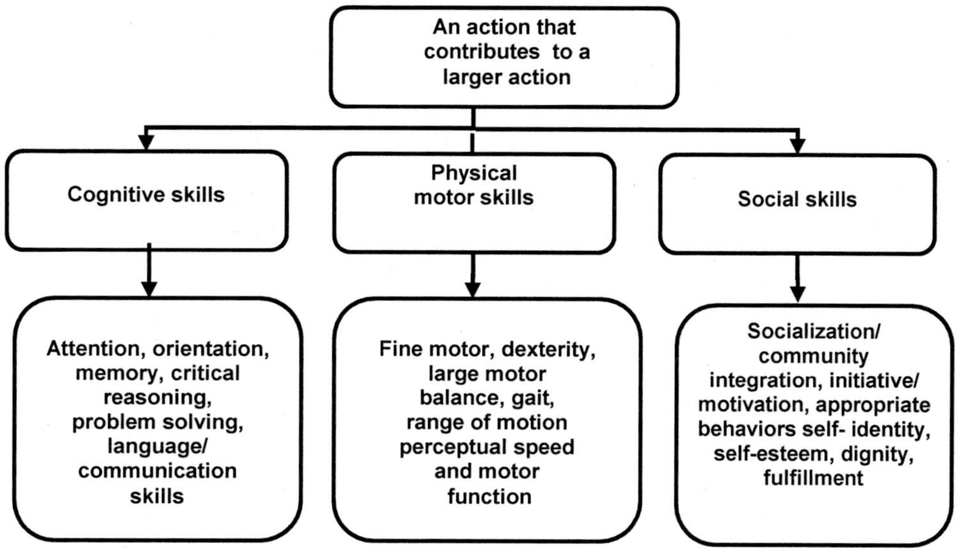

Figure 3.0-Functional Issues: needs, abilities and skills

UNDERSTANDING FUNCTIONAL SKILLS

Once one understands the physical, cognitive and socio-emotional aspects of aging one can begin to understand needs and abilities necessary for function. Function can simply be explained as one action that contributes to a larger action, a capacity, or a mechanical action.

While there are certainly even more skills that can be named within each domain of physical, cognitive and socio-emotional function, the ones listed are fairly common for need and purposes.

Cognitive function or needs and abilities include: memory, recall, recognition, attention, language and communication, abstract thinking, concrete thinking, orientation, attention, perceptual awareness, problem-solving, following patterns, and cognitive stimulation.

The physical function or needs and abilities include: small-motor skills, dexterity, manipulation of materials, large motor skills, hand-eye coordination, range of motion, tactile stimulation, perceptual speed and motor function, coordination, gait, posture, flexibility, cardiovascular well-being, posture, and strength-training. When looking at the socio-emotional areas of function, or needs and abilities, we are looking at socialization, community integration, self-esteem, self-identity, dignity and pride, emotional gratification, toleration of stimulation, feelings of productivity, and reminiscing/ semblances of past routines.

Psychological/behavioral well-being includes the abilities to adapt or use "appropriate behaviors," awareness of others, initiative, and motivation.

Spiritual needs include the need to have opportunity for solace, nurtured care, healing therapies, and the chance to relax. The psychological components will be related to the ability to take in healing qualities/therapies, be nurtured, and be able to relax.

COGNITION TERMINOLOGY

Abstract thinking is a cognitive process requiring the ability to consider multifaceted/"far reaching" ideas while considering a problem. This is the opposite of perhaps concrete thinking, which is more direct, simple and understandable without complex choices or considerations.

Alzheimer's patients do much better with concrete thinking, questions, or without complex need of action.

Offer simple directions, facial cues or other hints to help them to understand what you are saying or doing.

Attention - Reactive focus to a task or information by a stimulus. The goal is to stay focused to the task at hand rather then "taking in" other stimulus. Further this information can then be processed.

Cognitive functions - The physical aspects of cognitive functions involve the brain as it has developed, continues to develop, "under develop", and/or declines as a result of physical condit-ions. It affects speed and ability to process information for sensory functions, motor functions, and perception based on neuro-physical abilities.

The knowledge aspects of cognitive functions include thought and reasoning, problem-solving, memory, and comprehension of written and spoken language.

Cognitive thinking involves thought, reasoning and the abilities to gather and sort incoming information.

Cognitive stimulation involves stimulating an intellectual process for cognition. An example might be offering a resident a music box (preferably one with music from their time era) the music will be good to stimulate hearing, nurturing qualities of music, and it may also bring up memories.

Disorientation may be the result of many factors, such as dementia, delusional episodes and delirium. An example of being disoriented might be a patient suffering from Alzheimer's disease that has progressed to a point where he or she cannot remember earlier details of the day, such as having had lunch, not recognizing this, and asking for it at four o' clock. They may not even recognize it is four o'clock, or what day or year it is, or even their location. A temporary disorientation might be someone who is depressed and becomes unaware of external happenings in the world, and therefore may be unaware of what day or time it is.

Following patterns is the ability to maintain attention, understand and follow a set course for problem-solving. After you make the plans, need to be able to remember where you are going and stay focused on your direction and follow the plan though.

Language and communication is the ability to recognize letters and words and understand their meaning, or/as in the example of the older adult with hearing problem, the ability to distinguish sounds. To communicate means to be able to give a response in such a way that others can interpret/comprehend what you are trying to state **or** the ability to interpret/comprehend what others are trying to state to you.

Memory is the ability to store and retain information for a short or long time and be able to recall and recognize based on retention.

Perceptual and motor development - The level of development whereby perceptual and motor development are coordinated to complete a task.

Perceptual speed and motor development involves coordination of the speed of processing information, and perceptual/sensory and motor function to complete a task.

Problem-solving-An example might be making a list to take to the grocery store. You need to be able to consider what you need, write it down, figure out how much it might cost, and how you will get to the store. All of these thoughts must be solved in order to go about the action desired. Problem solving requires comprehension, memory and processing information.

Retention is the ability to store and retain information for a short-term or long-time.

Recall is the ability to repeat information stored to memory using short or long term memory. Without the ability to recall information, we can not process information or follow through adequately on a task.

Recognition is the ability to perceive and mentally respond/register a situation, person, place, or thing as known and stored in memory.

PHYSICAL TERMINOLOGY

Fine motor skills- the skills needed for movement and control of the extremities. Mastering of these movements facilitates dexterity, flexibility, and manipulative skills of the hands and fingers. Fine motor skills for dexterity are required for tasks such as grasping objects, snapping snaps, buttoning clothes, and forming dough to cook bread.

Hand-eye coordination - The goal and ability to successfully coordinate perceptual input and fine motor skills to complete a task. Some examples include the ability to draw, write, throw a ball, play darts, and play golf. All of these activities require coordination of both hand and eye movement.

Gait is the way one goes about the mechanical process of balance, steps and coordination involving the ability to walk. Gait requires quite a few skills all at once, including balance, coordination of movement, posture, and strength in weight-baring limbs. Gait requires the ability of tone, and can be affected by neurological issues, such as complications from disease.

Gross motor skills– The skills needed for movement and control of the proximal muscles. Mastering of these movements facilitates agility, flexibility, and control of the whole body as well as legs and arms. This includes the ability to walk, run, bend, reach for an item, pick up a heavy item, toss an item, and dance.

Range of motion is the ability to have full range and movement of the extremities and the proximal muscles. There are various types of range of motion therapies. For example:

Active Assistive Range of Motion-This range of motion exercise is done with a therapist's assistance, when the patient may be limited to doing the exercises without assistance. It is used to promote stretching and strengthening.

Passive Range of Motion- This range of motion exercise is completely done by the therapist, when the patient is completely unable to do the exercise. This involves patients who have paralysis of the body part or other issues of immobility.

Stretching exercises are used to lengthen the muscles/connective tissue to help loosen tight muscles/spasms. The exercises can increase range of motion and lessen pain or spasms.

Tactile stimulation requires the use of a material, human touch, and machine to cause a sensation and promote neurological, muscular, and physical response/awareness. Some types of tactile stimulation include lights, vibration, sounds, smells (like aromatherapy), special foods, and varied texture items.

Socio-emotional Terminology

Community integration involves being integrated or brought together for a group activity for the expressed goal of interaction and adaptation to people, places, and experiences. It may also be beneficial in helping the older adult to feel a part of life in and of itself.

Culture is described as the shared values, traditions, norms, customs, arts, history, folklore and institution of a group of people. Understanding culture helps us to understand how others interpret, perceive, and function. Culture shapes the individuals and the group attitudes, ideals, goals, and values.

Productivity is to produce, stay productive, to contribute something to others for feelings of worth and value to others. It also is important for a sense of belonging. Some examples of ways to stay productive include helping out at home and in the nursing home, offering a skill to the commu-nity, or being a foster grandparent.

Reminiscing is used to exercise the memory for recall and recognition, Reminiscing is also a therapeutic activity used to help residents share a bond or share and recall one's own life-time of valuable experiences, joys, and history. An example is offering older adults from specific time frames activities that reflect that time frame. This type of activity is certainly good for memory stimulation. It is also good for identification with others and self–identity.

Self-esteem- There are two types:

- how one feels or relates to their individual abilities and worth; - how one interprets others' feelings about them and their abilities/worth.

Self-identity- A reflection of how we view ourselves in terms of who we are and what we have to offer as an individual within the world. It is based on such issues as interests, views, values, and passions.

Socio-emotional needs- A term used for meeting the needs of personal well-being in conjunction with changes in life conditions such as the loss of a spouse, a change in living arrangements, the loss of work, or problems with finances.

DEMENTIA/ALZHEIMER'S DISEASE

UNDERSTANDING DEMENTIA/ ALZHEIMER'S DISEASE

Dealing with issues of dementia in older adults creates unique and extremely challenging circumstances for all caregivers. Those suffering from dementia/Alzheimer's disease will require a much higher degree of time, encouragement, sensitivity, and ingenuity from the caregivers or staff. Going about daily activities or the use of activities as a way to help the Alzheimer's patient will be of tremendous benefit.

Dementia can be caused by a variety of reasons. Some causes of dementia are the result of vascular and other diseases. Some disorders and diseases associated with cognitive decline include Parkinson's disease, Multi-infarct disease, and Pick's disease.

A large percentage of dementia is the result of Alzheimer's disease. Dementia is defined as the loss of cognitive function in thinking, remembering, and reasoning. It also includes changes in personality, mood, and behavior. Dementia can be helped if the problem is with medication, the use of alcoholic beverages, depression, or the result of other conditions that are reversible. Intensive research continues to try to understand and someday possibly cure Alzheimer's disease.

However, presently, Alzheimer's disease is not reversible. Due to different causes of dementia and even different areas affected by dementia, not all patients will have all the same symptoms.

Dealing with circumstances that patients exhibit can influence the ability to implement activities. Remember, when we talk about activities we are not just referring to leisure or recreational activities but also daily living experiences.

The challenge to the caregiver (recreational) activity personnel will be to understand the patient's diagnosis and how to enhance and nurture activities for overall well being. Due to the high percentage of Alzheimer's patients and the full spectrum of cognitive losses, it is important to point out how to go about activities for the Alzheimer's patient.

Alzheimer's disease is a progressive brain disease that causes neuron-cognitive chemical changes, plaque buildup, and global wear and tear to cells and tissues within the brain.

Due to problems associated with inadequate neurotransmission/messages within the brain, there will be problems in thinking, memory, and communication/language skills. There will be changes in personality and behaviors. The life expectancy and duration of Alzheimer's disease patients is on average eight years, with a range of anywhere from 3 years to 20 years. Each patient case is unique, and the speed of progression/decline will vary. Not all patients will exhibit all symptoms, and the degree of symptoms will vary.

Not all patients will go through all the stages of Alzheimer's disease. They may have other diseases or medical concerns and succumb to death as a result of these complications.

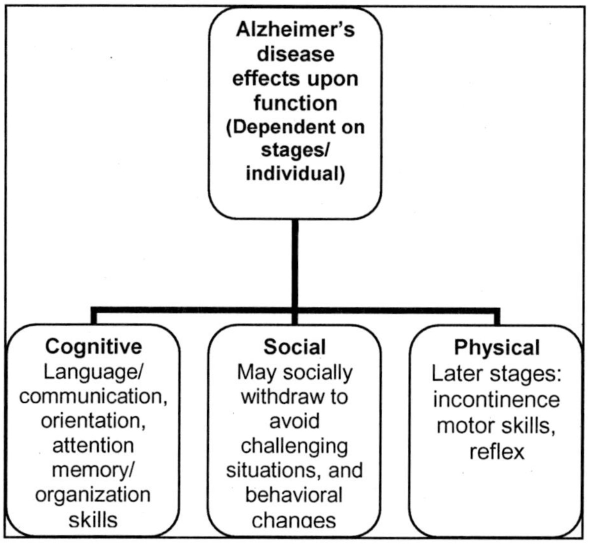

Figure 4.0-Alzheimer's disease: Effects on function

Functional Changes and Dementia/ Alzheimer's Disease

The primary affects of Alzheimer's disease/ dementia on function include changes in cognition. These changes include language/communication skills, attention, orientation, short-term and working memory and long-term memory and problem-solving.

Some affects to Alzheimer's disease regarding social/psycho-social issues may include social withdrawal to avoid challenging situations, behavioral/mental issues, sun downing, hoarding, repetitive movements, wandering, paranoia, hallucinations, and abusive behavior to self or others.

Towards the last stage of Alzheimer's, the patient will experience physical effects such as incontinence, motor skills deficits, and changes in reflex, muscle coordination and strength.

Stages of Alzheimer's Disease

Charts/scales are used to measure the degree and stages of a disease or disorder. Alzheimer's scales can help the patient and family to understand and prepare for Alzheimer's symptoms and stages. Reference charts or scales are also used to help researchers focus on the details of what takes place in the patient within the disease process. The charts give a general idea of what happens at each stage of the disease.

One scale measuring Alzheimer's disease is the FAST scale. Dr. Reisberg and associates studying Alzheimer's disease developed this scale. The functional assessment staging scale (FAST) is scale used to measure Alzheimer's patients' stages of disease by examining ADL skills and behaviors.

There are seven stages of Alzheimer's disease in this scale.

1. Normal and completely independent.
2. Normal with some personal awareness.
3. Early A. D.
4. Mild A.D. -Diagnosis of Alzheimer's usually is defined.
5. Moderate - A.D.
6. Moderate severe -A.D.
7. Complete dependence.

In stage one the patient is considered completely normal.

In stage two the patient may notice problems, but maintains normal capabilities. A physical exam would not show any signs of the disease.

In stage three, early Alzheimer's disease, short-term memory loss "will begin to emerge". Some examples of cognitive effects will be forgetting proper words and terms and trouble remembering the names/faces of those one has just met well begin to emerge. The patient may have trouble retaining information he or she has just learned or read. The patient may lose items or put them in the wrong place. An example of this might be putting their wallet in the refrigerator. Slight declines will be seen in the ability to plan, organize or complete a task they were able to without earlier problems. The presence of Alzheimer's may be questioned, but may be too slight to actually make a clear diagnosis.

In stage four, mild Alzheimer's disease, the patient will show measurable findings of Alzheimer's disease. At this point, a diagnosis is usually defined. The patient will begin to need mild assistance. By the fourth stage, the patient will have trouble remembering recent events and may struggle with letters, words, or number comprehension and doing calculations. Planning, or-ganizing, and taking care of money/household responsibilities will become more difficult and one will begin to see agitation and frustration while the patient tries to perform these tasks. They may even begin to avoid or withdraw from situations that they previously enjoyed to avoid the struggles they are experiencing.

In stage five, moderate Alzheimer's disease, the patient will begin to have moderate trouble answering questions regarding critical information, such as where they live, their phone number, birthday or other personal information. They may not be able to tell you what day, month, or year it is. Along with continued decline in short-term memory, comprehension, and calculations, critical thinking will become more difficult. Alzheimer's patients do much better with concrete thinking. Using simple gestures and forms of visual instructions becomes a more suitable method of communication with the Alzheimer's patient. Critical thinking and judgment will begin to be effected. They may have trouble choosing appropriate dress, and may mix, match or put on wrong layers of clothing when dressing. They may lack good judgment regarding their funds, and may donate or purchase unnecessary items or engage in other actions dangerous to their well-being.

In stage six, moderate-severe Alzheimer's disease, the patient will need a moderately high degree of assistance with activities of daily living skills. They will need help when dressing, bathing, and with using proper hygiene.

Short-term memory problems will become more severe, and patients will struggle remembering recent events, which may cause them to become disoriented. They may become confused regarding the timeframe they are in. An example may be that they may think it is ten years earlier and get ready to go to work or prepare for some other event they would have done in that time period. Wandering may become of concern, as they may actually prepare to (try to) leave the unit as if they going to work.

Long-term memory will also be affected. Patients will have trouble remembering personal information and background as well as recognizing those who have strong ties with them. This will include family members and caretakers. They will seem to have some recognition, and may drift from remembering to forgetting with inconsistency.

Behavioral issues and behavioral problems will become more evident around the sixth stage. Issues regarding sleep patterns, disturbances, sun downing, and agitation will develop. Behavioral and emotional issues may include wandering, repetitive behaviors, paranoia, hallucinations, screaming, self-abuse, and abuse to others.

Between the sixth and seventh stage, the Alzheimer's patient will not be able to use the toilet without assistance and will have urinary and feces incontinence. Behavioral issues will also become more prominent. Again, not every patient will display all symptoms or behaviors. Dependant on each patient there will be also be varied degree of symptoms, behavior and methodology to handle the behavior by staff.

In stage seven, severe Alzheimer's disease, the patient's communication skills will deteriorate significantly. Little by little, their vocabulary may slowly regress from an ability to talk in paragraphs, then sentences, a few words and eventually only noises. They may also exhibit echoing sounds and repeat them over and over.

By this point, the areas of the brain affected by chemicals that relay messaging and neuron motor abilities including reflex and movement will be affected. At first the patient may lose the ability to walk. This may be followed by the ability to sit up, hold one's head up, eat, smile, and swallow.

Research and Realism Regarding Alzheimer's Disease

Dr. Reisberg and his associates have also developed a scale showing the connection and parallels seen between the progression in child developmental stages for children up to the age of 12 and the regression patterns seen in Alzheimer's patients. Starting around the third stage of progression of the disease, by using the scale one sees that the Alzheimer's patients exhibit a decline in skills. This has been likened to a backward slide from the development normally seen in developmental stages of an average 12-year-old child. The Alzheimer's patient's skills and function level may continue to decline downwards to that of an infant. Watching these declines and the stresses, frustrations, depressions, fears, and losses of Alzheimer's disease can be overwhelming to the patient and the caregiver.

In the book, *House on Beartown Road*, Elizabeth Cohen talks about this very real parallel she witnessed while caring for her father, who suffers from Alzheimer's disease.

She talks about the similarities of watching her child go through the progress and developmental stages that a healthy child will, and watching her father go through a regression of developmental skills. In caring for her father, and at the very same time raising her young child, she notes how very similar they seem to be, both contented and capable of the same functions, interests, and joys, and both relying on her to meet their needs. Elizabeth's frankness and openness to recognize these similarities is both a testament to her observation skills and her ability to face this issue head on.

Many families are very sensitive to any correlation's made between their loved ones and the regression regarding correlations to child development. This is understandable. Most certainly, it is ext-remely important to remember that Alzheimer's patients are adults and should be respected and treated with the dignity of an adult. However, if we focus too much on labels and age brackets, we might miss out on the most important ele-ment of this research and the importance of recognizing the realism of what takes place for the Alzheimer's patient and their caregivers. Only then can we truly offer the Alzheimer's patient proactive care and institute the mag-nitude of support services the Alzheimer's patient and their family may need.

While many illnesses and topics can be uncomfortable, many steps and advancements in healthcare, involving physical, mental and social issues have made great strides by bridging the gaps surrounding "uncomfortable topics" and meeting the issues with openness, respect and dignity.

We need to be able to find a balance of respecting the Alzheimer's patient and understanding the high needs of these patients and their families. Perhaps, by recognizing needs without labels or age attachment, and focusing on skills and needs, we can help understand the higher goals of realistic support and respect for this population.

Elizabeth Cohen goes on to write about her own journey and thoughts as she comes to terms with the impact of the disease and its effects on memories, history and role reversals: changing from a daughter who looks to her father for answers and care into the role as her father's caregiver.

Her use of humor and her honesty regarding the struggles experienced as a "full fledged" member of what has been termed the "sandwich generation" (those who care for their children and aging parents at the same time), coupled with the extreme challenges of caring for her father and the impact of Alzheimer's disease, gives us a true insight of how families struggle and cope on a daily basis.Recognizing the full scope of issues that take place for these patients and their caregivers can help us to offer the potential for top quality research and care.

Communication, Behavior Issues, and Helpful Techniques

Generally, visual, tactile or facial gestures work better when one is trying to communicate with Alzheimer's patients. Language skills are not only harder to interpret, but the patient may also have trouble understanding what is being said in terms of reasoning and the retention of information. They may take what you are saying literally and have trouble with abstract thinking. Messages should be concrete, short, simple, and direct.

It is also important to remember that as older adults age they may experience varied hearing loss. They may have trouble distinguishing words or sounds. Older adults' vision can also be affected by other visionary problems. For these reasons, a complete examination should be included addressing these issues. The compounded problems of language compre-hension, psychological issues, critical thinking, and physical wear and tear visionary and auditory problems are all extremely challenging issues for Alzheimer's patients.

Dementia (and Alzheimer) patients will exhibit behaviors such as wandering and engage in compulsive, repetitive behaviors such as echoing, screaming, rocking, hand watching, and other behaviors. They may take on behaviors such as hoarding or rummaging through items. It is important to note that unless this behavior is an infringement on other's personal items, it may be okay to allow them to do this. Sometimes they need to be able to have the freedom to explore or engage in an activity without restriction. As long as what they are doing is safe and does not infringe on the rights of others, patients should be free to explore.

It is important also to be sure the environ-ment is safe and appropriate.In the case of a patient engaging in an inappropriate behavior for others to witness such as self-stimulation, this does warrant additional measures and the patient should be directed to a private area.

Never allow and never dismiss the behavior regarding a patient touching other patients inappropriately. This is a sensitive area of concern, but it is extremely important to remember. Even if an Alzheimer's patient is incapable of understanding their behavior, abuse is abuse and the situation must be addressed and taken care of with serious solutions. In some cases, repetitive or disruptive behavior will require intervention or redirection to another activity.

Some suggestions for behaviors may include: distracting the patient from the behavior by offering another activity they like. If the patient is hoarding or rummaging though another's private possessions, setting aside a crate, bag or special place containing their own items may be helpful. If you notice they tire of these items, you can change the items from time to time.

Dementia/ Alzheimer's patients may suffer from paranoia or confusion about what you are doing. They may accuse you of being an imposter or of trying to poison them. In either case, try to talk calmly with them. Use a calm, gentle voice with short simple language terminology.

Do not use baby talk. Slowly explain what you are doing. Use visual, facial or tactile methods to accent your point. If the patient is delusional or is having visual or auditory hallucinations, talk softly and nod so they know you hear what they are saying. Try to reassure them, but don't demand they believe you, as this may only aggravate them. If reasoning does not work, you may need to distract them or get them engaged in another activity. If the patient is exhibiting sun downing/agitation, arrange for an early afternoon nap. Make sure the area is very quiet with no stimulation. Sometimes, soft music may help the patient to stay calm and relaxed.

Wandering is a serious concern for Alzheimer's patients. There are various types of wandering behaviors. The term elope is used when referring to when a patient leaves the premise without permission. Then there is a **safe wander or the "safe wanderer"**. This is a person that might walk up and down the halls, but does not go into other residence rooms or try to leave the building. An **unsafe wander or an "unsafe wanderer"** will walk the halls and go into other peoples' room. They may even try to get into bed with them (another resident's bed) or some other aberrant behavior.

The Alzheimer's patient may become confused regarding time periods, and, as a result of disorientation, they may set out to complete a task with no relevance to the present time period. An example might be getting up to go to work for a prior job. They may try to leave the unit. If they are at home, they may decide to leave the house. Alzheimer's patients can be at extreme risk if they do leave the house, unit, or even when on a community trip. Because of their lack of orientation, their inability to communicate effectively, and a lack of ability to interpret/comprehend communication, they may not be able to help themselves. They may not be dressed appropriately for the weather. They may lack judgment in terms of safety. For all these reasons, they will be extremely at risk.

Whether in a unit or in their home, Alzheimer's patients may forget where they are, the timeframe they are in, or where things are located. Putting signs and pictures around the unit or house may be of help. Pictures, cues outside of each room, and their purpose may be helpful. For example, placing a picture of a chair and table by the dining area or making bathroom signs may be helpful. Labeling items with visual/picture cues will also be of help.

IMPLEMENTING ACTIVITIES FOR ALZHEIMER/DEMENTIA PATIENTS

Implementing activities for those suffering from dementia will require a much higher degree of time, encouragement, sensitivity, and ingenuity on the caregivers/activities personnel behalf. Using activities as a way to help the dementia patient, will be of tremendous benefit

The use of activities to help Alzheimer's patients will not stop the progression of the disease, however maintaining skills that have not been affected by the disease will allow the older adult to continue activities that are still possible. Activities will help maintain skills that otherwise may deteriorate simply as a result of lack of use, rather then any real clinical deficits.

Activities will allow the older adult to be monitored for any changes that may need further attention. Activities can also be satisfying at any level of quality care.

When you begin an activity, it will become important to not only speak but also offer cues along with your words. When communicating, speak slowly and use visual, auditory and tactile gestures. Make eye contact, use hand gestures, and gently guide them. You will need to go very slow with directions. If necessary, demonstrate or perform the actions you would like them to do.

You may need to do a project one step at a time. The degree of communication struggles will dictate the degree of need to use communication cues. As the disease advances, this will require much more time, redundancy, physical help, and encouragement.

Due to problems associated with color discrimination, depth perception, visual acuity and visual-spatial ability/discrimination, having items that show a clear distinction in colors will help them to see objects more clearly and distinctly.

On a unit with higher needs and lower function, there will be a need to plan individual patient time. This will afford time for individual patients to complete a task with support. When activity time must be done with larger groups, ask staff members to help with activities. You may need to work in smaller groups.

If you have to do an individual activity and have other older adults who will need your attention at the same time, it will be helpful to know what items keep each older adult calm and engaged in an activity. This will be of help as you work with each individual.

If you can find an activity that they know from past routines and tailor it to their present abilities, this can be very useful and pleasurable for them. They are reassured when they can do something for themselves. Unfortunately, as time goes by, they may not remember what they liked but this will depend on the stage of illness. As stated earlier in the book under "special needs," activities at any level can have a therapeutic value.

Keep activities simple and similar

Keeping routines are crucial for the comfort factor as well as basic memory abilities for the patient. They may do best with tasks that have a routine.

Choosing activities that are simple, familiar and repetitive will be helpful.
Activities need not be elaborate to be satisfying and beneficial. It will depend on the older adult's level of skill.

They may still be able to do many tasks, but more time may be needed. As mentioned under Special Needs, you can also have some activity steps completed earlier by someone else.

As the disease progresses, these activities will need to be tailored down. A task that they did in their home may work well. Folding towels, sorting nuts from bolts in jars, sorting colored buttons into jars, polishing silverware, painting small pre-built birdhouses, etc. are suitable examples. At each stage of decline, you will have to again tailor the activities to the stage of Alzheimer's disease for the older adult.

Activity ability is a question of skill level not ages level. By using ingenuity many items can be modified to reflect honor, dignity, and age of the patients

Many of the issues brought up here are everyday concerns for the Alzheimer's patient.
The caregiver/activities personnel can be critical to the overall well-being of the older adult. Giving the Alzheimer's patient activities that help them feel contented and also help them maintain the highest function levels possible are key to enhancing the older adult's quality of living.

ADDRESSING SAFETY AND HEALTH CONCERNS

Falls

Falls are a major safety issue when working with older adults. In 2001, more than 1.6 million seniors were treated in emergency departments for fall-related injuries, and nearly 388,000 were hospitalized (CDC, 2003).

Falls account for not only injuries and factors that decrease mobility, but falls have been associated with a high likeliness of needing care in a long-term care facility. Studies have also shown correlation to deaths not just attributed to the fall but, as a secondary cause, such as the exposure to disease, infections, or pneumonia while inpatient or immobilized.

Anytime you are working with older adults, use caution regarding the potential danger of a fall. Be sure you know your residents' abilities. Before and during activities assess the circumstances and be alert to times the older adult may require additional support.

There should always be adequate staff present to assistance the older adult in case they require help with standing, or monitoring while walking. Safety precautions also include proactive prevention measures such as being sure the floors are clutter free, residents have the ability to maneuver around the room freely without disruption, and rooms are well lit. If a spill happens, clean it up immediately. Put up caution signs if the floor is still drying. Be careful with older adults on stairwells. If they must use a stairwell, make sure they hold on to the railing at all times.

A good assessment should include:

1. A history of fall circumstances, medications, acute or chronic medical problems, and mobility levels
2. An examination of vision, gait and balance, and lower extremity joint function
3. An examination of basic neurological function, including mental status, muscle strength, lower extremity peripheral nerves, and ability of movement and reflexes
4. An assessment of basic cardiovascular status including heart rate and rhythm, postural pulse and blood pressure and, if appropriate, heart rate and blood pressure responses. You also need to assess any other particular concerns for individual residents. (Adapted from the Department of Health and Human Services, DHHS 2003).

CPR, First Aid, and Heimlich Maneuvers

All staff must attend training workshops for CPR, First Aid and the Heimlich maneuver. Studies have shown a decline in the ability of staff members to remember details, techniques for initiation of CPR procedures, as the time span between class instructions of CPR widens. It is suggested that staff stay updated frequently.

Anywhere food will be served there must be signs with instructions for choking and initiation of the Heimlich maneuvers, First Aid, other emergency procedures.

Sanitary factors

There will be occasions when older adults will be engaging in activities such as cooking. In a nursing facility or day care center, nutritional guidelines, sanitary conditions, infectious disease control, and any pertinent mandatory regulations must be followed. All staff should be aware of these regulations.

Be sure to disinfect surface areas after cooking, eating, or any activity time.

A solution that meets OSHA/NIOSH approval should be used for cleaning using protocol and NIOSHA guidelines.

Employees and patients should wash hands as often as needed. Hairnets should be worn. Many germs and toxins can enter the body through contact on the skin, inhalation of the lungs, or though the mucus membranes of the eyes, nose or mouth. There is also the possibility of germs caused by injury from a sharp object or needle. Because of the frailty of an older adult's skin, every precaution should be made to beware of potential for injury. Residents and staff should be treated immediately for any injury.

You may at times also be working with an older adult who has infection control measures in place. You may need to go to their room to offer activities. Be sure to wear a proper gown that covers you adequately. Also, wear gloves if needed. You must remember to wash after each visit. Also wash any items that you used during the activity time. This is appropriate after any activity time.

If during activity time or an outing an older adult needs to use the toilet, make sure both the older adult and yourself wash your hands thoroughly after.

If the older adult wears undergarment pads and there is an accident, avoid contact with the skin, use gloves, and clean up the spill immediately. Discard the pad properly.

Understanding individual patient special needs and safety concerns

It is important to read the resident's chart regarding dietary/nutritional concerns and food consistency plan. This includes awareness of the resident's ability to swallow, chew, sit up, etc.

Choking is a serious concern for older adults. This is particularly a high concern for those with disorders that effect swallowing ability .Be aware of any special drink consistencies. Some older adults may only be capable of drinking fluids with special additives that thicken the drink consistency.

Positioning is also an important safety issue. Be sure residents sit upright while eating or drinking.

Be sure food temperatures are within a safe temperature range for eating, as well as for safe handled of dishes.

Be aware of all restricted diets such as diabetics, low-salt restrictions, or any other notations on medicines and foods. Some foods can contradict or impact the effects of medicatons.

Whether you are working in a facility, a family member or a family caregiver, you should learn all you can about medication administration and the effects.

Be sure you are aware of any resident's allergies. Be aware of the ingredients you are using when cooking. This includes awareness of various materials the residents will be exposed to during any activity. For example: allergies to peanut butter, or in the case of an activity, an allergy to wool.

You should have a clear understanding of all of your older adult's special needs and safety concerns. Be aware of individual special positioning needs, lifting techniques, skin concerns, infection transmissions, restricted diets, allergies and medications.

Safety and Health Concerns, Fire Safety, and Emergencies

In the event of an accident (environmental danger such as fire, smoke, or chemicals) or if there is a hostile situation or any other emergency situation that threatens the safety of an older adult, if necessary immediate evacuation to a safe designated area. All facilities should have fire, accident, disaster, and hostile preventive and response plans. If cooking or engaging in activities that require electrical components, be sure the electrical equipment are secure and away from water. Be sure residents are in flame retardant clothes that do not have fray or items that may catch fire. Be sure you know where all fire extinguishers are and how to use them. You should also be aware of where all exits and alarms are located as well as fire safety procedures.

The majority of fires are the result of smoking or other factors in an individual resident's room or the personnel coffee room. This is followed by faulty equipment including appliances that are left on, old defective toasters, coffee pots, etc.

If you feel the fire is small enough that you can put it out, do so with extreme caution. If you have doubts about your ability to put out even the smallest of fires, it will be best to pull the alarm immediately or follow fire procedure for your unit/facility.

If you need to use a fire extinguisher, pull out the pin on the fire extinguisher, aim the extinguisher just below the flames, squeeze the trigger, and spray back and forth in a sweeping motion.

If you are on the phone getting emergency help, stay on the line until the dispatcher has all needed information.

Try to move the residents along in a quick and timely fashion, but calm voice. If you remain calm, the residents will do the same and you will actually be able to get out more quickly.

If you can exit, stay as close to the floor as you can to avoid toxins and smoke. Be very cautious of oxygen tanks. Try to keep residents away from the tanks. You need to be aware of the procedure for safety/fire and oxygen concerns for your residents.

Evacuate ambulatory patients first and try to move as close to the exit as possible. .If you must use the stairs, try to move in a calm, orderly fashion. Do NOT use an elevator. If the electrical system shuts down you may be trapped inside.

After any emergency, you must fill out documentation stating what happened and all relevant information within a set period of time, depending on regulations.

(Fire Safety, Department of Health and Human Services (DHHS, 2003). Fire safety (NIOSH 2003)-http://www.cdc.gov/niosh/2003.

ELDER ABUSE

Older adults are very vulnerable to abuse. They may be limited to respond when in a physical, mental, or emotionally abusive situation. Abuse can be verbal, physical, or emotional. If you are working in a facility, abuse training is a mandatory course. If you are concerned of abuse, or if you suspect abuse of an older adult, you can contact your local social services or other community resources to ask for help.

The 1998 National Elder Abuse Incidence study funded in part by AoA found the following:

- 551,011 persons, aged 60 and over, experienced abuse, neglect, and/or self-neglect in a one-year period;
- Among known perpetrators of abuse and neglect, the perpetrator was a family member in 90 percent of cases. Two-thirds of the perpetrators were adult children or spouses.

Elder abuse is an umbrella term used to describe one or more of the following:

Physical abuse is the willful infliction of physical pain or injury, e.g., slapping, bruising, sexually molesting, or restraining.

Sexual abuse consists in the infliction of non-consensual sexual contact of any kind.

Emotional or psychological abuse is the infliction of mental or emotional anguish, e.g., humiliating, intimidating, or threatening.

Financial or material exploitation is the improper act or process of an individual, using the resources of an older person, without his/her consent, for someone else's benefit.

Neglect is the failure of a caretaker to provide goods or services necessary to avoid physical harm, mental anguish or mental illness, e.g., abandonment, denial of food or health related services. Self-neglect is characterized as the behavior of an elderly person that threatens his/her own health or safety.

It is also important to be aware that older adults who show signs of dementia may become abusive as part of the disease process, and the object of the abuse may be another older adult, for example, a spouse who is caring for the impaired elder.

The abuse may take the form of hitting or gripping the caregiver to the extent of causing bruises, or creating hazards such as sett-ing furniture on fire. Although the behavior can be explained by the impairment, it is still unacceptable.

Signs that abuse might be taking place

It is important to point out some medicines and diseases may cause some of these symptoms, but not all.

Physical Abuse:

- Bruises or grip marks around the arms or neck
- Rope marks or welts on the wrists and/or ankles
- Repeated unexplained injuries
- Dismissive attitude or statements about injuries
- Refusal to go to same emergency department for repeated injuries.

Emotional/Psychological Abuse

- Uncommunicative and unresponsive
- Unreasonably fearful or suspicious
- Lack of interest in social contacts
- Chronic physical or psychiatric health problems
- Evasiveness.

Sexual Abuse, Financial Abuse or Exploitation may include factors in which:

-Life circumstances don't match with the size of the estate;

- Large withdrawals from bank accounts, switching accounts, unusual ATM activity;

- Signatures on checks don't match elder's signature.

Neglect signs include:

- Sunken eyes or loss of weight;
- Extreme thirst;
- Bed sores.

To report elder abuse, contact Adult Protective Services through your state's hotline. The APS agency screens calls for potential seriousness, and it keeps the information it receives confidential. If the agency decides the situation possibly violates state elder abuse laws, it assigns a caseworker to conduct an investigation (in cases of an emergency, usually within 24 hours). If the victim needs crisis intervention, services are available. If elder abuse is not substantiated, most APS agencies will work as necessary with other community agencies to obtain any social and health services that the older person needs.

The older person has the right to refuse services offered by APS.

The APS agency provides services only if the senior agrees or has been declared incapacitated by the court and a guardian has been appointed. The APS agency only takes such action as a last resort (DHHS, 2003).

Website:http://www.elderabusecenter.org

Phone: (202) 898-2586.

Fax: (202) 898-2583.

E-mail: NCEA@nasua.org

Mail: 1201 15th Street, N. W. Suite 350 Washington, D. C. 20005-2800.

Elder Abuse Resources:

National Center on Elder Abuse (NCEA) Six partner organizations that make up NCEA:

National Association of State Units on Aging

ABA Commission on Law and Aging

The Clearinghouse on Abuse and Neglect of the Elderly

The National Committee for the Prevention of Elder Abuse

National Association of Adult Protective Services Administrators

Other Elder Abuse Resources:

1998 National Elder Abuse Incidence Study

National Center for Elder Abuse (NCEA). (2003). www.elderabusecenter.org.

Administration on Aging, Department of Health and Human Services (DHHS, 2003).

The National Elder Abuse Incidence Study, Final Report, http://www.aoa.gov/. Adapted from the Department of Health and Human Services (DHHS, 2003)

Some factors that may lead to abuse

Family situations and elder abuse are usually related to a higher level of stress in the home as a result of the household changes. There may be other factors behind the abuse and/or additional circumstances such as an adult child struggling with an ailing parent or unre-solved issues. There can be a high need for help with a respite care. This is particularly so for families dealing with an elderly person with Alzheimer's disease or intensive medical care.

Caregiver issues and elder abuse are generally related to personal problems of the caregiver. The caregiver may also become overwhelmed with caring for an older adult with chronic illness.

Cultural issues and elder abuse are very sensitive areas. Due to cultural upbringing, the elder may not even recognize they are being abused or even believe it is abuse due to culture customs and elder issues. If you find yourself overwhelmed, take a break, count to ten, and ask for help/support. Try to focus on understanding the patient's perspective/needs.

Remember: empathy, support, and patience. Avoid blaming or shaming messages. If you find yourself saying things in an angry or shameful manner, it is time to step away. When you are stressed or overwhelmed, it is your job to recognize you need a break. When you are away from the situation, talk with staff about additional support or ways to help the resident's behavior. Discuss the stress you may be under and support services you may need to seek. Be alert to verbal or physical abuse from others as well. Never ignore a coworker's abuse of a patient or stay silent to protect the elderly, as they are mandated reporters and are required under state law to report abuse.

DOCUMENTATION

The following is the Title 1 Older Adult American Act.

Figure 5.0
Title 1, OlderAmericans Act

The Older American Act has been instrumental in improving the quality of care for all older adults. To obtain further information please visit aoa.hhs.gov 2005

Title I, Older Americans Act

The Congress hereby finds and declares that, in keeping with the traditional American concept of the inherent dignity of the individual in our democratic society, the older people of our Nation are entitled to, and it is the joint and several duty and responsibility of the governments of the United States, of the several States and their political subdivisions, and of Indian tribes to assist our older people to secure equal opportunity to the full and free enjoyment of the following objectives:

(1) An adequate income in retirement in accordance with the American standard of living.

(2) The best possible physical and mental health which science can make available and without regard to economic status.

(3) Obtaining and maintaining suitable housing, independently selected, designed and located with reference to special needs and available at costs which older citizens can afford.

(4) Full restoration services for those who require institutional care, and a comprehensive array of community-based, long-term care services adequate to appropriately sustain older people in their communities and in their homes, including support to family members and other persons providing voluntary care to older individuals needing long-term care services.

(5) Opportunity for employment with no discriminatory personnel practices because of age.

(6) Retirement in health, honor, dignity - after years of contribution to the economy.

(7) Participating in and contributing to meaningful activity within the widest range of civic, cultural, education and training and recreational opportunities.

(8) Efficient community services, including access to low-cost transportation, which provide a choice in supported living arrangements and social assistance in a coordinated manner and which are readily available when needed, with emphasis on maintaining a continuum of care for vulnerable older individuals.

(9) Immediate benefit from proven research knowledge which can sustain and improve health and happiness.

(10) Freedom, independence, and the free exercise of individual initiative in planning and managing their own lives, full participation in the planning and operation of community-based services and programs provided for their benefit, and protection against abuse, neglect, and exploitation.

Documentation and Regulations

The Joint Commission on Accreditation of Healthcare Organizations (JCAHO) has the following specific documentation standards (JCAHO, 2004):

When an older adult is initially assessed, an educational assessment is required. This assessment must show the resident's ability to understand and answer questions. If the patient is not capable of answering questions, someone must be present to help the resident understand as well as possible, or someone must be present who can show consent as the resident's legal representative. A nutritional and rehabilitation assessment must also be done. Generally, it is required that the head/registered nurse fills out the initial forms of resident assessments. You need to check on the type of entry that you will be allowed to make at your particular center. All paperwork must include the resident's name, the date and your signature.

Documentation Forms and Styles

There are a variety of documentation forms and styles used within different facilities. Some documentation programs are used following a pattern that use an acronym and intention focus, such as the Data Action Response/Result Plan focus charting method. The goal is to help direct care plans in a format that includes the major areas of concerns and goals.

Traditional documentation includes the narrative notes along w/ additional charts and data. A newer format is Charting by Exception, where the focus is primarily on critical needs being addressed. This type of system can be hard for staff to adjust to; it shows less documentation of what goals/tasks are being done throughout the day and only focuses on special concerns. This system is much different then the older standard practice of full documented patient care. However, as long as all other goals are met and procedures followed emphasis on critical needs can eliminate unnecessary paperwork and allow the staff to focus on patient care. Some facilities use continuing flow chart systems/clinical pathways and computer programs that only require input information on the patient and will actually assist the staff with suggestions on care plan concerns, or additional input. Some facilities use a combination of all these documentation styles.

A major factor is the essential need for full staff training to ensure adequate use of programs and documentation.

Each system has pros and cons. The success or failure of any documentation system may be more related to additional issues regarding documentation and protocols methods.

Be sure that you write clearly and check for grammatical errors. This will ensure information is interpreted correctly. Those who may be involved in medication administration should follow guidelines regarding format for proper words or symbols to ensure medication accuracy without medical errors or to ensure medical instructions are accurate. Do not eat or drink around the paperwork and keep the area clean. Papers need to be clear and any smudges could be a potential danger for misread documentation and errors. Use black/blue permanent ink. Be sure all writing material is legible and adequate for copy/transfer purposes

Some other general rules include being sure to follow procedure of caution if working on a computer. Be careful where information is stored. Paper documents should be filed in a secure area. Use locked cabinets. You need to ensure the patient's records are protected and private. If you use a computer make sure a hard copy and or paper copy is filed. This will ensure confidentiality of patient records and that important resident's records are safe, permanent and available.

Protection and legal protection

Except in special circumstances of acceptable practices and protocols that meet state/ government regulations never fillout documentation for other employees'. Never allow others to fill in your documentation. If someone else is filling out a report and information you were involved in, be sure to read the document if asked to do so, and initial your approval. Always be sure any instructions that will involve your directions are in writing and signed.

When finished entering your inform-ation, put a line through any empty spaces. If you make an error put a line through the error and initial it. Be sure to do your paperwork as soon as possible to avoid forgetting important details. Be sure to take the proper time to do your documentation. Documentation is extre-mely important for the patient, staff, facility and government procedures.

Patient Care

Documentation ensures that the older adult is re-eiving the utmost quality of care. Be sure you have all paperwork updated and completed and that you include all data and information requested by the facility. Be sure you are aware of all information and services your patient is receiving. It is important to continuously read the patients' data and stay updated between treatment plan meetings. Whenever you have concerns or information that impacts the client's care, make sure you update the file as needed. This will ensure all staff is alert to current information, needs and goals for the patient.

Following professional standards /code of ethics are essential for your professional conduct and commitment to older adults or others in your care. You should be sure to stay updated and informed of your particular profession code of ethics and standards. It is your responsibility to read the standards/code of ethics for your profession.

Standards found in every profession will include maintaining professionalism and boundaries, staying objective and impartial and following treatment plans according to regulations not personal feelings. Following directions regarding patient's rights is the responsibility of the professional as well as the patient. Advocacy is a wonderful thing, but it does not include disregarding the rules, regulations or others rights or laws that are in place.

Facility's Quality Control/ Compliance

Documentation is essential for Facility's Quality control/compliance and ensures that standards, responsibilities, and continuing challenges are met to increase the goal of facility quality, compliance, and excellence. It is also required for federal and state regulations. For example, in the case of an accident, if documentation is omitted, the facility will be heavily fined. If paperwork is not filled out, funding will be held until requirements are met. Even then there will be fines. The purpose of these actions is to ensure the facility is following regulations. Fines may be given if requirements are not met.

Reimbursement

Documentation is necessary to obtain reimbursement and support services. Documentation validates needs and spending and shows how you are implementing effective programs, following regulations and ensuring quality guidelines. Be sure to stay updated to changes or additional regulations that may affect your facility or your particular job requirements.

Statistics show that the majority of older adults live at home or with family members. Many times the older adult will either have his or her own private or supplemental insurance. If the older adult has financial hardship and can not meet their medical costs, they may be eligible for Medicaid services.

Older adults are eligible for help with medical bills through The Center for Medicare and Medicaid services.

The Prospective payment system is used by CMS to determine costs and reimbursements for outpatient services. These medical expenses are covered under Medicare B. There are guidelines and papers that must be filled out for a determination of reimbursement. Beginning in January 2006, older adults receiving Medicare are now eligible to receive help with prescription drug costs. Information on understanding the new prescription drug program can be obtained by contacting Medicare or by calling a senior resource center in your area. Older adults who meet eligibility requirements may qualify for both Medicare and Medicaid to cover the costs of medical services and prescription drugs.

The first government intervention and support program for older Americans, the Social Security Administration, was created in 1935. In 1965, the Social Security Act established both Medicare and Medicaid.

The Prospective Payment System

The Prospective Payment System was created as a result of *The Balanced Budget Act of 1997. This bill mandates the implementation of a per diem prospective payment system (PPS) for skilled nursing facilities (SNFs) covering all costs (routine, ancillary and capital) related to the services furnished to beneficiaries under Part A of the Medicare program.

Major elements of the system include: Per diem payments for each admission are case-mix adjusted using a resident classification system (Resource Utilization Groups III) based on data from resident asses-sments (MDS 2.0 or updates)) and relative weights developed from staff time data. Geographic Adjustment: The labor portion of the federal rates is adjusted for geographic variation in wages using the hospital wage index. In the skilled nursing facility, in order to meet Medicare/Medicaid funding, the Social Security Act specifies that each state must use the RAI or compatible equivalent format.

One element of the RAI (Resident Assessment Instrument is the MDS. We will talk about the MDS when we talk about facility assessments. The second required forms/procedurals are used for maintaining utilization management.

The Combination of factors for PPS is: The RAI (resident assessment intake or continued resident assessment plan)/ MDS, RUG III classification system, and Staff time Geographic Adjustment.

Rugs- III

Rug-III is a 44-group model to classifying nursing home residents. It includes health characteristics, amount and type of resources the older adult uses. Residents are classified based on the residents' clinical conditions, extent of services used, their functional status, the general order of costs associated with caring for residents in this bracket. This is information gained from the Minimum Data Set (MDS) and the wage-weighted staff time.

The RUGS are broken down into level of needed care for rehabilitation. They include extensive services, special care, clinically complex, impaired cognition, behavior problems and the lowest need, reduced physical function.

Rehabilitation is measured by five levels of intensity, based on: the total minutes of therapy received per week, the days of therapy per week and the number of different types of therapy received. Residents whose clinical conditions do not require skilled therapy are classified into lower categories, which descend in order of severity, the number of services used, and the amount of time and resources required to care for the resident.

F248

(f) Activities

Activity Regulations OBRA 1987 Clinton Healthcare Initiative

1. Understanding the Activity Regulations Clinton Healthcare Initiative
Survey Process
-What will the surveyors want from the Activity Department?

Quality Indicator Reports
-Facility Characteristic Report
-Facility Quality Indicator Report
-Resident Level Summary Report

Abuse and Neglect

Regulations Pertaining Specifically to Activities
-F 248 Activity Program
-F 249 Qualifications
-F 272 Assessments
-F 279 Care Planning

Other Activity Related Federal regulations Tags;
–Resident Rights; F-tags # 151, 155, 164-166, 169-171
-Resident Behavior; F-tag # 223-225
-Quality of Life; F-tag # 240, 246
-Resident Assessment; F-tag # 271-281, 284-285
-Quality of Care; F-tags # 309-311, 319-320
-Infection Control; F-tag # 444
-Physical Environment; F-tag # 464
-Administration; F-tag 492, 499

Common Areas for Activity Deficiencies
-Red Flag Areas
-Plan of Action; What will you do?
-Guidance to Surveyors

2. Federal Activity Regulations

(1) The facility must provide for an ongoing program of activities designed to meet, in accordance with the comprehensive assessment, the interests and the physical, mental, and psychosocial well-being of each resident.

Guidelines 483.15 (f)(1)

Because the activities program should occur within the context of each resident's comprehensive assessment and care plan, it should be multi-faceted and reflect each individual resident's needs. Therefore, the activities program should provide stimulation or solace; promote physical, cognitive, and/or emotional health; enhance, to resident's self-respect by providing, for example, activities that support self-expression and choice.

Activities can occur at anytime and are not limited to formal activities being provided by activity staff. Others involved may be any facility staff, volunteers and visitors.

Probes: 483.15 (f)(1)

Observe individual, group, and bedside activities.

1. Are residents who are confined or choose to remain in their rooms provided with in room activities in keeping with life-long interests (e.g., music, reading, and visits with individuals who share their interests or reasonable attempts to connect the resident with such individuals) and in-room projects they can work on independently? Do any facility staff members assist the resident with activities he or she can pursue independently?

2. If residents sit for long periods of time with no apparently meaningful activities, is the cause: (a) resident choice; (b) failure of any staff or volunteers either to inform residents when activities are occurring or to encourage resident involvement in activities; c) lack of assistance with ambulation; d) lack of sufficient supplies and/or staff to facilitate attendance and participation in the activity programs. e) Program design that fails to reflect the interests or ability levels of residents, such as activities that are too complex?

F249

3. Must be directed by a qualified professional

Who (i) is a qualified therapeutic recreation specialist or an activities professional
Who A) is licensed or registered, if applicable, by the State in which practicing; and B)
is eligible for certification as a therapeutic recreation specialist or as an activities professional by a recognized accrediting body on or after October 1, 1990;

(ii) Has 2 years of experience in a social or recreational program within the last 5 years, 1 of which was full-time in a patient activities program in a health care setting; or (iii) Is a qualified occupational therapist or occupational therapy assistant; or (iv) Has completed a training course approved by the State.

The Geriatric Observable Activities Program

Many agencies prefer that Certified Recreational Therapists or those with particular certification/clinical expertise be involved in the assessment of activity choice, interpretation of assessed skill level/ treatment plans.

It is hard to know what the rules will be in your center regarding ability to choose activities. You will have to follow the requirements of your particular center. Because safety is an issue that must be considered when doing any activity, this issue does need to be addressed whether you are working in a facility or at home.

RECREATIONAL/LEISURE ACTIVITY PROTOCOL MODEL

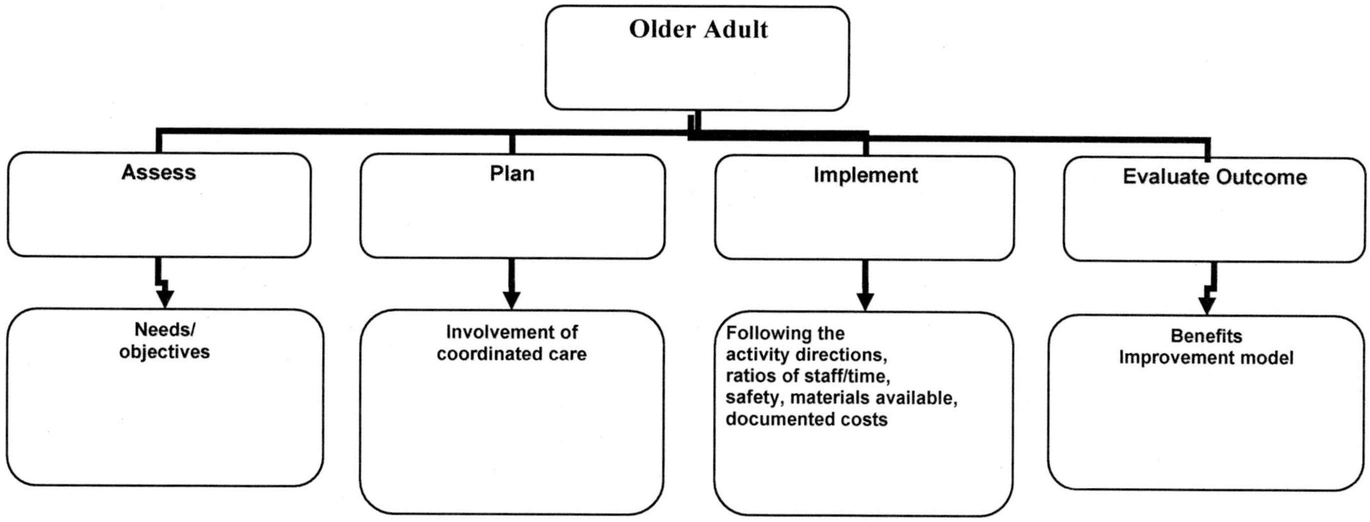

Figure 6.0
Recreational/Leisure Activity Protocol Model

What we are looking at is the Recreational/ Leisure Activity Protocol Model. (Fig.6.0)

In this section of the book we are going to use the four basic steps of effective activity programming and learn how to implement full use of the Geriatric Observable Activities for Longevity program.

1. Assess
2. Plan
3. Implementing Activities
4. Evaluate Outcome/Reassessment

ASSESSMENTS

Patient Charts, Tests, and Assessments

Data submitted on the resident can be found in the facility's patient chart. Along with personal information, the patient chart will include information regarding standardized tests and a facility wide assessment form.

Standardized tests allow licensed clinicians within specialty fields to use tests and make a diagnosis. Some examples of standardized tests include; The Folstein State Mini-Mental State

Examination, Katz Index of Activities of Daily Living, Instrumental Activities of Daily Living,

Modified Barthel Index, Performance Assessment of Function, Revised Memory and Behavior Checklist, Norbeck Social Support Questionnaire, and the Tinetti Balance and Gait.

The set of standards that go into these tests are immense, respected, and of great value. The tests use the most up-to-date studies and testing tools to make accurate clinical diagnoses.

In turn, the clinical assessment allows the clinician to make the staff aware of a patient's diagnosis, abilities, and needs so the appropriate treatment may be implemented. In nursing facilities, along with the use of standardized tests, facilities must also use specific protocols and paperwork to ensure overall quality care.

Understanding Nursing Facilities and OBRA Regulations

The Omnibus Budget Reconciliation Act (OBRA) regulations were enacted to ensure quality of care for patient's to ensure patients are given the best possible opportunities to maintain or reach their highest potential of function levels. This act also includes issues pertaining to fiscal rehabilitation and resource management. Nursing Facilities must use various assessment programs depending on reason for usage. The RAI/MDS is an assessment tool used by the Center for Medicaid and Medicare Services.

The RAI (Resident Assessment Instrument)/ MDS (The Mini Data Set) is an 18 item checklist used to examine patient status and needs regarding health care and quality care concerns as well as additional data. The Joint Commission on Accreditation of Healthcare Organizations requires that the nursing supervisor or another specialist that meets qualifications initially fill out these forms.

The Resident Assessment Protocol (RAP) Form

The RAP form is a continuum of the RAI; it is used to implement "action" within the eighteen areas of attention regarding overall healthcare concerns. This data is used as a tool to examine, classify and develop ongoing treatment goals for the resident.

This instrument/data sheet/flow-chart will become the "base" form. This data will initially be used to assess a patient's present condition in eighteen areas of function, abilities and needs. This information will then be implemented for ongoing treatment plans, goals and care. The RAPS form is reassessed quarterly.

The treatment team will use this information in the patient's chart to carry on each department's responsibility to quality healthcare.

As a recreational or activities personnel member, you will use the information you have been given by the physician or the treatment team and data notes to decipher where a resident would fall within the range of ability to take part in an activity, and gain therapeutic value in recreation.

The final step is to integrate the patient data, clinical diagnosis of assessed abilities found in the patient's chart, MDS/RAI (if in a nursing facility) recreational assessments, and treatment plans involving activities.

Implementing the Geriatric Observable Activities Program

The Geriatric Observable Activity for Longevity program was designed to run smoothly with other flowchart systems

The Recreational Goals: Initial Assessment and Mastery Checklist

The Recreational Goals: Initial Assessment and Mastery Checklist is for your **initial** recreational assessment. You will use the information you gain from this initial assessment to begin planning activities based on the resident's abilities and goals.

The checklist will also serve as a "graph"/checklist, showing progress and steps towards complete **mastery/attempt** for a particular skill within a specific domain (cognitive, physical, socio-emotional domains).

For example, cognitive function involves various types of mastery of skills for cognitive function. Cognitive function includes abilities such as attention, orientation, language skills, problem-solving, etc.

If we break this down even further and concentrate just on the factors regarding attention, we can see that attention involves or includes various steps towards obtainment in the mastery of attention.

We have broken down the steps for mastery of attention into five steps or levels of function, ability or need. The steps range from total dependence (one) to total independence (five). Sample objectives have been included to give you an idea of how to obtain the immediate goal and move onto the higher level of skill obtainment and mastery of the function. You can then check off each step as you move higher up the scale.

The Recreational Goals: Initial Assessment and Mastery Checklist meets three goals. It allows you to get an immediate assessment of the resident's needs and abilities, to see where your resident falls within mastery of the steps, and to begin your planning considerations to place on the Recreational Objectives Observational Form.

The Recreational Objectives Observation Form

The Recreational Observation Form (R.O.O.F.) can be used after you have done the initial checklist/assessment. The Recreational Objectives Observation Forms coincides with the Recreational Goals: Initial Assessment and Mastery Checklist. You can also use it along with any initial assessment and tests by your facility.

Each Recreational Objectives Observat-ion Form includes an optional score section for various assessments instruments. The Recreational Objectives Observational Form (R.O.O.F.) also includes the AMA current procedural codes for professionals who may submit bills and receive reimbursements for patient services. You can follow the entire format of the program and insert your facilities rating/score system or use the rating system included with this program.

If you use a center-based assessment or tests for initial skill levels, you will need to cross-reference the scale between the standardized test, MDS or other assessment instruments. You can then cross-reference your facilities initial assessment and where it coincides with the Recreational Objectives Observational Forms.

Both the Recreational Goals: Initial Assessment and Mastery Checklist and The Recreational Objectives Observation Forms include skills, goals, methods, and objectives. However, the Recreational Objectives Observation Forms (ROOF) also include empty spaces to implement your own specific goals, objectives, and methods unique to individual resident's needs.

You can use the information you have obtained from the Recreational Goals: Initial Assessment and Mastery Checklist to immediately fill in your first Recreational Objectives Observational Form. However, the Recreational Goals: Initial Assessment and Mastery Checklist is really meant to be your initial observation. It is also a tool to chart ongoing mastery of functions. This will allow you to implement a format based on abilities, goals, long-term considerations and planning for your resident.

Therefore, it is suggested that you use the Recreational Goals: Initial Assessment and Mastery Checklist first and follow this with three specifically targeted activities based on your goals. You can then use the Recreational Objectives Observation Forms to assess three full activities and the measurable outcomes.

Objectives, Goals and Methods Charts

Each activity in the book contains three matching forms: one cognitive, one physical, and one socio-emotional form. Directly before each form you will find a sample chart that you can use as a guide to help you fill out the particular activity forms. This will help you to understand the types of skill, goals, objectives, and methods you can use to obtain full benefits of the activity.

Each category of cognitive, physical, and socio-emotional areas is distinguished for the specific skills and goals of that domain.

The breakdown into these specific areas will help you to understand the types of skills needed for full mastery of the particular domain, as well as depict a clearer picture of strong and weak skills in the individual older adult. This information can be extremely valuable in helping to understand your resident's abilities and needs.

The Recreational Objectives Observation Form can be done over a set period or as often as needed. A set number of patients can be assessed with rotating observations. This procedure then rotates at a continuous flow or flowchart, with quarterly reviews.

An ideal method of choosing the sample of older adults per assessment is to group patients according to needs and observe these particular residents doing the particular types of activities over a three-month period. For example, choose the number of clients you feel need more physical activities, needing more cognitive observations, etc. You could then observe them during times you have scheduled these types of activities or as part of planning considerations.

Incorporating the use of activities and the Recreational Objectives Observation Forms

Each activity lists the skills and functions that can be gained from the activity, the time needed to do the activity, the staff and residents ratio, the instructions on how to do the activity, and any additional considerations.

You will use the matching Recreational Objectives Observation Form to chart increases or declines in function levels of physical, cognitive, and socio-emotional skills noted while residents are engaged in the activity. You will use this information to run a quality activity program inclusive of enhancing therapeutic recreational methods and observations. During quarterly RAPS assessments and team meetings, you can share this information and the charts with the treatment team.

The Recreational Observation Form is designed to show quarterly recorded skill levels. The last column will be the most current, level of function observed during activity times. You can also add up scores at the bottom of each column to see an overall score for each skill area. Being able to see set intervals of function levels will help to observe the older adult's progress, decline, or abilities maintained during ongoing activities and care.

The Recreational Objectives Observation Form (R.O.O.F.) also allows you to assess the resident behavior over a period of time during activities. It documents the amount of assistance or amount of time the behavior is observed and will allow you to show unique consistency of need or behavior, as well as where this amount of assistance/exhibiting of behavior is in proportion to the goals, objectives and skills level of your resident. The forms include codes for those professionals who can submit bills to insurance or agencies.

Using the Recreational Objectives Observation Forms

---

1. Information obtained from the MDS, the Recreational Goals: Initial Assessment and Mastery Checklist and Facility assessments, data, are used to understand the resident's abilities and needs.

2. Activities are chosen according to which activities will support the patient's needs/goals.

3. Find matching activity Recreational Objectives Observation Forms that coincide with the activity. You could also do activities in groups with residents needing the same skills observed. This can be helpful if you can only assess on days when you have a volunteer.

4. For initial score, begin by using the Recreational Goals: Initial Assessment and Mastery Checklist, and facility test assessments

5. Plan activity according to needs and goals

6. Institute use of the Recreational Objectives Observation forms and observe resident doing activities over a three-month observation period

7. As observing, fill in skill-level observed

8. At the end of the day, tally score for all three areas (physical, cognitive and socio-emotional) skills observed.

9. Tally the final score you have for all three observations in all three areas.

10. Bring the assessment reviews and documentation to treatment team/staff attention.

By using the recreational goals: initial assessment and mastery checklist and the Recreational Objectives Observational Forms, we hope you are able to get a strong assessment of the needs and skills exhibited by the older adult involved in an effective recreational therapeutic activity program.

Our purpose and the ultimate goal of these assessment tools are to assess individual needs, so that the adult is able to engage in recreational activities for function and fulfillment.

It is also our expressed hope that these activities can be an asset to the team of professionals working together with the older adult, for an inclusive betterment of treatment plan goals and the older adult's quality of life.

Interpreting Skills

One important factor regarding the use of assessments includes the system used to interpret the skills. Some assessments are self-assessments, and therefore are measured by the resident's answers.

When one is doing an observation or assessment of a resident, we know that certain skills are quantified, and therefore our residents will fall within a range of ability assessed for older adults doing this particular type of task.

The use of a tier-style checklist such as the Recreational Goals: Initial Assessment and Mastery Checklist can also be of help to gauge ability levels.

Doing an assessment on skill levels with clear-cut abilities is fairly simple. If we know that an independent resident can completely cook a meal or bake a cake without any assistance, we know they would be considered independent.

In this type of activity we can observe them making a "product." But how do you interpret emotional gratification and self-esteem?

In this case, we have to be part intuitive, part investigative, and at the very same time, factual.

One way to assess "abstract" behaviors is to use the clues of the resident's reactions, verbal expressions, facial expressions, perseverance, and tolerance of situations.

We can observe their physical behaviors to discern cognitive and socio-emotional abilities/needs.

For example, a resident who consistently joins in on dance classes and smiles and laughs while dancing and socializing could safely be assessed to be showing high emotional gratification. Even still, we might have to really know this patient to make this assessment. But, if this observation is fairly accurate and this same resident suddenly stopped joining dance classes or rarely joined dance or other classes, or never smiled or laughed, we could safely say she does not seem to be able to obtain emotional gratification during dance class.

In another type of example, not washing or showering, brushing hair, or putting on clean clothes, despite availability and support of these supplies, can be a sign of lack of initiative. This could also be a sign of depression, disorientation, etc. During a recreational or leisure activity, a lack of initiative or motivation would show up when the patient barely does the project, or has to be cued at least three times. But, it's important to be sure that the resident did not have cognitive deficit or medication issues that might be mistaken as motivational problems.

In a further challenging situation, how do we interpret attention? How do we interpret a measurable outcome when normal cues may not be available? Again, in this case, we have to be part intuitive, part investigative and, at the very same time, factual. If the resident falls asleep often, needs repetitive cues and physical help, seems confused, doesn't make eye contact, doesn't follow directions, and doesn't respond, we could say they are having trouble with remaining attentive or have a short attention span.

Dependent on a resident's condition, they may show they are paying attention differently than what is considered the norm. They may be incapable of verbal communication. Sometimes, you may be able to tell they are paying attention and are oriented by other forms of communication. They may respond by using eye contact or producing a slight movement of a limb, which may alert you to the fact that they hear you and are paying attention. While you may be accurate, you must back this up with concrete evidence. You must be able to show that this is a true form of their communication, attention, and orientation. You must be able to show this behavior is a consistent reaction for this situation. You must show a measurable outcome.

One way of doing this is to document a pattern. You must get to know the patient before assessing their individual signs of attention, behavior, and skill levels. You must be careful not to assume you know what they are communicating. You must show a pattern, including consistent circumstances that show why this assessment has validity. This must include the stated task and measurable outcomes.

Measurable objectives

When initiating an activity, remember to insert the resident's personal measurable objectives or "demand" for the task being sought. Some examples include: The resident will engage in an activity which require fine motor skills, *two times* (2x) per week, or the resident will maintain attention for up to *five minutes* per activity. You need to show pre-measurable objectives in order to demonstrate a change and a clear outcome of the resident's ability.

To measure a skill, meet the objectives and observe the outcome, you will need to consider your particular resident. The value or number you insert for your set goal will be determined by the resident's needs and progress. For example: once Tillie has mastered walking 10 steps, we would increase her physical function (if approved by her doctor) level to 20 steps a week. We might then increase that to twice a week. Every activity in the book can be matched with the particular goals, objectives of the particular resident. You will need to fill in the amount of time, etc. dependent on your resident. As you increase the task level, you will observe mastery of this particular task for your quantitative task ability and outcome.

Understanding the Rating Scale and Skill Numerical Levels

When addressing the issue of skill levels, resident abilities are measured by level of individual rate of ability or support needed to complete the task. For example, those requiring support of three or more cues and at least three or more physical supports are considered to possess up to, but not more than, 25% of ability, and are scored totally dependent.

Those requiring two-to-three cues and two supports during the activity possess at least 25% + ability, and are scored having high assistance. Those requiring one or two cues and one physical support need a moderate amount of support, and possess up to 50 % + ability. Those requiring one-to-two cues need a mild amount of support or possess up to 75% ability of the skill. Those requiring only occasional cues or just a general encouragement, and can show they are able to do the activity 75% or more of the time, are considered to be independent.

Cues can be described as a method of encouragement, the use of simple or complex stimulating questions, visual guides or the use of clues. All are used in order to support the resident in their obtainment of the needed task.

Cues do not include any type of physical or "mechanical" support. For example a staff member might point to a place a resident needs to sit, a staff member might show the resident some ribbon to knit with. This type of assistance differs from actual physical support which affects the resident's personal ability.

Actual physical support ranges from the simple act of gently guiding a resident to an activity and any higher actual physical support needed for the resident to complete the activity.

Let's use our case study of Tillie. The recreational therapist/activity professional assesses Tillie's skill levels using the Recreational Goals: Initial Assessment and Mastery Checklist for the initial evaluation. His goal is to help Tillie pursue meaningful and fulfilling activities and maintain function levels though the use of activities.

He begins his observation by observing how well Tillie adjusts to the center and meets other seniors. Tillie comes to the senior citizen center on Monday. She walks around the center and becomes familiar with the various programs, rooms, etc. He notes that Tillie hesitates to walk over to the activity table and introduce herself, or join in on the activity.

The recreational therapist walks up to Tillie and then gently (physically) guides her over to the table. He offers a cue by saying "Tillie, I would like to introduce you to Mary," "Tillie, this is Mary," "Mary, this is Tillie," etc. Tillie then says hello to Mary, and they sit down and continue to get to know each other, etc.

In this scenario, Tillie required one cue and one physical intervention. Because she required one physical intervention, Tillie would score a three or moderate skill-level observed.

After using the Recreational Goals: Initial Assessment and Mastery Checklist for the initial assessment, the recreational therapist/activity professional can use this information to understand where Tillie scores in the area of socio-emotional abilities (in this case, socialization skills). He could then use this information to fill in her first month on the Recreational Objectives Observation Form or use the information to begin formulating goals, objectives, etc. In either case, he can use this information to understand Tillie's initial intake ability or her skill-level within the range of ability, and how to help her obtain mastery of independent socialization skills.

Recreational Goals: Initial Assessment and Mastery Checklist

We will now look at various skills within the domain of cognitive, physical, and socio-emotional development, and consider the levels, steps, or goals sought to reach mastery of skills for each domain.

Cognitive Development

Attention

Goal	Objective	Method
Show increased attention span, attend to task for function, and to engage in meaningful, recreational/fulfilling activities	Will make eye contact with swim staff, will verbalize with staff/ instructor, will read/listen to swim rules, will say yes/no to show they understand or by actions. 1x week	Staff will instruct, state rules, or stand in front of resident, make eye contact, ask questions or use others forms to get resident's attention or show the resident is listening during a swim event

Problem: needs encouragement, cues or physical guides to increase attention span; attend to task for function, and to engage in meaningful, recreational/fulfilling activities.
Goals: show increased attention span; attend to task for function, and to engage in meaningful, recreational/fulfilling activities;
(1) ____makes eye contact for up to 15 seconds;
- will look at a staff member and vocalize or communicate in some form for 15+ seconds;
(2) _____ makes eye contact and maintains attention for more then 30 seconds - will make eye contact with staff, family member, or object for 30+ seconds and will engage in swim activity/ task;
(3) _____ follows simple directions and maintains attention for one minute and up to five minutes;
- will engage in swim activity/task and complete 50+% of task;
(4) ____can follow simple directions and maintains attention for five minutes or more - will engage in swim activity/task and are attentive 75+% of time;
(5) ___can follow sustained attention throughout activity (independently);
-will follow and complete swim instructions to complete a task (independently)

Orientation

Goal	Objective	Method
Show increased awareness of time/ "timeframe," people, circumstances, and past experiences vs. present experiences, to engage in present-time activities, or for a reminiscing intended activity	Will respond w/correct answer to two choice questions Or yes/no, will state place, time, present company of people, or past experiences on own during activity 1x a week	Staff will ask residents a series of questions to stimulate focus to the present setting (Ex: "Are you at the mall or at the swimming center?") Or past if a reminiscing exercise (Ex: "Have you swum before? With who? What is your swim partner's name? Mary or Karen?"

Problem: needs encouragement, cues, or physical guides to increased awareness of time/ "timeframe," people, circumstances, past experiences vs. present experiences; to increase awareness in present-time activities or reminiscing ability.

Goals: Increased awareness of time/"timeframe," people, circumstances, past experiences vs. present experiences; to increase awareness in present-time activities or reminiscing ability

(1) _____ is oriented to the environment for up to 15 seconds - will be engaged in present time activities or for a reminiscing intended question engaged in conversation /questions regarding past orientation during activity

(2) _____ shows a "consistent" acknowedgment through verbal communication, actions in context to situation for 30 seconds

-will be engaged in present time activities and asked questions to gauge present orientation or for a reminiscing intended question engaged in conversation/questions regarding past orientation for 30+ seconds____ time(s) this week

(3) _____ comes to activity at appropriate time, answers questions in context to the present environment and circumstances or for a reminiscing intended question engaged in conversation /questions regarding past orientation for 30+ seconds- and correctly responds 50% of the time

-will be engaged in present time activities or for a reminiscing/oriented awareness intended question for up to 50+% of time

-will come to group on time, and for example: mark individual calendar, state where she is____ time (s) this week

(4)_____ comes to activity at appropriate time, answers questions in context to the environment and circumstances or for a reminiscing intended question engaged in conversation /questions regarding past orientation and correctly responds 50+% of the time

-will be engaged in present time activities or for a reminiscing/awareness intended question for up to 75% of time

-will state date, month, year, birthday and important personal information or events in correct context.

(5)______ is orientated to surroundings, circumstances, people and timeframes (independently)

-will be engaged in present time activities or for a reminiscing intended question for 75+ of time /all of the time

-will state place, time/"timeframe", present/company of people or past experiences on own during activity.

-will continue to be involved in activities to stay oriented to environment, circumstances, people and timeframes of present/past.

Language and Communication

Goal	Objectives	Method
Show increased ability to communicate/ comprehension use of words phases, sentence structure, comprehension, interpretation	Will reply to interpret a question ex: states color swim board, favorite swim form, yes, no etc. will interpret instructor's request and shows understanding by initiating task.	Staff will ask questions to stimulate communication. Ex: "What color float do you like?" Or make a demand to observe interpretation or language skills.

When using the Recreational Goals and Mastery Checklist or the Recreational Objectives Observational Forms, verbal communication is only scored for actual resident ability to speak/express/comprehend. The use of assistive devices involving speech and language therapy is out of the range of recreational therapy, and therefore was excluded beyond ordinary communication to engage in activities.

Physical interventions, communication boards, etc. are included under written communication/written language tools, but only to assess the resident's ability to communicate within a limited scope of the activity. While the use of activities can enhance communication skills, and communication should be

Problem: needs encouragement, cues, or physical guides to increase verbal communication skills during activity)
Goals: show increased ability to communicate use of words, phases, sentence structure, comprehension, interpretation.

Verbal Comprehension

Problem: needs encouragement, cues, or physical guides to stimulate communication interpretation/comprehension skills of verbal language during activity (can be non-verbal response; the intent is to show language comprehension)
Goal: Increase language comprehension

(1) _____ unable to comprehend verbal language, staff terms, and requests, due to language deficits
-will attempt to interpret staff communication by showing understanding and initiating one response to a statement or demand. (Can be non-verbal response; the intent is to show language comprehension)
(2) _____ can interpret a few words and/or verbal statements
- will attempt to interpret staff communication by showing understanding and initiating two or more responses to statements or demands. (Can be non-verbal response; the intent is to show language comprehension)
(3) _____ can interpret/comprehend language forms and understands 50% of the time
- will comprehend/interpret stimulating and consistent conversation with staff/others 50+% of time and show comprehension by following direction of demand (can be non-verbal response; the intent is to show language comprehension)
(4) _____ can interpret/comprehend language and understands uses of proper words 75% of the time
(5) _____ comprehends proper words/terminology and order of words of verbal language independently (can be non verbal-

encouraged, speech therapy is a specialty area reserved for licensed specialists. If scales are used by a licensed speech pathologist, it is suggested that notations include your own relevant information.
response; the intent is to show language comprehension)
-will understand game rules through interpretation of words, word order, terms, sentence structure _____ time(s) this week.

Verbal Expression

Problem: needs encouragement, cues or physical guides to increase verbal communication skills during activity)
Goal: increase verbal communication
(1) _____ unable to verbalize; express needs, desires, etc.
- will attempt to vocalize/express to staff and attempt to respond with any sound____ time(s) this week
(2) _____ can express/communicate, speak a few words coherently
- will maintain or try to increase expression of vocabulary of five words or more, and continue to increase vocabulary and verbal expressive forms by use of matching word/picture associations and repeating sounds to increase communication skill during activity _____ time (s) this week
(3) _____ can speak/use language expression, and is coherent or uses proper words 50% of the time
- will engage in a stimulating and consistent conversation with staff/others, and is able to express needs, desires, etc. 50+% of time _____ time(s) this week
(4) _____ can verbally express and is coherent or uses proper words, sentence structure, etc. 75% of the time
(5) _____ speaks clearly, fluently, and uses proper word/sentence structure/terms and is able to express independently
-will continue to engage in conversations; name, describe use, and make a sentence during a game/etc. using proper word order, terms, sentence structure _____ time(s) this week.

Written Comprehension

Problem: needs encouragement, cues, or physical guides to stimulate comprehension of written language, symbols, numbers, during a recreational activity, as part of recreational activity (not as a form of speech therapy, unless done by licensed speech pathologist).

Goal	Objectives	Method
Show increased ability to write, use keyboard or use symbols to communicate/ comprehension use of words phases, sentence structure, comprehension, interpretation	Will write, draw or use devices to show comprehension of a question, etc. ex: states color swim board, favorite swim form, yes, no etc. ,will interpret instructor's request and shows understanding by initiating task	Staff will ask questions to stimulate communication (Ex: "What color float do you like?" Or make a demand to observe interpretation or language skills

Goals: show increased ability to communicate use of words, phases, sentence structure; comprehension, and interpretation of written forms of communication.

(1) _____ needs total support to stimulate comprehension/interpretation/recognition of symbols/pictures, numbers and/or associations to written words.
(2) _____ cans comprehend/interpret/recognize symbols or a pattern to make a simple picture/design
(3) _____ comprehends/recognizes letters, numbers, and symbols
- will understand/recognize simple-to-moderate written language forms, explore arts, sciences, and varied educative materials; and shows comprehension by written forms, letters, etc.
(4) _____ comprehends written language and explains meaning, etc.
(5) _____ can understand correlation of words formulates language abilities and does crosswords puzzles/word games (independently) during a recreational activity as part of recreational activity
- will understand/comprehend, explore arts, sciences, and varied educative materials; do more challenging crossword puzzles, word games; show understanding (verbal or written form) ____ time this week.

Written Expression

Problem: needs encouragement, cues, or physical guides during a recreational activity as part of recreational activity (not as a form of speech therapy, unless done by licensed speech pathologist) _____ time(s) this week.

Goals: show increased ability to communicate through use of words, phrases, sentence structure, and expression using written forms of communication.

(1) _____ needs total support to draw a simple picture, number, letter or symbol - will form simple symbols _____ time(s) this week
(2) _____can form or use simple written expression to make letters, numbers, and symbols
- will write explore arts, sciences and varied educative materials
(3)_____can write short words and numbers
____ Time this week – will write a short story, do crossword puzzles/word games
(4)___can write sentences do simple crosswords puzzles/word games (independently) - will use written expression to tackle science and varied educative materials, use written forms to do higher challenging crossword puzzles, word games independently during a recreational activity as part of recreational activity.
____ Time this week.
(5)_____can create (through written expression) own ideas, themes, crafts, and stories (independently) during a recreational activity, as part of recreational activity.
- will create (through written expression) own ideas, themes, crafts, and stories using written language or communication. Boards, etc. to communicate order, terms.

Memory

Goal	Objectives	Method
Show increased memory skills of recall, recognition, retention of information, working memory	Will retain/repeat how to float1x wk, will repeat/recall how to freestyle (or) will remember lesson at next class.	Staff will show step, actions on how to ex: float, do free style, etc Or game: teach steps of game

Problem: needs encouragement, cues, or physical guides to use memory skills of recall, recognition, retention of information, working memory

Goals: Show increased memory skills of recall, recognition, retention of information, working memory

(1) ____ needs support/cues to show small or long-term memory, recall
- will be engaged in memory activities, will bring or (staff will bring) one personal item (to spark memory associations, recall, recognition, and for identification) to share with the group ____ time(s) this week

(2)_____can locate own items identify items
- will verbally state family members, staff's name or use eye contact to acknowledge recall, recognition

(3) _____can state important dates, events, or items to master task
- will state marriage date, birthdates or world event during current event hour or at other setting ____ time(s) this week

(4)_____knows what day it is
- will state the day and knows the daily schedule

(4)_____knows the daily schedule
- will describe an event that took the prior day

(4)_____knows what happened yesterday and is happening tomorrow
- will talk about a past or future event

(4)_____knows events past or coming up
-will describe an event that took place in consistent sequence

(5)_____arranges events in sequences from first to last (independently)
- will describe an event that took place in consistent sequence

(5)___________recognizes items by association (independently) (a baseball, a baseball ticket, a bat-are all associated w/ baseball)
- will match/categorize at least two items with associated relevance

(5)_____can recall items named and repeat when asked (independently) - when presented with items after a set time period, will repeat names of objects, will answer correctly

(5)____ can do basic math (independently) - will gather a set number of items and verbally or physically write down the appropriate answer to math calculation, can plan events/multi-task

Problem-solving

Goal	Objectives	Method
Increase problem solving ability, processing of information/ thinking, reasoning, and use of good judgment, decision making	- Will do a synchronized swim w/ a partner, will follows synchronized rhythm of music and recognize change in music rhythm as the signal for a team player to toss the ball at the net. - Will consider strategies of water game.	Staff will place a musical tape with a steady rhythm in the tape player. Staff will support/ encourage residents to dance/swim in a synchronized swim w/ a partner, or staff will instruct residents to toss the ball at the basket net when music tempo changes.

Problem: needs encouragement, cues, or physical guides to problem solve.

Goals: Increase problem solving ability, processing of information /thinking, reasoning, and use of good judgment, decision making;

(1) _____ needs total support/cues to problem solve even basic needs

- will let staff know when wants something though eye blink, verbal statement, behavior etc.
(2) _____ can use "simple reasoning decisions" or "show need" regarding immediate basic needs Or imitate a simple direction (ex: - understands and imitates action, swim class example: tap hands in water or makes noises, behavior to get staffs attention
(3) _____ can problem solve to master task). Ex: will tap hands in water and create splashing, if swim can swim to where wishes and shows understanding by repeating and laughing or increasing behavior;
(3) _____uses reasoning to understand two actions/ or request.

Ex: will verbalize what is being req-uested, attempts/ imitates action that requires thinking to meet the need (ex: will splash in water (paddle), then swish in water (push down with hands to push forward on own, shows und-erstanding that pushing on water moves body, shows awareness by repeating and laughing or increasing behavior. Is able to interpret and problem solves concrete directions ex: und-erstands a request and does the actions when asked "Please give me your wet towel". Or if swims will do a two step problem, shows awareness by repeating and laughing or increasing behavior.
(4) _____ can understand steps and outcome, can consider, implement own short plans, problem to maintain attention/problem solve during activity). Ex: when requested or wishes to do activity will understand or begin process of making own short plan _____ time(s) this week ex: makes a plan to swim using technique learned ex: shows understanding by verbal and initiation of action (paddling);
(4) _____ can make higher level decisions, such as appropriate clothing choices. Ex: will choose own outfit, or make increased level decisions, awareness of the swim time, swim rules, choice of swim _____ time(s) this week;
(5) _____ can put together facts (abstract ability) and solve a problem (independently). Ex. will join a group council to address unit issues _____ time(s) this week;
(5) _____ can follow directions (recipe, task, game rules, etc.) independently. Ex: will make a cake, write mail, do gardening and challenging activities _____ time(s) this week.

Completes task

Goal	Objectives	Method
Increase ability to complete a task.	Will recall/retain and sort/gather information, problem-solve, and complete the bowling activity or game, will follow through on steps of bowling.	Staff will show the resident the step-by-step actions to bowl, encourage, and make use of adaptive devices, if needed, and supply necessary materials and support.

Problem: needs encouragement, cues, or physical guides to increase ability to complete a task
Goals: Increase ability to complete a task
(1) _____is unable to do task without full supp-ort
- will do as much of task as possible with full staff assistance
(2) _____ 25 % of the time to complete task)
- will do as much as possible 25 +% or more of the time
(3) _____ 50 % of the time to master task
- will do as much as possible 50 +% or more of the time
(4) _____ 75 % of the time to master task - will do as much of the task as possible 75 +% or more of the time
(5) _____ can complete the task independently (independently) - will follow and complete instructions to complete a task independently _____ time(s) this week

Perceptual awareness

Goal	Objectives	Method
Show increased awareness of depth perception, visual-spatial, acuity for discrimination, comparison, and categorize safety, function, meaningful activities.	Will stay in own lanes will stay within own space next to others. 1x week, will maneuver around peers, during game-grab the water basketball and toss at the net.	Staff will instruct the residents on where they need to stay in their lanes, or game; -Staff will use a game to have residents swim and toss ball to peers or the net during the game.

Problem: needs encouragement, cues, or physical guides to increase awareness of depth perception, visual-spatial, acuity for discrimination, comparison, and categorize safety, function, and meaningful activities.
Goals: Show increased awareness of depth perception, visual acuity for discrimination, comparison, and categorize safety, function, and meaningful activities.

(1) _____ needs total support to fit objects to object, discriminate, etc.;
(1-2) ____ -will place objects into a large box, put objects on ring stand, sort objects with similar type objects (very basic items ex: match colors);
(2) _____ can place objects into large puzzle, put objects on ring stand, sort objects with similar type objects (very basic items ex: match colors);
- will place objects on a slightly smaller puzzle. Ring stand ____ time(s) this week ____ time(s) this week
(3) _____ can place objects on a slightly smaller puzzle/ring stand
- will maneuver, around objects, compare, discriminate/ categorize objects
(4) _____ is able to maneuver, around objects, compare, discriminate categorize objects consistently;
- will maneuver around objects, compare, discriminate, categorize, objects consistently and independently ____ time(s) this week;
(5) ____is able to maneuver, around objects, compare, discriminate categorize objects consistently (independently)

Cognitive stimulation

Goal	Objective	Method
Increased stimulus/exposure for visual/ motor memory, cognitive experiences/awareness and brain stimulation to enhance (function, pragmatics, and neuro-plasticity).	Will interact with peers while in the pool; -Will engage in a game of water basketball and consider strategies. 1x week.	Staff will set up a water basketball game and have residents toss the ball to each other and into the basketball net.

Problem: needs encouragement, cues, or physical guides to increased stimulus/exposure for visual/ motor memory, cognitive experiences/ awareness and brain stimulation to enhance (function, pragmatics, and neuron-plasticity.
Goals: Increased stimulus/exposure for visual/ motor memory, cognitive experiences/awareness and brain stimulation to enhance (function, pragmatics, and neuron-plasticity)

(1) _____ will accept or engage in a cognitively stimulating activity for 15 seconds with total support;

-will join group and accepts or engages in a cognitively stimulating activity verbal response for 30+ seconds etc.);
(2) _____will join group and accepts /engages in a cognitively stimulating activity for 45 seconds (shows awareness through eye contact, verbal response, etc.);
- will show awareness through eye contact, verbal response for 45+ seconds etc.)-
- will interact with peers while in the pool;
- will engage in a game of water basketball;
- will join group and accepts /engages in a cognitively stimulating activity;
(3) _____ engages in stimulating activities offered at group time;
- will engage in a game of water basketball;
(4) _____ shows increasing participation in stimulating activities;
- will engage in a game of water basketball;
(5) _____ actively seeks and participates in cognitively stimulating activity (independently);
- will engage in a game of water basketball or for other activities;
- will read, watch a movie, go for walks, do puzzles and other challenging activities, partake in massage and touch/tactile stimulating activities and any experiences that choose _____ time(s) a week.

Physical Development

Fine motor skills

Goal	Objectives	Method
Increase fine motor skills	Will place fingers in ball or pick up sm. ball or use to hands to push ball ____ time(s) this week	Staff will give residents instructions on the steps to bowl including use of the fine motor skills

Problem: needs encouragement, cues, or physical guides to increase fine motor skills.

Goals: Increase function and independence, increase fine motor skills:
(1) _____ can grip/hold large puzzle pieces, objects - will wash own hands and face- will brush own hair _____ time(s) this week;
(2) _____ can brush own hair - will manage own toiletries;
(3) _____ can manage own toiletries/bathroom needs (Be sure this resident's chart assessment shows ability to do this and it is documented) - will mix, knead dough, clay or other;
(3) _____ can use medium size tools (medium size paint tools), puzzle pieces, video games and computer games with regular equipment and engage in activities - will do a small motor project (Ex: collage, pick up bingo chips) _____ time(s) this week;
(4) _____ able to use smaller type activity tools, play video games and computer games with regular equipment, use baking equipment;
(5) _____ can do all activities requiring fine motor skills compare, discriminate categorize objects consistently (Independently) (fine art painting, small bead work, handling coins, keys, etc. - will use computer keyboard, other higher level fine motor skills _____ time(s) this week.

Hand-Eye Coordination

Goal	Objectives	Method
Increase hand-eye coordination, function, ADL skills, independence, ability to partake in meaningful activities and fulfilling experiences.	Will use hand-eye coordination to complete a task ex: writing, attaching pins to the board or other activities requiring hand-eye coordination.	Staff will use various types of items requiring the use of hand-eye coordination to increase resident's function for activities and enhancement of ADL skills.

Problem: needs cues, encouragement, physical guides to increase hand-eye coordination, function, ADL skills, independence, ability to partake in meaningful activities and fulfilling experiences.

Goals: Increase eye-hand coordination, function, independence, and ADL skills:

(1) _____ unable or able to make marks, move an item and place it somewhere with assistance;
- will work together with staff assistance and place an item where it belongs, etc. _____ time(s) this week, will turn cap/lid and open toothpaste without assistance _____ time(s) this week;

(2) _____ can turn cap/lid and open to complete task);
- will paint, draw with large handled items _____ time(s) this week;

(2) _____ can paint, draw with large handled items-will practice pouring drinks, objects into bins;

(3) _____ can pour a drink for self-will pour a drink for self;
-will show ability to control and coordinate writing, drawing ____ time(s) this week;

(4) _____ has ability to control and coordinate writing; drawing;
-will hold and control kitchen tools for cooking, small paint brush, etc. _____time(s) this week;

(5) _____ can hold and control kitchen tools for cooking, small paint brush, etc.-will hold and control kitchen tools for cooking, small paint brush, etc. (Independently)____ time(s) this week.

Dexterity

Goal	Objectives	Method
Increase dexterity, function, ADL skills, independence, ability to partake in meaningful activities and fulfilling experiences	Will use fingers to manipulate buttons, maneuver objects	Staff will use various types of items requiring the use of dexterity (buttoning, snapping, maneuvering items to increase residents function for activities and enhancement of ADL skills

Problem: needs encouragement, cues, or physical guides to increase dexterity, function, ADL skills, independence, ability to partake in meaningful activities and fulfilling experiences.

Goals: Increase dexterity, function, ADL skills, independence, ability to partake in meaningful activities and fulfilling experiences:

(1) _____unable to do activities requiring dexterity/small-motor skills - will engage in activities that require small motor dexterity skills with staff support

(2) _____ able to manipulate larger Velcro tabs
- will practice/manipulate Velcro tabs _____ time (s) this week;
- will work with smaller Velcro tabs or more difficult small-motor activities (buttoning/ unbuttoning (large to sm., snap etc.

(3) _____ can button, snap, and unsnap clothing or large tool manipulations;
- will practice/manipulate zipping and unzipping own clothing _____ time(s) this week;
(3) _____ can zip and unzip own clothing - will handle a pen/writing utensil;
(4) _____ can handle average size pen, writing utensil;
- will handle a pen, writing utensil;
-will practice/manipulate tying own shoes ____ time(s) this week;
(5) _____ can do activities requiring high level ability of fine motor skill (Independently)
____ ex: knitting, embroidery, drawing-will practice/manipulate/attempt an activity requiring high level ability of fine motor skills ____ time(s) this week.

Perceptual Speed and Motor Development

Goal	Objectives	Method
Increase speed and motor ability for function, safety, meaningful/ fulfilling activities	Will react and throw ball down lane in coordinated movement and speed (within one minute; Will join in on a bowling race game)	Staff will encourage residents to increase pace of actions while bowling, sliding bowl down the aisle by decreasing time between standing to bowl and release of the ball

Problem: needs encouragement, cues, or physical guides to increase speed and motor ability for function, safety, meaningful/ fulfilling activities.
Goals: increase speed and motor ability for function, safety, and meaningful/ fulfilling activities
(1) _____ needs total support to do activities
- will be supported and peruse activities involving perceptual speed and motor function (ex: hands guided computer game);
(2)_____can initiate gesture, contact, action too engage in an activity requiring "own paced" object (playing cards) or very slow movement of object;
-will engage in an activity that includes hand movement with some response time and played with another (ex: playing cards, chess, table bowling)
(3)______Has moderate perceptual speed and motor function;
-will catch a slowly moved object, larger ball/balloon and throw it to other residents;
(4)______Has adequate perceptual speed and motor function for games; ex: will catch a ball and throw it to other residents;
(5)______Has normal or slight perceptual speed and motor function and pursues activities (independently);
-will play in a slightly toned down or normal pace sport/game of volleyball, catch, tennis computer game etc. to increase perceptual speed and motor function ____ time(s) this week.

Tactile Stimulation

Goal	Objectives	Method
Increase sensory processing and enhance awareness of sensations and toleration/adaptation of sensory stimulation and demands	-will join in on class, share items/tools, listen and follow instructions, use appropriate behavior for the setting; will wait turn, stand in line quietly; will quiet down when asked	Before class begins, staff will discuss the rules, appropriate behaviors, respect of property, safety, and respect of fellow peers/staff

Problem: needs encouragement, cues, or physical guides to increase sensory processing and enhance awareness of sensations and toleration/adaptation of sensory stimulation and demands.

Goals: Increase ability to recognize sensations:
(1) ____ attempts to touch or exhibits touch, smell, taste, visual, hearing item
-will be given sensory experiences (needs total support);
(2) ____ shows some form of acknowledgement
-will touch, smell, taste, see, or hear a sensory stimulating "item" and responds;
-will blink eyes, move a toe, laugh or exhibit some form of acknowledgement/or verbal statement 25+% of time;
(3) ____tolerates and responds to tactile stimulation 50+% of time;
-will show a tangible acknowledgement or verbally to state sensation 75+% ____ time(s) this week;
(4) ____seeks out and responds to stimulation during activity;
-will find stimulating activities and do activity for at least 5 min.;
(5)_____ can name, state, show clear recognition of stimulation (Independently);
-and increase exposure to more stimulating activities ____ time(s) this week.

Due to frailty of the elderly, an array of issues that impact balance, gait, bones, tissue, joints, heart, lungs, senses/ sensations, vision and other important functions, as well as, diseases and disorders

NO OLDER ADULT should be engaged in an exercise program without full medical approval, as well as doctor assessed and documented allowance of type of exercise and amount of individual exercises. You need to follow guidelines set by your facility or government guidelines related to physical activities and inclusion of recreational activities.

Those with complete dependence or high need of assistance during any physical activity will most likely require a degree of monitoring and therapy that fall out of the range and scope of recreational therapist/activity professionals.

Therefore if you are a recreational or activity professional scores of 1 and 2 on the scale will just require filling in the score-1(complete dependence and score 2- high assistance-as per residents chart) If scales are used by a licensed physical, occupational therapist, it is suggested that notations include your own relevant information.

Gross Motor Skills

Goal	Objective	Method
Goal: Increase function, ADL skills, independence, and ability to partake in meaningful activities and fulfilling experiences and function Increase strength, endurance, agility and flexibility.	-will engage in large motor/ gross motor activities using arms, legs trunk ex: volleyball, exercise programs (to capacity-set by clinician).	Ex: Staff will perform or give residents instructions on full swing of arms for bowling mechanics(if approved by Dr./ clinician).

Problem: needs encouragement, cues, or physical guides to increase function, ADL skills, independence, and ability to partake in meaningful activities and fulfilling experiences and function, increase strength, endurance, agility and flexibility.

Goals: Increase function, ADL skills, independence, and ability to partake in meaningful activities and fulfilling experiences and function. Increase strength, endurance, agility and flexibility:
(3)_____ can do mild –moderate large motor /active range activities (as documented/approval by physician);
-will join mild stretch exercise classes' to increase strength, endurance, agility and flexibility (as documented/approval by physician);
(4)_____ can do moderate-moderate high large motor activities (as documented/approval by

physician);
-will join moderate stretch exercise classes' to increase strength, endurance, agility and flexibility (as documented/approval by physician) _____time(s) a week;
(5) _____can do all large motor activities (as documented/approval by physician) independently);
-will join regular stretch exercise classes with increased intensity strength, endurance, agility and flexibility (as documented/approval by physician) ____time(s) a week
(5)______can join in on a dance class, or strength building exercises or physical sports (as documented/approval by physician) ____ times a week
-will join dance class, or strength building exercises or physical sports _____ time(s) a week

This section is for licensed clinical professionals wishing to use the activities in this book within the scope of their field and practice.

*****Balance ***** All older adults even with approval to participate in any activity, should be supervised when engaging in an activity requiring balance and gait.

Posture and balance

Goal	Objective	Method
Increase improve body alignment, flexibility	-when ready to bowl, will stand straight using proper body alignment/posture as stand to bowl	Staff will show residents proper posture and asked to hold body in straight alignment/posture (with device/support if needed)

Problem: needs cues, encouragement, or physical guides to increase improve body alignment, flexibility
Goals: maintain body alignment, continued activities (with physician's approval) ____ time(s) this week
(1) ____can not maintain posture and balance on own;
(2) ____maintains posture and balance 25% of time;
(3) ____ maintains posture and balance 50%of time;
(4) ____ maintains posture and balance 75% of time;
(5)____can maintain posture and balance (Independently);
-will maintain posture and balance during activity time (with physicians approval) ____ time(s) this week;

Range of Motion Activities

Goal	Objective	Method
Increase function, ADL skills, independence, and ability to partake in meaningful activities and fulfilling experiences; Increase strength, endurance, agility and flexibility	Will lift arms, legs, turn truck, bend (to capacity -set will extend and flex (to capacity - set by clinician)****	Ex: Staff will perform or give residents instructions on full swing of arms for bowling mechanics (if approved by Dr./clinician)

Problem: needs cues, encouragement, or physical guides to increase function, ADL skills, independence, and ability to partake in meaningful activities and fulfilling experiences; increase strength, endurance, agility and flexibility.

Goals: Increase function, ADL skills, independence, and ability to partake in meaningful activities and fulfilling experiences and function.
- Increase strength, endurance, agility and flexibility (as documented/approval by Dr.).
(3)_____ can do active range activities (as documented/ approval by physician);

- will join mild stretch exercise classes' to increase strength, endurance, agility and flexibility (as documented/approval by physician to master task).
(4)_____ can do moderate active range of motion activities (as documented/approval by physician);

____

-will join moderate stretch exercise classes' to increase strength, endurance, agility and flexibility (as documented/approval by physician)

____

______time(s) a week

(5) _____can do all range of motion activities (as documented/approval by physician) independently) ____
-will join regular stretch exercise classes with increased intensity strength, endurance, agility and flexibility (as documented/approval by physician) ______________________
___time(s) a week
(5)______can join in on a dance class, or strength building exercises or physical sports (as documented/approval by physician) ____ times a week
-will join dance class, or strength building exercises or physical sports_____ time(s) a week

Gait

*******Balance and gait ***** All older adults even with approval to participate in any activity, should be supervised when engaging in an activity requiring any balance and gait!**

Goal	Objective	Method
-Increase gait	Increase gait /mechanics of walking, steps, balance while walking	-Staff will have residents walk to/from lane, etc. (with device/support if needed) -Staff will support /show proper, including proper balance, steps, and holding body in alignment

Problem: needs encouragement, cues, or physical guides to increase gait/mechanics
Goal: Increase/maintain gait
(3) _____ can maintain gait and during activity time (as assessed by balance assessment in chart) and capable of maintaining balance and exercises. (As documented/approval by physician)
-will engage in basic large motor activities ____ time(s) this week _____

(4)___ has gait and use good mechanics when walking (as documented/approval by physician)

____

-will join in on exercises that help maintain balance and coordination _____ time(s) a week
(5)______can follow step patterns through dance routine or other type of step program (Independently)
-will engage in a dance class, step pattern program ____ time(s) this week _____

Muscle stimulation (*Must be done by a licensed/certified clinician*)

Goal	Objective	Method
- Increase muscle stimulation, circulation, etc.	- Will relaxes tight muscles, -will revitalizes skin, exfoliates skin, -will stimulates lymphatic system, -will stimulates nervous system, -will stimulate circulation,-will stimulates nerve endings, help misaligned bones, detox the body,-will improves sleep patterns	- Massage therapist/pt. or licensed appropriate specialist will use massage techniques, or methods below to increase muscle stimulation and benefits of massage techniques(with device/support if needed)

Goals: to stimulate muscles for overall health benefits (to be used by a licensed therapist only)

(1) ____unable, done by medical staff;

(2) ____does mild activities to stimulate muscle, circulation, etc. (with doctor approval);
- will engage in activities that stimulate active muscle movement) (with doctor approval) ____ time(s) this week;
(3) ____does moderate/slow activities to stimulate active muscle movement, circulation, etc. (with doctor approval)
-will engage in activities that stimulate active muscle movement) ____ time(s) this week;
(4) Does moderate level activities to stimulate active muscle, circulation, etc. (with doctor approval);
-will engage in activities that stimulation active muscle movement) ____ time(s) this week
(5)____ Does all/any activities to stimulate active muscle movement, circulation, etc. (Independently) (with doctor approval)-will engage in activities that stimulation active muscle movement) (with doctor approval) ____ time(s) this week

Socio-emotional Development

Socio-emotional needs are based on addressing the changes the elderly are going through while assisting them in meeting these requirements.

Socialization

Goal	Objective	Method
Increase social interactions, meaningful/ fulfilling activities	Will interact with peers for pleasure, belonging needs, etc. ,will engage in community integration experiences, uses manners, social practices at swim 1x wk	Staff will take residents to swim center 1x week and supported/encouraged to socialize, through community integration and being paired w/ swimmers/ group games

Problem: needs encouragement, cues, or physical guides to increase socialization.

Goal: Increase social interactions, meaningful/fulfilling activities:
(1)______ needs total support to socialize /form relationships with friends, family and staff, -staff, family, friends, volunteers
- will engage resident in some form of socialization
(2) ____hesitates to socialize;- will socialize with one person or seek out another's company with encouragement
-will sit in the sitting room with another resident and join in on conversations ___ times a week
(3)_____ socialize with one person; seek out another's company with encouragement
-will seek out group activity with support 50% of time ___ times a week
(4)________ will engage in group activity
-will continue to seek out friends, time with family, etc.
(5) _____socializes with staff, residents, family (Independently)- will invite others to visit or write, -will be exposed to socialization activities and community integration.

Self-esteem

Goal	Objectives	Method
Increase self–esteem, feelings of belonging, dignity, self-worth, integrity	Will state/communicate positive feelings about self and ability to swim, will join swim class to take an active role in maintaining health though exercising, will join the swim class based on own choices 1xwk.	Staff will educate residents on the value of swimming /exercise and encouraged to swim/ exercise, staff will design a wall chart showing swimmers names and personal swim time and endurance

Problem: needs cues, encouragement or physical guides to increase self–esteem, feelings of belonging, dignity, self-worth, and integrity.

Goals: Increase self –esteem, feelings of belonging, dignity, self-worth, integrity:
(1) _____needs total support to recognize/ express self-esteem. (needs 3 or more cues and two or more physical guides to complete task) - will have hair done, treated with dignity, etc
(2)_____ unable to share feelings, history, likes, dislikes;
– will be encouraged and supported to share feelings, history, likes, dislikes ____ times a week;
(3) ____shares feelings, history, likes, dislikes opinion if asked 50% of time - will share feelings, ideas 50+% of time
(4) ____ shares feelings , history , likes ,dislikes 75% of time- will share feelings, ideas 75+% of time will share feelings, ideas
-will voluntarily share an opinion
(5)____has a positive self–esteem (Independently)
-will share a project they made or a story, idea etc. ____ times a week
(5)____takes an active role in living circumstances
(Independently)

____

-will help to decorate the unit for monthly themes or an activity involving unit "happenings" ___ times a week

Self Identity, Sense of belonging

Goal	Objectives	Method
Increase self-identity, feelings of belonging, productivity	-will state/communicate positive feelings about self and will join swim class to take an active role in maintaining health/making choices though exercising, will join the swim class based on own choices 1xwk.	-Staff will educate residents on the value of swimming /exercise and encouraged to swim/exercise, staff will design a wall chart showing swimmers names and personal swim time and endurance

Problem: needs encouragement, cues, or physical guides to increase self-identity, feelings of belonging, productivity
Goal: Increase self–esteem, feelings of belonging, dignity, self-worth, integrity, and increase self-identity.

(1) ____ needs total support to express own self –identity
-responds to activities, based on past likes, passions, etc.
(2)____ can choose or gravitates towards activities relating to own likes, values, background association
-will be encouraged and supported to share customs, values, etc.
(3)_____has own cultural beliefs, chooses, spiritual/religious beliefs and shares them (if states desire to attend service, be offered books, visitors, etc. to foster identity) will demonstrate a choice of activity or make a decision to foster own identity and practices of faith, beliefs
(3)_____ makes own choices and decisions regarding morals, values, likes, dislikes-attends services, etc.
-will demonstrate individuality by choosing an activity and sharing it with the unit or times a week, -will stand up for own rights, beliefs
-will demonstrate an act of standing up for own self or be motivated to do so if needed.
(4)_____ stands up for own rights, beliefs
-will express personal feelings, opinion on a subject matter with a staff member or resident ___ times a week.
(5)___ has a good self –identity (Independently)
-will engage in activities and honors own ethnic and cultural background____ times a week (if wishes to)-will share information, stories etc, involving ethnic cultural history ___ times a week

(5)______Continues to engage in activities that are related to cultural background independently) times a week

*_____joins small groups but not larger group activities, only socializes with own visitors or small group of residence –is personal choice.

Fosters appropriate behavior

Goal	Objectives	Method
Increase social interaction, social opportunities/social adjustment, safety, using appropriate behaviors during an activity, for a calm environment and fulfilling experiences	Will join in on exercise class, will listen and follow instructions, will use appropriate behavior for the setting, will wait turn, stand in line quietly -will quiet down when asked during swim class 1x wk.	Before swim class begins, staff will discuss the pool rules, appropriate behaviors, respect of property, safety, and respect of fellow swimmers while swimming.

Problem: needs encouragement, cues or physical guides to increase social intera-ction, social opportunities/social adjustment, safety, using appropriate behaviors during an activity, for a calm environment and ful-filling experiences or : lack of or a need to increase appropriate be-havioral skills
Goals: Increase social interaction, social opportunities/social adjustment, safety, using appropriate behaviors during an activity, for a calm environment and fulfilling experiences

(1)____ needs total support, is unaware of environment and behavioral issues
-Staff will help support patient if behavior/vocal noise is an issue
-will wait patiently while staff hands out activity materials for ____ minutes ____times a week
(2)______ sit and wait patiently while staff hands out activity materials -will be respectful to self care and feelings/ care towards others, will control behavior)
- will control outbursts, engaging in a be-havior that are safe for self and others ___ times a week
(3) ______ is able to control behavior, fost-ers appropriate behavior for the environment
(3)______ accepts or adapt well to enviro-nment
-will follow rules, join groups, keeps room clean; share table at lunch, handle a fair amount of stress and control behavior ___ times a week
(4)______can handle a fair amount of stress (Independently)
-will stay in the dining room area during a busy hour ___ times a week
(5)_____ expresses emotions and behaviors appropriately
-will demonstrate by vocal statements or show appropriate reaction to the setting, -will show appropriate reactions to emotional circumstances ex: cry when sad, laughs when happy or something funny happens according to the setting ___________
times a week.

Emotional gratitude

Goal	Objective	Method
Increase emotional gratification/wellness, fulfillment and quality of life	Will state that the swim class is a gratifying experiences or will show pleasure by smiling, laughing, deep focus on swimming 1x wk.	Staff will ask residents if they enjoyed the swim class and what they liked through verbal discussion, group discussions

Problem: needs encouragement, cues or physical guides to increase emotional gratification/wellness, fulfillment and quality of life: lack of ability or a need to increase emotional gratification
Goals: Increase emotional gratification/wellness, fulfillment and quality of life

(1)____is unable to show emotional grati-tude by smiling, verbal or other form of communication (needs 3 or more cues and two or more physical guides to complete task) -will express when emotionally gratified by a smile, eye blink or verbal statement will express something they like at least one time a week ___ times a week
(2)_____ can experience or expresses emotional gratification if prompt
- will express something they like at least two times a week ___ times a week
(2) _____ expresses emotional gratitude
–will list things that they find emotionally gratifying
(3) _____ is able to express or identify things they are grateful for or verbalize needs
(4)_____seeks emotionally gratifying experiences with support or encouragement
(5) _____ seeks, obtains emotional grat-ification independently)

Teamwork/sharing

Goal	Objective	Method
Increase teamwork/sharing, meaningful /fulfilling activities	-will join in on a water sport game or water exercise with others and share, wait turn, support peers, show compassion and patients to team members (listen, wait, positive comments)	Staff will place a basketball floater in the pool and residents will be encouraged to play, share floats, form teams, strategize together, consider peers

Problem: needs encouragement, cues or ph-ysical guides to increase teamwork/sharing, meaningful /fulfilling activities: lack of ability or a need to increase teamwork
Goals: Increase teamwork/
sharing, meaningful /fulfilling activities

(1) ____ struggles or refuses to play as a tea-m player
-will be encouraged to get to know, help one other member of the team, will be given instructions on game, will list rules of conduct-will share wait turn with full assistance for ___ minutes of the game
(2) ____ Will share; wait turn with assis-tance and other appropriate actions
-will list rules of conduct- will share; wait turn with full assistance for ___ minutes of the game
(3) ____ can share; wait turn with assistance and other appropriate actions
- help another member of the team-will offer an idea to the team
(4) ____ can offer ideas to group or share game
- works with a group to do a project ___ times a week
(5)____shows self to be a team player. Shows compassion and empathy (In-dependently)
-will help/wait patiently or offer verbally support to a slower resident while playing a team sport
-will share magazines while making a coll-age ___ times a week
-will show concern and empathy and helps others_____________________
-will demonstrate an act of concern, em-pathy by listening to another struggle, help someone else ___ times a week

Initiative and Motivation

Goal	Objective	Method
Increase Initiative and motivation	will choose if wishes to swim or not, will choose if wishes to join in on team water	Staff will support /encourage the resident to prepare to swim(change, shower

Problem: needs encouragement, cues or physical guide to increase initiative and motivation: lack of ability or a need to increase initiative and motivation.
Goals: Increase initiative and motivation.
(1) _____does not do the activity unless given cues/encouragement or physically gui-ded;
-will be encouraged to do one task towards goal ___ time(s) a week;
(2) _____ will do activity but needs support 75% of the time;
-will be encouraged and do two or more steps of the task ____ time(s) a week;
(3) _____shows interest in environment but needs prompting at least 50% of the time.
-will demonstrate the action by asking questions or voicing an opinion during a current event activity or unit based activity ___ times a week
(4) _____ takes initiative and is self-motivated to do activity
-will set up own project materials or other type of action for positive outcomes
(5)_____is enthusiastic takes initiative and is motivated to do things for self (inde-pendently);
-will choose an activity ___ times a week;
-will choose and complete a project as well as able ___ times a week;
-will gather own supplies when picking out materials for an activity, will join the group for an activity of own imitative ___ times a week.

Sense of Accomplishment

Goal	Objectives	Method
Increase feelings of self worth, pride, feelings of productivity, dignity	- Will look at the chart showing swimmers and personal bests, will use gestures to express pride in self, will talk about swimming ability to staff/peers1x wk.	A chart on the unit wall or a paper handed to the residents reflecting swim time, etc. will be available for residents to see their personal best/increased swim time

Problem: needs encouragement, cues or physical guides to increase feelings of self worth, pride, feelings of productivity, dignity: lack of ability or a need to increase feelings of self worth, pride, feelings of productivity, dignity.
Goals: Increase feelings of self worth, pride, feelings of productivity, dignity:
(1)____ Makes comments counterproductive to self worth;
- will do a task to increase sense of productivity, self-esteem___ time a week;
(2) ____ begins to acknowledge capabilities and partake in activities;
- will engage in an activity; help perform a task ___ time a week;
(3) ______shows sense of accomplish-ment/pride using verbal statements/ some form of communication stating own value, ex: "Look, I made a bookmark"; "I finished the project!"
(4)______can show staff or others an activity they did.
- will display or offer works to someone,-will display pride through smile, beaming (relevant to circumstances)-will continue to show, display work ___ time a week;
(5)____Does a job independently, with diligence, pride (Independently);
- seeks out tasks that promote challenge, value, dignity and staying productive___ time a week.

Tolerates Stimulation

Goal	Objectives	Method
Increase awareness of sensations and toleration/adaptation of sensory stimulation/demands	Will show adjustment to the smell of the pool, put hand or foot in the water to slowly adjust to water/water temperature, will enter water and adjust to the pool (2-4 min.) temperature (read memo on temperatures)	Staff will take residents to the pool and exposed to sensory stimulating experiences. Staff will support residents as they adjust to the stimulus a step at a time

Problem: needs encouragement, cues, or physical guides to increase awareness of sensations and toleration/adaptation of sensory stimulation/demands
Goals: Increase awareness of sensations and toleration/adaptation of sensory stimulation/ demands

Due to the various reasons or causes of sensory problems, all residents must have clearance before introduction to sensory integration/sensory stimulation. Or a decision made by the physician/clinical team. Even with permission, you must also listen and respect the resident's choice. No or no more is No or No More. For suggestions, please read the section on encouragement and support.
(1)_____has a difficult time tolerating stim-ulus (sound, visual, smell, taste, touch,)
–will be introduced to sensory integration during one activity for ___ minutes___ times a week
(2) _____ tolerates stimulation up to ____ minutes
–will increase stimulus up to 25%
(3) _____ tolerates stimulation up to 25+% ___ times a week? during activity
-will tolerate increase stimulus up to 50+ %___ times a week/ during activity
(4) _____ tolerates stimulation up to 50+% ___ times a week/ during activity
-will increase/tolerate stimulus up too 75%+ ___ times a week/ during activity
(4) _____ tolerates stimulation up to 75%
-will increase/tolerate stimulation up to 75+%
(5)_____ tolerates stimulus (Independently)
-will join, partakes in project etc. ___ time(s)week

Relaxation

Goals	Objectives	Method
Increase ability to relax.	Will sit and relax for 15 minutes at a time. Will do projects or read books, etc .while relaxing.	Staff will provide a calm, "orderly transitional "and calm environment to support residents ability to relax.

Problem: needs encouragement, cues, or physical guides to increase ability to relax: lack of ability or a need to increase rel-axation capability
Goals: Increase ability to relax

(1)_____is unable to relax, do quiet projects, calm self down
-will sit, relax for 2 min .at a time-will sit and relax for 2 min. at a time___ times a week
(2) _____ can sit do quiet project/relax for two min. at a time
-will sit and relax for 5 minutes at a time
(3) _____ can sit do quiet project/ relax for 5 minutes at a time
-will sit and relax for 15 minutes at a time-will find projects or books, etc. to enjoy while relaxing
(4) ____ can sit, do project and relax for 15 minutes or more

(5) ____ is able to relax, sit quietly and do activities/relaxing activities (Independently)

-will relax; do quiet activities at leisure___ time(s) a week.

Solace

Goals	Objectives	Method
Increase ability to obtain solace.	Will do a meditation or quiet reflection/ take a break, relax 5 min. ___ time(s) a week.	Staff will provide a place on the unit where resident can sit in a quiet area/ sanctuary.

Problem: needs encouragement, cues, or physical guides to increase ability to obtain solace

Goals: Increase ability to obtain solace

(1)_____ is unable to obtain solace, peaceful /moment's

- will accept experiences/help finding brief moments/at least 15 minutes of solace every day

(2) ____accepts help finding brief moments/at least 15 minutes of solace every day will accept experiences/help finding brief moments/at least 30 minutes of solace every day

(3) ____accepts help finding brief moments/at least 30 minutes of solace every day

-will seek solace on own for at least 30 minutes everyday

(4) _____seeks solace on own for at least 30 minutes everyday

-will actively pursue solace through experiences, or seeks solace on own for at least 30 minutes everyday

(5) _____is very active in pursues solace through experiences, reminiscing, or own space for solace-(Independently) will do a meditation or quiet reflection/ take a break, relax 5 min. ___ time(s) a week

Healing/Nurturing

Goals	Objectives	Method
Increase ability to accept/ experience nurturing, healing experiences	Will engage in self nurturing activities- will continue to accept nurturing from others and to nurture self	Staff will offer activities and materials used to promote healing qualities, nurturing experiences

Problem: needs encouragement, cues, or physical guides to increase ability to accept/ experience nurturing, healing experiences

Goals: Increase ability to accept/ experience nurturing, healing experiences

(1) _______is unable /rejects nurturing from others or nurturing self

-will accept one act of being nurtured or nurture self ____ times a week

(2) ______ has difficulty much of the time, accepting nurturing from others or giving/doing self nurturing activities

-will accept two acts of being nurtured or nurture self ____ times a week

(3)______ allows others to help or comfort her/him in words, can nurture self-50%% of the time

-will accept nurturing or nurture self three times a week

(4) ______allows staff or other resident to give a hug, sit by, will accept healing/nurturing) ___ times a week/as needed

-will continue to accept nurturing and to nurture self

(5) ______voluntarily go and talk to a resident, accepts hugs, engaging in self nurturing activities (Independently)

- will continue to accept nurturing and to nurture self___ times a --week/as needed

Reminiscing

Goals	Objectives	Method
Increase memory, feelings of belonging, self-identity	-will engage in an activity that reflects age/time period	Staff will offer activities from residents time period or past experiences for pleasure, sense of belonging, memory enhancement, healing qualities

Problem: needs encouragement, cues, or physical guides to increase memory, feelings of belonging, self-identity
Goals: Increase memory, feelings of belonging, self-identity

(1)_____ unable to recall, recognize, retain memories, or has a lack of/opportunities or desire for reminiscing
-If desires to partake in reminiscing-will be stimulated with activities of aromatherapy, and other objects from past to stimulate, soothe
(2) _____shows some form of recognition or is affected by sensory stimulation (2-3 cues and at least one physical guide by being visually guided and shown item, face or actual physically guided) to complete task)
-will verbally or physically, show emotional reaction to stimulus
(3)_____ is comforted by familiar music, activities related to past time fame, semblance of past routines
-will state information of past -will join in and share a story from past, will join an activity from generation
(4)_____ enjoys/joins in on reminiscing therapy/activities
(5)_____ pursues activities related to own generation/ lifespan activities (Independent-ly)
-will share an item, help with theme parties, or other form of interaction related to reminiscing times ___ times a week

Self-Expression

Goals	Objectives	Method
Increase self/emotional expressions, wellness	-will engage in an activity and uses self expression to show own creativity, desires, feelings	Staff will offer activities that include the ability to express creativity, personal expressions of desires and feelings

Problem: needs encouragement, cues, or physical guides to increase self/emotional expressions, wellness
Goals: Increase self/emotional expressions, wellness
(1)____has trouble expressing, requires total assistance
-will be offered an environment rich in materials based on past self expressions,
-will show self –expression through facial cues, role-play,
(2) ____will offer ideas, express through art, music, etc. to group
(3)____will offer and share an activity idea, music, talents-with cues and encouragement (2x or less)
- will offer one item that shows a form of self expression (poem, art. etc) when enc-ouraged 50% of time
-will show two forms of self-expression (poem, painting, etc.) ___ time(s) a week
(4)_____seeks activities of self expression through various mediums and expressions

-will ask for art paper and draws a picture showing art expression of feelings, desires

(5)____actively uses self-expression through various mediums (Independently)

-will vocalize or express self through an art, music, and story ___ time a week

Aquatics/Swimming

***Cognitive Challenges*:** attention, memory, language, orientation, following patterns, keeping rhythm, perceptual awareness, and cognitive stimulation

***Physical Needs*:** fine motor skills, gross motor skills, coordination, range of motion, flexibility, posture, balance, backward and forward movement, gait, following step pat-terns, circulation, cardio-vascular workout

Socio-emotional Needs: socialization, community integration, initiative and motivation, emotional gratification, sense of accomplishment, self-esteem, tolerating stimulation, fostering appropriate behaviors

Supplies: Availability of swimming pool, qualified supervision provided by facility or other qualified/certified lifeguards and staff.
Time: 20–30 minutes
Staff/older adult ratio: 1:2 or as assessed per needs of individuals or group
Instructions: Generally, an aquatic therapist or swim coach/instructor would teach the actual swimming program. Have them warm up for swimming by leading them in a sub maximal active warm-up first. This will gradually increase their body temperature, blood flow to the muscles, and synovial fluid to the joints. You may then lead them in a three to five minute stretching exercise. The swimming could be done as a freestyle activity that allows older adults to get adjusted to the water and swim at their own pace. It may also be a set water workout.
Many older adults will have to adjust to the water temperature.

Generally, many facilities in the community will have a water temperature in the range of 85-86 degrees. You should, however, inquire what each facility's temperature is, so as not to cause distress or over-stimulation. It should be a moderate temperature. Due to medications, or falling potential, older adults should be supervised very carefully. Older adults with restrictions may be able to use special equipment available for the use of the physically challenged. It might be helpful to ask the facility what they have available to enhance swimming activities.

Aquatics/Swimming
Cognitive Goals Objectives and Methods

Skill	Goal	Objectives	Method
Orientation	Show increased awareness of, time/"timeframe," people, circumstances, and past experiences vs. present experiences, to engage in present-time activities, or for a reminiscing	-will respond w/correct answer to two choice questions Or yes/no, will state place, time, present company of people, or past experiences on own during activity 1x a week	Staff will ask residents a series of questions to stimulate focus to the present setting (Ex: "Are you at the mall or at the swimming center?") Or past if a reminiscing exercise (Ex: "Have you swum before? With who? What is your swim partner's name? Mary or Karen?"
Attention	Show increased attention span, task for function, and to engage in meaningful, recreational/fulfilling activities	-will make eye-contact with swim staff, will verbalize with staff and instructor, will read/listen to swim rules, will say yes/no to show they understand or by actions	Staff will address or stand in front of resident, make eye-contact, ask questions, or use others methods to get resident's attention, and then observe or ask the residents questions to see if they are listening and understand
Memory	Show increased memory skills of recall, recognition, retention of information, working memory	-will retain/repeat how to float 1x a week, will repeat/recall how to freestyle (or) will remember lesson at next class	-Staff will show steps on how to float, do free-style, etc. -Staff will teach steps of game and then ask questions to gauge memory skills
Language	Show increased ability to communicate use of words, phrases, sentence structure, comprehension, interpretation	-will reply to a question (Ex: states color of the swim board, favorite swim form, yes/no etc.), will interpret instructor's request, will initiate task	Staff will ask questions to stimulate a communication (Ex: "What color float do you like?"), or make a command to serve interpretation skills
Cognitive Stimulation (awareness, seeks information in)	Increased stimulus/exposure for visual/ motor memory, cognitive experiences/awareness and brain stimulation to enhance (function, pragmatics, near-plasticity)	game -will interact with peers while in the pool, will engage in a game of water basketball, will accept challenge of input information and engage/interact in swimming	-Staff will show the resident the step-by-step actions to swim -Staff will give instructions on water basketball game -Staff will instruct residents in the step-by-step procedure for games, encourage, make use of adaptive devices if needed, and supply necessary materials and support
Perceptual Awareness	Show increased abilities of depth perception, visio-spatical awareness, and acuity (for discrimination, comparison, and categorizing), safety	-will stay in own lanes, will stay within own space next to others, will maneuver around peers during game, will grab the water basketball and toss at the net	-Staff will instruct the residents on where they need to stay in their lanes -Staff will use a game to have residents swim and toss ball to peers or the net during the game
Problem-solving	Increase problem-solving ability, processing of information, thinking, reasoning, and use of good judgment /decision-making	-will do a synchronized swim w/ a partner, will follows synchronized rhythm of music and recognize change in music rhythm as the signal for a team player to toss the ball at the net. -will consider strategies of water ball	Staff will place a musical tape with a steady rhythm in the tape player. Staff will support/encourage residents to dance/swim in a synchronized swim w/ a partner, or staff will instruct residents to toss the ball at the basket net when music tempo changes
Complete a Task	Increase ability to complete a task	will recall/retain and sort/gather information, problem-solve, will do the required swim, will play the water basketball game and complete the task	Staff will set up a water basketball game to stimulate visual/motor memory, thinking, etc. and cognitive awareness and encourage residents to participate in the game

Table 1.1

Recreational Objectives Observation Form
Aquatics/Swimming-Cognitive Skills

Patient	Dependent (Totally dependent)	High Assistance (25+ ability)	Moderate Assist. (50+ ability)	Mild Assistance (75+ability)	Independent Totally independent
	1	2	3	4	5
See codes below use optional codes if appropriate	3 cue/ 2-3 physical	2-3 cues/ 2 physical	2-3 cues/ 1 physical	1-2 cues	Encouragement

(Code 97113)-if actual Aquatic therapy	Skill	Goal	Objectives ____times per ____	Method	Outcome Date			
97532 Cognitive skills or if using Therapeutic Activity code-9753o	Orientation							
97532 Cognitive skill[s]	Sample							
97532 Cognitive skill[s]								
97532 Cognitive skills	Problem-Solving							
97532 Cognitive skills	Complete a Task							
97139 Speech Therapy /97532 Cognitive skills	Language							
97533	Sensory Stimulation /Cognitive Stimulation							
97532	Perceptual Awareness							

97532-Development of cognitive skills to improve attention, memory, problem-solving, includes compensatory training and/or sensory integrative activities, direct (one-on-one) patient contact by the provider, each 15 minutes; 97530-Therapeutic activities, direct (one-on-one) patient contact by the provider (use of dynamic activities to improve functional performance), each 15 minutes; 97533-Sensory integration techniques to enhance sensory processing and promote adaptive responses to environmental demands, direct (one-on-one) patient contact by the provider, each 15 minutes; 97150-Therapeutic procedure(s), group (2 or more individuals); 97139-Unlisted therapeutic procedure (specify) minutes	Staff initials				
	Add total score here Maximum Score 40 pt. each form per activity				
	See scale below or use own/facilities optional score system				

(Score 1-8)=1 (9-16) =2 (17-24) =3 (25-32) =4 (33-40) =5 If w/device add d if wish, If using 1-7 scale (42-48) =6 (49-56) =7

 ********Actual charts are larger to allow for completion of areas*********

Background and Interests Form

Resident's Name: Residents room:

Date of Assessment: Diagnosis:
Staff: ________________________________

Diagnosis/affected skill level: abilities to participate/functional capabilities to engage in activities

Physical impediments:

Social impediments:

Allergies or special concerns regarding safety

Social information (examples: marital status, children, grandchildren, friends, and ability to visit/frequency of visits)

Special friends:

Prior or current pets:

Personal background regarding prior living area, birth place:

Primary language (ability to interpret/communicate):

Spiritual/Religious affiliations:

Cultural or ethnic customs:

General interests:

Reading/book interests:

Music interests:

Sports interests:

Favorite foods:

Favorite television shows, movies:

Favorite past times /hobbies:

Work history:

Special talents:

Associations to civic groups, heritage:

(Can the resident attend association meetings? Can the association send a volunteer or hold a meeting at the facility?)

Volunteer work:

Goals to ensure continued interaction/activity: Resident's schedule, medication times, etc.

Goals to ensure continued interaction/activity: to ensure full staff awareness of activities and timeframes

GOALS AND OBJECTIVES

Goals are generally broken down into a systematic process or steps. We start out with the goal. Once the objectives of the short-term goal are met, we then increase the rate of complexity with higher level of our goal/objectives. We continue to seek out objectives and methods that lead to our long-term goals.

We use activities to meet our goals. Activities are the actions, tasks and methods used to create responses, reactions or results.

When we are talking about something that should be obtained for the older adult's well-being, rights, fulfillment and comfort, we are referring to their needs. When we are working for a purpose towards a particular goal we wish to obtain, we are looking at the objectives of the activity. When we talk about purpose and striving for optimum outcomes we are referring to our goals.

This is generally gained though steps or a method that includes: implementing a series of actions/ tasks inclusive of assistance or support, and ultimately obtaining the objectives, goals or outcomes/results.

Needs are obtained through improvement and ability to gain well-being, rights, fulfillment and comfort. We explored Maslow's theories of needs and motivation when looking at physical and psychosocial issues. We also explored research stating what older adults felt were important to their quality of life.

Objectives are a means to meet the goal. Generally the objectives include *what the resident will do* to obtain the goal.

The method is a means to meet the objectives or *what the staff member will do* to enhance the resident's ability to obtain the objectives, to then meet the goals.

Let's use an example:

The recreational therapist/activity professional first assesses Tillie's skill levels using the older adult individual assessment form.

Goal: Increasing social interactions, community integration and pursuing meaningful/fulfil-ling activities.

Objective: *Tillie (what the resident will do)* will explore the senior citizen center and introduce herself (with support, if needed) to the other seniors.

Method: Staff (*what the staff member will do*) will invite Tillie to the senior citizen center and support her as she becomes familiar with the senior center, meets the other residents and engages in a craft activity.

Staff member will observe Tillie's ability to adapt to the environment and her ability to socialize with the other seniors.

Outcome of observation/assessment: Staff member introduced Tillie to a group of seniors. Staff member invited Tillie to join the seniors who where sitting at a craft table.

Tillie hesitated to walk over to the table and sit down. Staff member physically guided Tillie to the craft table. Staff member invited Tillie to sit next to Mary. Staff member then introduced Tillie to Mary. Mary said hello and started to initiate a conversation. Tillie responded.

When prompt, Tillie continued to reply and engage in conversation throughout the activity time.

Using, the Recreational Goals: Initial assessment and mastery checklist, the staff member assessed and entered a check on the checklist reflecting **Tillie's skill level as a three (moderate) Tillie needed 2-3 cues and a physical guide to join in on an activity.**

Use of the Recreational Objectives Observation form

After the staff member has done his initial assessment using the Recreational Goals: Initial Assessment and Mastery Checklist, he institutes use of the Recreational Objectives Observational Form. He uses the information he obtained from the checklist to then initiate his plans and considerations of the goals, objectives and method. For example:

Certified Recreational Therapist/Activity Professional

Problem: Lack of meaningful activities and moderate level of community integration and socialization skills

Goal: Increase social interactions, community integration and pursuance of meaningful-/fulfilling activities

Skill: Socialization/Community Integration (will also observe initiative and motivation skills to gauge if hesitance is more related to socialization/community adaptation or initiative and motivation)

He begins with a short-term goal

Goal: to increase Tillie's socialization skills, adaptation to community integration

Objective: *Tillie (what the resident will do)* will continue to explore the senior citizen center and introduce herself (without physical support) to the other seniors. Tillie (*what the resident will do*) will initiate a conversation and socialize.

Method: Staff (*what the staff member will do*) will announce the type of activity the residents will be doing for the day. Staff will invite all of the residents to sit at the table (Knitting activity).

*Staff member intervention: If Tillie hesitates; Staff will verbally encourage Tillie to sit at the table. Staff may encourage Tillie by re-introducing her to the other residents or by encouraging Tillie, "Tillie, you remember Mary, I see a seat next to her, perhaps you can sit there, if you would like". Staff will give adequate time (one minute) for Tillie to go to the table without physical guide

Outcome: Tillie sits by Mary and gets reacquainted. Tillie initiates a conversation with Mary.

Outcome: skill level four: Tillie engages in the activity and is able to engage in an activity/ able to socialize and join the other residents at the table with 1-2 cues and but without need of a physical guide. Tillie initiates a conversation with Mary.

Once this goal, objective is met, the staff member challenges Tillie with higher level, more challenging objective to be met

Goal: Increase socialization skills and pursue meaningful/fulfilling activities

Objective: Tillie will join in on an activity 2 times a week and will interact/socialize with peers and staff without the need of physical guides, cues. Tillie will initiate 2 or more conversations during the activity time.

Method: Staff- will offer an activities area and ongoing activities (ex: cooking, crafts, etc.) to promote opportunities to socialize and encourage residents to engage in socialization and community integration.

Tillie will continue working on the long-term goal of increasing social interactions, and pursuing meaningful/fulfilling activities. The staff will help her obtain this goal with increasing levels of challenge and experience.

PLANS AND CONSIDERATIONS

Skill Levels/ Needs of the resident

To begin planning, we need to take many considerations into account. What are the skills being effected by the older adult's illness, disorder, or the aging process?

What skills are irreversible and adaptation necessary rather then restoration? (This includes those who may be under total care and other residents who need additional assistance.) What are the particular skills we are looking to enhance, and which activities have the highest benefits to meet our need? (For example, sports usually promote a high level of physical potential and gains.) Games and puzzles usually have a higher benefit for cognitive goals. Community get-togethers usually have a high benefit for socio-emotional activities.

It is important to point out that, while you focus on one particular type of skill that requires attention, you need to remember all the domains important for activities and well-being.

Ability to appraise ratios of staff and time needed per activity

Generally, if you are working in a facility and do not have qualifications to assess staff ratios, this issue will and should be assessed by qualified staff. You should not assume you can judge staff/patient ratio without guidance and clear guidelines. This is for client safety. The amount of staff will be determined by the needs of your clients. If you have high need clients who need assistance quite often, need to be prompt, need supervision, or even patients who require two staff members, this will impact the amount of older adults you can attend to adequately for safety factors and to complete a project.

This will also have an impact on the timeframe necessary to complete activities. You will need to follow the guidelines of your facility. The ratio and time frames mentioned in each activity presented in this book are based on high-functioning clients. Be sure that you have the appropriate staff on hand to ensure all older adults are safe. Also, an adequate amount of staff can be a factor in how well the activity goes. When making a choice of the activity, you will need to consider some factors that will enhance the use of the activities.

Safety

Safety must always come first. It is better to be cautious and always be sure your planning will allow you to do the activity and ensure safety. Also, make sure you have sufficient time to do the activity along with helping residents. You want to be sure the residents get to finish their project.

Understanding Specific Skills Obtained through Different Activities

The activities in this book are broken down into five sections. The lists of sections are Sports/ Physical Activities, Games/Educational Activities, Expressive Art Forms, Tangible Expressive Art Forms, and Relaxation, Self-Nurturing Activity or Sensory Integration Activities.

These sections were designed specifi-cally to include a balance of physical, cognitive, and socio-emotional type activities. While each activity can generally promote skills in physical, cognitive, and socio-emotional areas, particular activities are known to enhance particular skills.

Sports activities generally provide a high level of physical benefits. Educational activities generally provide a high level of cognitive stim-ulation. Relaxation activities generally provide a high level of socio-emotional and healing qualities. Tangible Expressive Art Forms, generally offer an array of benefits geared towards functional components in all three aspects of physical, cognitive, and socio-emotional well-being.

Social, cultural, ethnic and group dynamics

You will need to gear your activities to the setting and clientele of those you are working with. It is important to use good judgment of what is appropriate and will have a positive outcome during activity times.

You need to consider the combination of older adults who are present, their personalities, likes, cultural concerns, religious practices, abilities, and any other factors that may have an impact on the group dynamics and activities. The book includes a personal background and interest's worksheet. This will help you to choose ideal activities for individual and group settings of older adults.

Creativity and the use of themes

Another important factor when choosing activities is how you present and implement creative, fun activities while addressing the needs, goals using various themes. The activities included in this program are specifically designed as "base" activities.

The activities promote different creative or themes focused activities and enhance function. For example, you can choose any type of cooking activity theme. The skills listed are the skills observed while cooking. This allows you to enhance function using a cooking activity, and also engage in many different types of cooking themes. Be as creative as you like.

Encourage a variety of cooking/baking routines designed around holiday themes, cultural events, etc. You can use the same forms for cooking when choosing any cooking/baking activity and still meet your skill objectives. Being creative will help you to foster strengths and abilities while creating an environment conducive to fun, function, and fulfillment.

Addressing Appropriate Activities for Older Adults

Activities should be appropriate and geared to the age of the older adult population. You need to be sensitive and use your ingenuity. For example, while you might give a child play dough to help with strengthening fine motor skills in the hand, you would never want to give play dough to an older adult. It might insult them (unless of course they request play dough, which is a different matter.) A better choice than offering play dough might be to buy colored clay. You still obtain the goal and you also show sensitivity, dignity, and respect for the age of the resident.

Be sure the activity allows the older adult to voice preferences on the types of activities they engage in. Because the activities are presented without naming a "set dance routine," you can gear the activities to the desires, sensitivities, religious affiliations, and cultural issues of the older adults. This book includes a Personal Interest and Background Experience Worksheet. The patient can fill this out himself or herself or you can help them to fill it out. You can use this form to get to know your patients' interests and background.

Understanding the Need to Work with Staff and Staff Schedules

It is important to make staff aware of your wishes for a resident to attend an activity. This is part of teamwork and recognizing and respecting the importance of each team member's work. This will also ensure residents' wishes to participate or need to participate in an activity are sought and obtained when possible.

It is your responsibility to give all staff a list of the residents who are on your schedule for an activity. This information will help the staff when they are preparing their schedule. The infrmation will make staff aware of your activity, the time frame you request, and, if attendance to the activity is possible, ensure the resident is available and prepared.

Activities throughout the Day

The ability to take advantage of activities can be utilized during leisure times. This includes music, favorite television shows, and movies. Magazines, books, art supplies, and other interesting items should be readily available throughout the day, as well as on weekends and other times when the adult would like to do an individual activity.

There will also be times when perhaps grandchildren or visitors will come to visit, and they may wish to share an activity together. Keep in mind the types of activities that may have special meaning to individual residents. This may include cultural types of activities, religious materials, access to the radio, computer availability, and having letter materials available to write a letter or card to a friend.

Having activities available throughout the day will also make the unit feel more natural and like a home setting. A resident's individual choice for preferred activities may actually also be more easily met in this way.

Many older adults don't wish to "bother" the family members, friends, and staff with their individual wants. They may have a hard time expressing their personal desires. There may also be particular times of the day when they may prefer to do an activity. Having an array of activities available will allow the older adult to feel like they have some control over the choices and schedule of their day.

Due to appointments and other factors, the older adult may be away during a time a favorite activity was presented and may wish to finish it at a time convenient to them. There may be factors such as medications they must take or treatments that may interfere with their schedule or capacity to do activities at particular times.

Older adults who take medications that affect their ability to participate in activities at a particular time may benefit from activity times when they are more responsive and alert; they may wish to do an activity when they are feeling up to it.

If you are a volunteer in a nursing home or homecare setting, including activities as an element during team/unit planning has many benefits. The preplanned scheduled use of activities during shift changes, setting up for meal times, medication times, etc. can help the staff to attend to their work and address the needs of the residents.

Depending on the time frame, you can decide on a short- or long-term activity. Doing something as simple as singing or reading a book can be a good choice. You may also allow them to take turns reading or offer a riddle or something to share if the unit is one in which older adults are capable of this skill. The main idea is to find something interesting for the older adults to do so they are fairly content and staff can complete their work.

For example, as older adults begin to come to the table for meals, you can plan activities during the wait. Items readily available in the dining hall are a beneficial source. Perhaps you can use this time to play games. This can even be an incentive to get to the dining hall and be seated for the meal.

An example of a table game is: Place 3 items on the table. Take one away. Let the residents guess which one you have removed. Be creative! The more enthusiastic you are, the more fun everyone will have.

This is helpful to other staff members when they need to concentrate on their work, as well as advantageous to the older adults. The environment will be less chaotic, with all needs addressed, and a calm and cheerful atmosphere.

Special Needs

Addressing the needs of those unable to attend to activities outside of their room or home

It is important to address the needs of those unable to attend to activities outside of their room or home. Older adults who can not leave their home, are too sick to attend a group activity, or choose not to join activities must still be given activities for their well-being. Be sure to offer reading materials, games, crafts, computer games, movies, paints supplies, knitting, crossword/word puzzles, or any other activities/therapeutic materials. Remember to include adaptable equipment, etc. if needed.

If the patient is not able to do an activity himself or herself, offer all the support you can. Have as much of the activity done as is geared to their needs. Remember, sometimes the activity may be more about the experience then about an actual produced item.

Understanding and Implementing Activities for those with Special Needs

Many activities can be modified to work well for the skill levels of special needs adults.

The blind and vision-impaired older adult may need modifications or extra help, but, unless the activity specifically demands vision, they may still be able to do the task. Many blind people are very good at adaptation.

The hearing-impaired can do most activities. If they wear hearing aids, be sure their hearing aids are on and to speak clearly and in front of them. You can visually guide the hearing impaired through the activities if they have trouble following directions. Older adults with mobility issues will need varied assistance based on their needs. The value may be more in the experiences and allowing them to do as much as they can.

Residents who suffer from Alzheimer, Parkinson, multi-infract dementia, or any array of brain impairments can also be involved to the degree they are capable. Activities should be very simple and easy to follow. If those with Parkinson's cannot control tremors, perhaps they can be given assistance; an aide can help steady their hands and guide them in the process. Those with Multi-infract dementia and other brain disorders can be given very simple projects or have some parts of the activity completed before activity time begins.

Activities for the patients with Alzheimer's will be determined by stages in disease development. In the beginning, they may be able to do many activities without assistance. Later, giving them picture books to look at when verbal or reading abilities begin to diminish can help them complete activities with only a bit of assistance. Eventually, it may be necessary to have activities that are very basic and repetitive with a lot of assistance available.

Activity time is supposed to be a fun and enjoyable time. Many older adults with and without dementia are very easily agitated.

All older adults should be allowed to do as much as they can, at a pace that allows them to do the activity without feeling hurried. The special needs of some older adults can be a challenge, but extra help and adaptations can make it possible for all older adults to benefit from recreational activities.

Adaptive Equipment

In every profession, awareness of support services can help enhance any services offered to the older adult. It is important to not only be aware of additional services available, but also to support the older adult in receiving all the benefits available to them, and to gain maximum benefits within the bio-psychosocial perspective.

It should also be pointed out that adaptive programming is not limited to groups or the nursing home setting. By using ingenuity, most activities can be used in almost any setting. For example, in a physical therapy setting, physical therapists can use an array of equipment to imitate an activity.

For example, equipment such as golf clubs, baseball bats, or small basketball machines are all examples of in-house physical therapy equipment. It adds a bit of fun to the routine and atmosphere, along with reaching the goals and objectives. These can apply to any professional who might use other activities, whether in an office, adult daycare setting, or even working with older adults who are homebound.

The ingenuity and availability of devices for disabled older adults has also gone through dramatic changes, particularly in the last five years. There is more emphasis and focus on making devices that adapt to the patient's interests. Some visionary supportive devices include: large print items, magnified/glare resistant glasses, magnified screen projection, and Braille items.

Hearing/ assistive devices include TTY, hearing aids, closed-caption television, sign language, vibration, and light equipment-/movement sensors (for example, lights that switch on when there is a knock at the door, smoke alarms that set off alarms by beeping and flashing light.)

Some assistive devices for communication include communication boards, sign language, and one-touch computer programs.

There are items that have been adapted for those who have past particular likes and interests, as well as for those interested in pursuing new activities. Some examples include fishing poles and gardening tools, which can be used by those with limited hand use.

Special devices and modifications allow those with varied abilities to complete tasks. Some of these items include lighter weights for those with muscle weakness, or braces to help hold an item in place or offer additional support. There are also heavier weights used to help those with spastic/tremor problems continue a task.

There are also adaptable items that support the coord-ination or manipulation of tools that curve and allow access and proper direction of an item wh-en a patient suffers from bone deformities and range of motion restrictions.

Amputee disabilities may create a barrier to obtaining an item or doing a task. Suction cups, Velcro, or tape are used to hold down items for these residents.

Mobility supportive devices include motorized all-terrain vehicles that can be ridden on sand and grass, and can even climb up hills. The list of adaptive equipment continues to grow. It is definitely worthwhile to send for a catalog of resources available.

Additional mobility items include stair climbers and adaptive car equipment that allows a person with limited mobility to get around.

Items that enhance or help with activities of daily living skills include reachers for grasping items out of reach, shoe tie assistance, shoe horns, buttoner helpers, back scrubbers, special feeding equipment, and hygiene helpers.

There are services that can be provided to modify, remodel, or install helpful items throughout the house for safety and accessibility.

Additional resources include employing the help of occupational therapists and obtaining catalogs for adaptive equipment.

The ability to engage in activities is vital to a quality-filled life, and the tools needed to do activities are priceless.

Adaptive Programming

Adaptive programming is an important element when the goals of particular activities are sought. Adaptive programming makes it possible for those with varied skill abilities to engage and have access to the same rights, opportunities, and types of activities as everyone else. Some important factors to consider are assessing and planning how to maintain the structure, objectives, goals, challenges, and enjoyment of the game.

The main goals are to maintain structure, safety, skills and satisfaction of the game. Some things to consider are the skills required for the game in standard play. You also need to know the skills of your client/group and your realistic expectations of goals and gains.

Some questions you need to ask are: "Can the game/equipment be modified?" "Is it safe enough for everyone?" "Will the game still retain its therapeutic value if you modify it?" "Will it be too hard or become too easy and unchallenging?" The goal is to find an intermediate balance through goal factoring.

This book includes activities that can be used for those with a full range of ability, as well as those with limited ability.

Some examples of games, sports, and activities that can be modified include: bowling/table bowling, chair basketball/table basketball, and balloon volleyball. Sports equipment can be adapted/modified. These are all ways to use resources and ingenuity to enhance adaptive programming.

Older adults are as diverse as any group. It's important to be aware of and address psychosocial issues and the group dynamics.

Will the group as a team be accommodating to others who may be slower at an activity or those who may actually hinder their personal success at winning? You need to remind players that they need to be respectful, caring, and understanding of others' feelings and abilities. Remember - the purpose of the game is to offer a nurturing environment combined with fun challenges..

An additional consideration is space availability. Will there be enough room for wheelchairs or other adaptive equipment? If there is not enough space, you may need to break the game down into two different activity times. This may be an option if a game would be avoided due to space.

Challenging and Encouragement

Challenging and encouragement are good. But listen to their choices, wishes, and rights. If they say no, no is no! Listen to their reasons; let them know you hear their fears. Try to see if you may be able to talk it out together, but never push, hurry, demand, shame or manipulate them. Be observant not to overtax/overexert them.

- Support those with socio-emotional struggles to do as much as they feel is safe and are willing to attempt.
- Support those with cognitive deficits to do what they can, and give them adequate time and support.
- Support those with physical deficits to do as much as possible, and increase activities a little bit at a time, if possible. But, again, never push.

Be observant and use care not to overexert them.

Following Directions and Implementing Activities

It is important to follow the directions when implementing activities to ensure the actual benefits that were the purpose are sought. Plan ahead for each activity. In the last week of the prior month you should usually have all your activities planned for the month.

If you are giving the residents choices of activities, make sure you get back the forms by this period. Read directions of activities so that you are aware of all the supplies you will need. Reread them at least a day before the activity. Have supplies available and set up or organized the day before.

Evaluation/Outcome Measurements

Scoring your Assessment

After the activity has been implemented, the final step is to evaluate the outcome scores of the residents in the skill levels observed during the activity. Scoring will depend on personal preference or facility choice.

You may choose to use the chart simply to observe an increase or decline gauged by looking at your scores from quarterly reviews. Then you can just add the last score of each assessment to the Reassessment Form included with this book. If you would like to do the accumulative tallied score you can follow the procedure below.

To calculate overall score you will need to total the older adult's score for the set number of activities used. Add the final total score listed on each activity sheet in the cognitive area.

After you have added the combined score you will divide this number by the number of activities you have done. This will give you an average score for cognitive function for the set number of observations done in the cognitive area. You will then repeat this same formula for the physical and socio-emotional categories

Ex: Cognitive scores
Baking 3
Computer 4, etc. x 30 activities

Total 120 divided by 30 (activities) = 4

Overall cognitive score = 4 (Assisted - mild assistance needed)

*** Repeat for physical and socio-emotional scores. Place these figures on the assessment/ reassessment form.

To calculate overall score for a measurement of combined cognitive, physical, and socio-emotional scores, you will need to add the overall score in each area and divide this by 3.

Ex: Cognitive score	4
Socio-emotional	4
Physical	4
Total	12 divided by 3 (3 areas of skills) = 4

**Overall score for all three areas for = 4 (Assistance - mild assistance needed)
Additional scoring

FIGURE 7.0
Scoring assessments

The following totals are a more detailed breakdown, and may or not be necessary. I have included them for you to use if you would like this further score breakdown.

To calculate overall cognitive score for a yearly review you will take the scores you have for each quarter and then divide them by 4 (4 scores) to get the overall score.

Cognitive score

June	4
Sept	4
Dec	4
Mar	4

Total 16 divided by 4 (months) = 4 (Assistance -mild assistance needed)

After you have totaled your scores, you can share this information with the treatment team you can take the actual Recreational Goals: Initial Assessment and Mastery checklist and the Recreational Objectives Observational Forms to the meeting, or you can fill in the short form-Recreational Activities Assessment Form.

Evaluation of Resident's Outcome Pertaining to the Use of Activities

After you have followed the program format, completed the activity, and added your scores for your resident's skill level, you will know whether the resident has shown an improvement, or in the case of a decline, a decline in ability. If the resident's skill level decreases, you may have to evaluate whether this is just a natural progression of the disease and/or aging process. You may consider that other types of activities may be more appropriate or helpful in improving resident's skill levels.

In this case, we can evaluate new goals, objectives, and methods to continue to promote activities. If the resident has improved, we will also write new goals, objectives, and methods to further increase ability.

Evaluation of Activities

When doing the activity programming evaluation, you need to consider what worked well and what did not. Was there enough time to complete activities? Where there adequate supplies on demand? Did the residents enjoy the activity? Once a month, it is a good idea to offer residents an evaluation form regarding the prior month's activities. This will allow residents to feel they have a voice regarding choices and feelings about the activity program. Additional questions might include:

Did the staff understand how to implement the activity effectively? Are there particular activities that the residents would like to include in the next month's activity program? All of these factors will help you to continuously improve and enhance your activities program.

Monthly Supply Form

It can be hard to be creative and produce a quality activity if you don't have the proper materials on hand. Be sure to do inventory checks and ensure you have enough materials available for activities.

At the beginning of the month, when you are ready to plan out your activities, have this supply list out and remember to update it, as well.

Your inventory should include enough materials for a month of activities and also back up activity supplies. It can also be helpful to have additional materials available in case of additional needs. This book includes a Monthly Supply Form inventory sheet; you can find this form in the back of the book.

Monthly Budget and Cost Sheet

You will need to fill in your supply and cost list. This is very important. This justifies how your money is being used. It also helps the facility to show the costs to run a quality program. Use the enclosed Monthly Budget and Cost Sheet to show need, justification, and documentation of spending costs. It is your responsibility to make sure your activity materials are on hand.

Recreational Objectives Observation Activities Assessment Form

Name: ____________________ Diagnosis: ________________

Staff Signature _______________ Date: ________________

Prior assessment level
Cognitive _____
Physical _____
Socio-emotional _____

Function Level
Cognitive _______

Recreational Skill Level
1-Dependent
2-Assistance - high assistance needed
3-Assistance - moderate assist. needed
4-Assistance - mild assistance needed
5-Independent

Function Level

Physical _______

Recreational Skill level

1-Dependent
2-Assistance - high assistance needed
3-Assistance - moderate assist. needed
4-Assistance - mild assistance needed
5-Independent

Function Level

Socio-emotional ____

Recreational Skill Level

1-Dependent
2-Assistance - high assistance needed
3-Assistance - moderate assist. needed
4-Assistance - mild assistance needed
5-Independent

Case Studies and Practical Uses of this Program for Specialists in the Community Setting

Primary Care Visit

To fully appraise the impact of activities and their observation value within various settings, let's look at a case study using the Geriatric Observable Activities for Longevity program.

Tillie is a 78 year-old elder living at home with her daughter. Tillie makes an appointment to follow up treatment for arthritis in her hands and hip discomfort. When the doctor is assessing Tillie, Tillie states her frustration, "The one activity I could do was knitting, and now I'm not even be able to do that!" She mentions that she can't even read because her vision has gotten so bad. She speaks about all the wonderful things she used to be able to do before she got so old, and asks, "What is the point of living when I just sit around all day doing nothing?" He notices that her voice seems flat. She keeps looking down, and he wonders if she may be suffering from depression. He notices her daughter also seems on edge and overtired/overstressed.

He asks some specific questions to perform a Geriatric Depression Scale Assessment on Tillie to check for depression. While he is doing his exam, he mentions that perhaps she needs to finally consider laser surgery for her cataracts. He then mentions the new magazine he started getting from an adaptive device company and the huge selection of adaptive devices they carry that allow older adults to carry on with all kinds of hobbies, even with limited use of arm/hand or wrist function.

He suggests that perhaps she might like to look into some programs like the local YWCA or senior center. Tillie's daughter speaks up and says this may be a problem because she works all day, and by the time she gets home her mom is winding down for the day.

The Dr. listens empathetically. He mentions that he'll send home some papers on services in the community. When he writes his notes on treatment for the arthritis, he also includes a quick memo to ask the nurse to send home a flyer from the adaptive device magazine. He also includes a note mentioning the possible needs for further evaluation of depression and a referral to the eye doctor, occupational therapist, and additional support services. When the nurse writes the instructions on the treatment, she includes pamphlets on adaptive devices. She also includes a list of organizations in the community that offer support services for seniors.

The truth is, Tillie could have made the comment, "What is the point of living when I just sit around all day doing nothing," at any point in treatment care, to any of the various professionals working with her.

Whether being evaluated by a doctor, nurse, physical therapist, case manager, or even a home health aide, Tillie's statement pertains to a very important issue. Tillie is struggling with aging and an inability to do the things she thrived on. She is stating a need so important to her essence and daily living experiences. Because she is no longer able to engage in activities that were once so important to her, she feels no sense of worth in living. We must consider ways to implement home modifications, help with activities of daily living skills (ADLs), medical benefits, and activities for successful aging and fulfilling experiences.

The following are some examples of the services Tillie might gain as a result of the doctor's assessment and that of various professionals using the observation forms to assess and implement successful inclusion of activities in quality of life issues and care.

Occupational Therapy

A recommendation is made for Tillie to see an occupational therapist. The occupational therapist performs a home assessment to see if Tillie will benefit from some home modifications or adaptive equipment.

The occupational therapist also assesses Tillie's cognitive skills and functional skills level. Tillie's past history of falls and her range of motion restrictions due to her arthritis.

She also is aware that Tillie takes blood pressure medicine, and knows this is a medical alert linked to a higher prevalence/danger of falls. Therefore, she makes a recommendation for safety bars in the bathroom. Because of Tillie's arthritis and agility problems, she makes some recommendations for kitchen modifications

/gadgets.

The OT has a copy of *The Bio-psychosocial approach to Therapeutic Activities and Successful Aging* textbook, which includes the Geriatric Observable Activities for Longevity program.

As part of her assessment, the occupational therapist includes the Interest and Background Sheet, the Recreational Initial Assessment and Mastery Checklist and the Recreational Objectives Observation Forms. She uses the forms to assess Tillie's skill levels and needs, as well as to assess ADLs needs. She also does a leisure/recreational assessment. Even if she will not meet with Tillie again, she will have a full assessment to document addressing Tillie's skill levels and validated needs.

If she were able to do follow up visits, she could assess Tillie at a later date to see if she has made progress or has further declined. If she does continue to work with Tillie, she could do set intervals of activities and tally scores to note decline or progress.

The occupational therapist asks Tillie about past activities regarding hobbies, past work, and interests. Tillie talks about the past events she did. She again mentions her frustration at not being able to do all the things she used to.

She mentions that when she saw the doctor he gave her a magazine on adaptive devices that can help her continue to knit. The occupational therapist shows Tillie some other great adaptive/ assistive devices made for the elderly and helps Tillie obtain the items. Some of these items are for activities of daily living. (ADLs)

The occupational therapist wants to be sure she addresses Tillie's needs from all three domains of physical, cognitive and socio-emoional factors. She also considers fulfillment issues, therefore she points out not just home modifications or help with ADLs for function/tasks, or even the medical benefits, but also activities (such as gardening and embroidery assistance devices) for successful aging and fulfilling experiences.

Support Services-
Social Worker/Counselor/ Case Manager

Tillie and her daughter also call the senior resource center. A case manager helps Tillie tap into resources in the community that can help her receive services. The geriatric case manager also helps Tillie and her daughter find a counselor. Tillie and her daughter talk about the many changes since Tillie's husband passed away and she has had to move in with her daughter.

Tillie talks about all the changes in her life and how happy she was when she was able to enjoy her life in the ways she chose. Tillie's dau-ghter talks about the changes in her life since her mom moved in. The counselor suggests Tillie's daughter may benefit from a support group for family caretakers.

Counseling/Therapy

During her sessions with Tillie, the counselor might choose to do some activities as a therapy in the office. She/he might use the activities to observe Tillie's cognitive/ psychosocial abilities, as well as assess/observe her physical abilities-/needs. This information may be of help to fully see the impact of Tillie's skill/need levels and help her meet her goals. She/he might also give Tillie some activities to do at home to guide her towards particular therapeutic needs).

The observation forms can be used over any time span. It is recommended that three assessments be done for a good reading. The scores should then be evaluated to chart progress or decline. These observation forms have been tested in a nursing home setting with the ability to show effective results for observation of changes.

If Tillie's was exhibiting signs of cognitive defects with a concern of Alzheimer's disease/Dementia the information obtained during activity observations could have been passed along to the psychiatrist/psychologist as additional information on Tillie's cognitive, physical and socio-emotional skills/needs.

Certified Recreational Therapist/ Activity Professional

This program includes procedural codes used for billing purposes. These codes are intended for licensed therapists.

However, an activity professional or certified recreational therapist can use the charts for either personal use or unit charting. In some circumstances, under some conditions a licensed professional may oversee the activity professionals' use of assessments and use the charts with supervision. An unlicensed professional must never submit a claim. You must be aware of your facility guidelines and the guidelines of government regulations.

If Tillie were a participant in an adult day care center where a certified recreational professional was present, the recreational therapist /activity professional would be able to implement this program.

When using this program a certified recreational therapist/ activity professional would have full use of the educational materials, activities and Recreational Objectives Observational Forms for personal use or as mentioned above, following regulations.

With continued follow up on how Tillie was managing, regarding her arthritis, vision and ability to enjoy aging activities, this information could be shared with her doctor or the counselor working with Tillie and her daughter.

If Tillie has shown early signs of Alzheimer's disease, any information gathered from the assessments could have been forwarded onto the appropriate supervisor as additional information gained on the patient's cognitive abilities during activities. This information can be helpful to all levels of care.

The recreational/activity professional could do continuous or quarterly assessments, as well as ongoing activities for successful aging, function and fulfilling experiences. She/he could also make referrals/report findings back to primary care. However, they must have patient release of information authorization.

Case Studies and Practical Uses of This Program for Specialists in a Long Term Care Facility

Shelly works in a long-term care facility. Shelly chose to observe a resident who had frequently declined activity invitations in the past.

The observational forms allowed Shelly to see growth in the resident's socio-emotional skills. The resident had recently begun to participate in bingo on a regular basis.

The patient went from requiring moderate assistance during the initial observation a month prior to now becoming independent in her motivation and initiative, and exhibiting emotional gratification.

The resident also improved in her socialization and community integration skills. She was now accepting a greater number of invitations to group activities, smiling more, and initiating conversations more frequently.

Shelly was also able to document the resident's abilities in cognitive and physical skills. There was documented improvement in the resident's attention throughout the month period. The resident had previously fallen asleep during activities. The resident was now staying awake the entire bingo hour.

A slight improvement in physical function was noted as well. The resident had highly impaired vision but was able to participate with the use of enlarged bingo cards. This same resident was observed during music and gardening activities.

In this case study the main emphasis of treatment goals centered on addressing the resident's socio-emotional needs. Now, let's see how the entire treatment team could use this information.

Certified Recreational Therapist

As noted by our example, in a nursing home setting activities professional can implement this program for personal use or use the procedural codes, following regulations and supervision. She/he will have full use of the educational materials, activities and Recreational Objectives Observational Forms.

For example, our previous patient Tillie was placed in a nursing home setting, continued follow up and information on how Tillie is managing regarding her arthritis vision and ability to enjoy aging activities, can be shared with the staff working with Tillie.

If Tillie has shown early signs of Alzheimer's disease, any information gathered from the assessments could have been forwarded onto the doctor/psychiatrist/psychologist as additional information gained on the patient's cognitive abilities during activities.

The therapeutic activity professional could do continuous or quarterly assessments, as well as ongoing activities for successful aging, function and fulfilling experiences. This information could also be shared with the treatment team.

Nurse/ Geriatric Case Manager/ Nursing Facility Administration

The nurse filling in the Mini Data Sets (MDS) would have information regarding skills assessed during activities to help with the patient's overall assessment. The case manager would have been able to assess that activities were part of the resident's needs and goals being met for ongoing care, and would have used this information accordingly.

This information could have also been shared with the resident's family to ensure them of high standards of care and fulfilling experiences of their loved one. This documentation would also be available to share with state or federal surveyors who assess the quality of programming and outcome measurements for facility compliance.

Geriatric Physical Therapist

In this case, the resident did not require physical therapy intervention. In fact, it was noted that the resident demonstrated slight improvements in physical abilities.

Due to HIPPA regulations, the observation forms were not returned with the participants scored recreational objectives observation forms. How-ever, if the resident had needed more intensive treatment by the Physical Therapy department, information in the chart noting skills observed during the activity times would have been a valuable addition. The physical therapist might also have been able to make some recommendations on activities that will help the resident.

Information to send on to the Physician/Psychiatrist/Psychologist

This information can be of use to the physician/psychiatrist/psychologist to assess the residents' cognitive/psychosocial needs, abilities, and behaviors during observation of activities. For example, as the resident exhibited more socio-emotional skills, her attention did improve, as opposed to a situation where her attention did not improve despite her own initiative and motivation. Questions regarding the reasons behind poor attention can be applied to instances such as this. Additional content areas within the cognitive recreational observational form might also become important information for ongoing cognitive/psychosocial information.

PROGRAM FORMAT

We will now follow the format and instructional training on how to implement this program effectively to ensure maximum outcome benefits.

We will use a sample case to fully understand the program method. After we have read the case study, we will further break each step down individually to explain the full benefits of the program.

SAMPLE USE OF THE GERIATRIC OBSERVABLE ACTIVITIES FOR LONGEVITY

Mary works in a long-term nursing facility. She is familiar with the Geriatric Observable Activities for Longevity. She read the educative materials and is able to understand the aspects of aging and various issues that are specific to her elder clients. She has looked at the activities section of the book and understands the variation of skills that are found in particular activities.

Mary understands that, to run a well-balanced program, she needs to include a variety of activities in all three areas of concentration. She makes sure that as she plans her activities for the month she has at least twenty-one activities with a rotation of physical, cognitive, and socio-emotional activities. She does a physical one day, a cognitive the next, and a socio-emotional the next.

All of the activities have benefits in all areas, but as she has seen by reading and understanding the program, each activity does have a concentrated area of focus. For example, exercise is good for physical, puzzles are good for cognition, and community outings are great for socio-emotional needs.

Mary is aware that her facility uses the MDS, which is an ongoing overall assessment chart of each resident's care. She understands that either a nurse will primarily fill out the mds or each discipline will fill in their own information on pertinent areas within the mds.

Mary works in a center where she will be responsible for filling in the mds report for the activity section. If she were another specialist, she would use the information to fill in her specialty section. She knows that, even if she was not responsible to fill in the mds, the information she gains can be given to the treatment team or for her personal use as a professional.

Mary will do her own assessment, using the Recreational Goals: Initial Assessment and Mastery Checklist for her initial assessment. She is also aware that any additional information she will need to understand her resident's skill levels is kept in the resident's chart. Mary reads the resident's chart regarding the information found on the MDS or other facility assessment forms and information.

After Mary has all of the information regarding the patient's chart, her own assessment, and the Interest and Background Sheet, she is ready to plan her activities and use the Therapeutic Recreational Objectives Observation Forms.

One of Mary's new residents, Lynn, shows a high need of help with physical skills. She decides that when she is doing physical activities she will do her observations on Lynn.

Mary considers the type of activities Lynn likes based on his background and interest form. She sees Lynn was an avid bowler, and decides she will observe him during bowling. She gets out her Recreational Objectives Observational Forms and goes to the sports activities. Mary makes a copy of the bowling activity, which includes a physical, cognitive and socio-emotional form).

Mary fills in Lynn's name and information regarding his initial skill levels in each area based on information she gained from her recreational goals: Initial assessment and Mastery checklist, the mds/facility assessment forms, and the treatment team meeting. Mary has already decided to observe Lynn on the day she does a bowling activity.

On bowling day, Mary does her activity program and observes Lynn during this activity. She fills in Lynn's physical, cognitive, and socio-emotional forms for the bowling activity.

On the day she observes Lynn, she takes a few minutes at the end of the day to tally his score. At the end of three months she compares the initial score and notes progress or declines. She adds the scores for Lynn in physical, cognitive, and social-emotional skills and puts this information on the Recreational Assessment Form. She then takes this information to the treatment team meeting and also makes sure a copy is in Lynn's chart.

This will allow all the staff to understand how Lynn is doing during activities. This information can be of benefit for all the professional caring for Lynn regarding his physical, cognitive, and socio-emotional skills and overall well-being.

Even tough she will observe Lynn in the physical aspect, because this is the most critical need for him, she also needs to fill in the cognitive and socio-emotional, so that she is sure he will continue to be okay in these areas. If not, she can explain her findings and be of help to those professionals looking at these aspects of care.

Mary puts a green tag on Lynn's forms. This helps her identify her residents whose highest needs are for physical skills areas. Mary does this because, when she is making her plans for activities throughout her month, during the activities with the highest physical potential, she will choose residents with high need of assistance in physical skills to observe during physical activity days. She uses yellow for those needing socio-emotional and red tags for those most needing to be observed for cognition. Each day, Mary chooses residents to observe at an activity that she has chosen to observe for that type of activity, whether for physical, cognitive, or socio-emotional needs.

Program Steps

1. Information obtained from the MDS/ Facility assessments, tests, personal interest and background form, and the Recreational Goals: Initial Assessment and Mastery checklist are used to understand residents' abilities and needs.

Mary is aware that the information she will need to understand her resident's skill levels, and other information on the individual resident, are kept in the resident's chart. Mary reads the resident's chart regarding the information found on the MDS or other facility assessment forms and information. Mary also does her own assessment. Mary keeps herself updated on any information for her residents.

One of Mary's new residents, Lynn, is 71-years-old. Lynn is a diabetic. He also suffers from hypertension. Two years ago, he suffered a mild stroke which left him with some mild cognitive deficits. He was able to stay at home until recently; his family could no longer give him the care he needed. Presently, his diabetes and hypertension are under control. He completed physical therapy and rehabilitation for his stroke a year ago.

Unfortunately, since this time period, he had very little activity. Due to his weight and lack of mobility, his function level is compromised. Lynn shows a high need of help with physical skills. Lynn's has a good family support system and quite a few visits from his friends. His psychosocial status appears to be high and he makes friends easily. His cognitive function status shows moderate-to-high independence.

Mary attended a treatment team meeting and is aware the team will be addressing dietary measures regarding Lynn's needs for weight maintenance to control his hypertension and diabetic. Lynn's physical assessment and status on the mds shows him to have moderate function level. He has decreased strength and endurance. Due to his hypertension and balance and gait concerns, Mary will need to use caution when Lynn is involved in activities.

Lynn's highest need presently appears to be for physical needs. Mary reads Lynn's Background and Interest form. She sees Lynn was an avid bowler and decides she will include bowling as an important activity for Lynn's likes. Because she needs to personally assess Lynn's abilities of balance and gait, she decides to start off with Table Bowling.

2. Activities are chosen according to which will support the patient's needs/goals.

Lynn needs physical activities to increase his activity level, his decreased strength and endurance (especially upper and lower right side extremities), and overall function level. She decides that when she is doing physical activities she will do her observations on Lynn.

Mary considers the type of activities Lynn likes based on his Background and Interest Form. She sees Lynn was an avid bowler, and decides she will observe Lynn during table/bowling activity time.

3. Find matching recreational observation forms that coincide with the activity.

Mary fills in Lynn's physical, cognitive, and socio-emotional forms for the table/bowling activity.

Mary gets out her Recreational Objectives Observational Forms and goes to the sports activities. Mary makes a copy of the bowling activity, which includes a physical, cognitive, and socio-emotional forms for the bowling activity.

4. For initial observation/score, begin with the Older Adult Individual Assessment Checklist and skill level from facility test assessments.

Mary fills in Lynn's name and information regarding his initial skill levels in each area. This information is based on her Recreational Goals: Initial assessment and Mastery checklist and information she gained from the mds/facility assessment forms.

5. Perform at least one observation of an activity over a three-month observation period.

Mary decides she will observe Lynn during table/bowling activity times, once a month for the next three months. If Lynn does not do bowling over the next three months, she knows she can substitute any physical activity because all the physical activities focus on the same skills. Mary makes a copy of the bowling activity, which includes a physical, cognitive, and socio-emotional form.

6. On bowling day, Mary does her activity program.

7. As observing, fill in skill level observed.

Mary fills in the skill level she observes as Lynn does the activity.

8. At the end of the day tally score for all three areas (physical, cognitive, and socio-emotional) skills observed.

On the day she observes Lynn, she takes a few minutes at the end of her day to tally Lynn's score.

9. Tally the final score you have for all three observations in all three areas.

After the three months (three activities), she compares the initial score and notes progress or declines.

10. Bring the assessment reviews and documentation to treatment team/staff attention.

Mary takes this information to the treatment team meeting and also makes sure a copy is in Lynn's chart. This will allow all staff to understand how Lynn is doing during activities. This information can be of benefit for all the professional caring for Lynn regarding his physical, cognitive, and socio-emotional skills and overall well-being.

Using the Recreational Objectives Observation forms

1. Information obtained from the MDS, the Recreational Goals: Initial Assessment and Mastery Checklist and Facility assessments data, are used to understand the resident's abilities and needs .

2. Activities are chosen according to which activities will support the patient's needs/goals.
3. Find matching activity Recreational Objectives Observation Forms that coincide with the activity.
You could also do activities in groups with residents needing the same skills observed. This can be helpful if you can only assess on days when you have a volunteer.

4. For initial score, begin by using the Recreational Goals: Initial Assessment and Mastery Checklist, and facility test assessments.

5. Plan activities based on needs and goals.

6. Implement the activity.

7. As doing activity observe and fill in skill-level observed.

8. At the end of the day, tally score for all three areas (physical, cognitive and socio-emotional) skills observed.

9. Tally the final score you have for all three observations in all three areas.

10. Bring the assessment reviews and documentation to treatment team/staff attention.

ACTIVITIES, CHARTS AND TABLES

Sports/Physical Activities

(High physical stimulation)

The CDC recommends that older adults participate in moderate-intensity aerobic activity 3-5 days a week for at least 30 minutes. This will help older adults to increase endurance, strength, and balance. It is also recommended that older adults engage in activities that include stretching everyday and strength training activities 2-3 days per week. (CDC, NCCDPHP. Special focus: healthy aging. Chronic Disease Notes and Reports 1999; 12(3): 10-11. Insert CDC recommendations obtained from aoa.hhs.gov 2005

* All older adults engaging in activities should have physician approval to engage in physical activities.

AQUATICS

Objectives and benefits

Cognitive Challenges: attention, memory, language, orientation, following patterns, keeping rhythm, perceptual awareness, and cognitive stimulation

Physical Needs: fine motor skills, gross motor skills, coordination, range of motion, flexibility, posture, balance, backward and forward movement, gait, following step patterns, circulation, cardio-vascular workout

Socio-emotional Needs: socialization, community integration, initiative and motivation, emotional gratification, sense of accomplishment, self-esteem, tolerating stimulation, fostering appropriate behaviors

Supplies: Availability of activity pool, qualified supervision provided by facility or other qualified/certified lifeguards and staff.

Time: 20–30 minutes

Staff/older adult ratio: 1:2 or as assessed per needs of individuals or group

Instructions: Generally, an aquatic therapist or swim coach/instructor would teach the actual activity program. Have them warm up for activity by leading them in a sub maximal active warm-up first. This will gradually increase their body temperature, blood flow to the muscles, and synovial fluid to the joints. You may then lead them in a three to five minute stretching exercise. The activity could be done as a freestyle activity that allows older adults to get adjusted to the water and swim at their own pace. It may also be a set water workout.

Many older adults will have to adjust to the water temperature. Generally, many facilities in the community will have a water temperature in the range of 85-86 degrees. You should, however, inquire what each facility's temperature is, so as not to cause distress or over-stimulation. It should be a moderate temperature. Due to medications, or falling potential, older adults should be supervised very carefully. Older adults with restrictions may be able to use special equipment available for the use of the physically challenged. It might be helpful to ask the facility what they have available to enhance activity activities.

The CDC recommends that older adults participate in moderate-intensity aerobic activity 3-5 days a week for at least 30 minutes. This will help older adults to increase endurance, strength, and balance. It is also recommended that older adults engage in activities that include stretching everyday and strength training activities 2-3 days per week. (CDC, NCCDPHP. Special focus: healthy aging. Chronic Disease Notes and Reports 1999; 12(3): 10-11. Insert CDC recommendations obtained from aoa.hhs.gov 2005

* All older adults engaging in activities should have physician approval to engage in physical activities.

Aquatics
Cognitive Goals, Objectives, and Methods

SKILL	GOAL	OBJECTIVES SAMPLE	METHOD SAMPLE
Orientation	Show increased awareness of, time/ "timeframe," people, circumstances, and past experiences vs. present experiences, to engage in present-time activities, or for a reminiscing intended question	-will respond w/correct answer to two choice questions Or yes/no, will state place, time, present company of people, or past experiences on own during activity 1x a week	Staff will ask residents a series of questions to stimulate focus to the present setting (Ex: "Are you at the mall or at the activity center?") Or past if a reminiscing exercise (Ex: "Have you swum before? With who? What is your swim partner's name? Mary or Karen?"
Attention	Show increased attention span, task for function, and to engage in meaningful, recreational/fulfilling activities	-will make eye-contact with swim staff, will verbalize with staff and instructor, will read/listen to swim rules, will say yes/no to show they understand or by actions	Staff will address or stand in front of resident, make eye-contact, ask questions, or use others methods to get resident's attention, and then observe or ask the residents questions to see if they are listening and understand
Memory	Show increased memory skills of recall, recognition, retention of information, working memory	-will retain/repeat how to float 1x a week, will repeat/recall how to freestyle (or) will remember lesson at next class	-Staff will show steps on how to float, do free-style, etc. -Staff will teach steps of game and then ask questions to gauge memory skills
Language	Show increased ability to communicate use of words, phrases, ntence structure, comprehension, interpretation	-will reply to a question (Ex: states color of the swim board, favorite swim form, yes/no etc.), will interpret instructor's request, will initiate task	Staff will ask questions to stimulate a communication (Ex: "What color float do you like?"), or make a command to observe interpretation skills
Cognitive Stimulation (awareness, seeks information in)	Increased stimulus/exposure for visual/ motor memory, cognitive experiences/awareness and brain stimulation to enhance (function, pragmatics, neuron-plasticity)	will recall/retain and sort/gather information, problem-solve, will do the required swim, will play the water basketball game and complete the task	-Staff will show the resident the step-by-step actions to swim -Staff will give instructions on water basketball game -Staff will instruct residents in the step-by-step procedure for games, encourage, make use of adaptive devices if needed, and supply necessary materials and support
Perceptual Awareness	Show increased abilities of depth perception, visual-spatial awareness, and acuity (for discrimination, comparison, and categorizing), safety	-will stay in own lanes, will stay within own space next to others, will maneuver around peers during game, will grab the water basketball and toss at the net	-Staff will instruct the residents on where they need to stay in their lanes -Staff will use a game to have residents swim and toss ball to peers or the net during the game
Problem-solving (goes beyond thinking/stimulus and initiates thinking process)	Increase problem-solving ability, processing of information, thinking, reasoning, and use of good judgment and decision-making	-will interact with peers while in the pool, will engage in a game of water basketball, will accept challenge of input information and engage/interact in activity	Staff will set up a water basketball game to stimulate visual/motor memory, thinking, etc. and cognitive awareness
Complete a Task	Increase ability to complete a task	-will do a synchronized swim w/ a partner, will follows synchronized rhythm of music and recognize change in music rhythm as the signal for a team player to toss the ball at the net. -will consider strategies of water game ,will grab the water basketball and toss at the net	Staff will place a musical tape with a steady rhythm in the tape player. Staff will support/encourage residents to dance/swim in a synchronized swim w/ a partner, or staff will instruct residents to toss the ball at the basket net when music tempo changes

TABLE 1.1

Recreational Objectives Observation Form
Aquatics - Cognitive Skills

PATIENT	Dependent (Totally dependent)	High Assistance (25+ ability)	Moderate Assist. (50+ ability)	Mild Assistance (75+ability)	Independent (Totally independent)
SEE CODES BELOW USE OPTIONAL CODES IF APPROPRIATE	1	2	3	4	5
	3 cue/ 2-3 physical	2-3 cues/ 2 physical	2-3 cues/ 1 physical	1-2 cues	Encouragement

(Code 97113)- if actual Aquatic therapy or	**SKILL**	**GOAL**	**OBJECTIVES** ____times per ____	**METHOD**	**OUTCOME DATE**			
97532 Cognitive skills	ORIENTATION							
97532 Cognitive skills	ATTENTION							
97532 Cognitive skills	MEMORY							
97532 Cognitive skills	PROBLEM-SOLVING							
97532 Cognitive skills	COMPLETE A TASK							
97139 Speech Therapy 97532	LANGUAGE							
97533	SENSORY STIMULATION /COGNITIVE STIMULATION							
97532	PERCEPTUAL AWARENESS							

97532-Development of cognitive skills to improve attention, memory, problem-solving, includes compensatory training and/or sensory integrative activities, direct (one-on-one) patient contact by the provider, each 15 minutes; **97530-Therapeutic activities**, direct (one-on-one) patient contact by the provider (use of dynamic activities to improve functional performance), each 15 minutes**; 97533-Sensory integration techniques** to enhance sensory processing and promote adaptive responses to environmental demands, direct (one-on-one) patient contact by the provider, each 15 minutes; **97150-Therapeutic procedure(s)**, group (2 or more individuals); **97139-Unlisted therapeutic procedure** (specify) minutes; **97003- occupational therapy evaluation**; **97004- re-evaluation**

Staff Initial				
Add total score here Maximum Score 40 pt. each form per activity				
See scale below or use own/facilities optional score system				

Score 1-8) =1 (9-16) =2 (17-24) =3 (25-32) =4 (33-40) =5 If w/device add d if wish, ex: 1d, 2d, or If using 1-7 scale: (41-48) =6 (49-56)

Aquatics
Physical Goals, Objectives, and Methods

SKILL	GOAL	OBJECTIVES SAMPLE	METHOD SAMPLE
Fine motor skills	Increase fine motor skills, including: using fingers, toes, hand-eye coordination, and dexterity	-will fan/cup hands, fingers, and toes to swim; for a game, will grasp ball and toss into the net, etc. 1x a week	Staff will give residents instructions on the steps to swim freestyle, or get involved in water game including use of the fine motor skills
Gross motor skills	or skills	-will bend, stretch, and do swim movements during water workout/game, will stretch, float, move arms, kick feet; will toss ball to others, throw ball at net	Staff will give residents instructions or get involved in an exercise workout/game in the pool, including use of the gross motor skills
Perceptual speed and motor function	Increase speed and motor ability for function, safety, meaningful/fulfilling activities	-will react and throw ball during activity in coordinated movement and speed (within one minute), will join in on a water ball race game (dr. approval)	Staff will encourage residents to increase pace of actions while engaging residents in a waterball game and will increase reaction time by decreasing time between tossing the ball
Following step patterns/backwards forward movement	Increase strength, balance, endurance, meaningful/fulfilling activities	-will walk forward in water, will turn, will take backwards and forwards steps while in the water	Staff will show resident the mechanics of bowling which require walking forward/backwards then forward and rolling the ball
For clinician/Dr. approved use only	For clinician/Dr. approved use only	For clinician/Dr. approved use only	For clinician/Dr. approved use only
Balance and Posture (approved by Dr. and capacity tests)	Increase balance and improve body alignment and flexibility	-will sit/stand up without losing balance, will hold on to pool ladder/handle and maintain posture for 3 minutes, will stand in water and maintain posture for 3 minutes	-While in the pool, staff will show residents the proper posture and ask them to hold body in straight alignment -Staff will help resident increase strength for balance by having them stand still in water (support if needed) and toss the ball into the net
Gait/Following Step patterns/ Backward/ Forward movement	Increase strength, balance, endurance, meaningful/ fulfilling activities	-will walk backwards in water, will walk ckwards, forwards, turn, move all ections 1x a week	Staff will ask residents to walk forwards/ backwards and turn in the water (support device if needed) while listening to music, and do these actions during a water basketball game (device/support if needed)
Cardio-vascular Workout*	Increase circulation, blood flow, stamina	-will swim at a safe pace (approved by Dr. and capacity tests), If approved by clinical specialist: _______________ 1x a week	Staff will have residents swim laps, participate in game (according to ability and approved amount of activity)

TABLE 1.2

Recreational Objectives Observation Form
Aquatics - Physical Skills

PATIENT		Dependent (Totally dependent)	High Assistance (25+ ability)	Moderate Assist. (50+ ability)	Mild Assistance (75+ability)	Independent (Totally independent.)
SEE CODES BELOW		1	2	3	4	5
USE OPTIONAL CODES IF APPROPRIATE		3 cue/ 2-3 physical	2-3 cues/ 2 physical	2-3 cues/ 1 physical	1-2 cues	Encouragement
(Code 97113)-if actual Aquatic therapy	**SKILL**	**GOAL**	**OBJECTIVES** ____times per ____		**METHOD**	**OUTCOME DATE**
97530 Therapeutic Activity	FINE MOTOR SKILLS					
97110/ 97530	GROSS MOTOR SKILLS					
97110/ 97530/	PERCEPTUAL SPEED/ MOTOR FUNCTION					
97530 or Gait training 97116-	STEP PATTERNS					
		Licensed/ Clinician	Dr. approved use only		Licensed/ Clinician	
97110- Therapeutic procedure	RANGE OF MOTION					
97112	POSTURE AND BALANCE					
97110 Or if Licensed clinician - Gait training 97116-	GAIT (INCLUDES STAIR CLIMBING)					
97110	CARDIO-VASCULAR WORKOUT*					

97110-Therapeutic procedure, one or more areas, each 15 minutes; therapeutic exercises to develop strength and endurance, range of motion, and flexibility; 97112-Neuromuscular reeducation of movement, balance, coordination, kinesthetic sense, posture, and proprioception; **97113-Aquatic therapy** with therapeutic exercises; **97116-Gait training** (includes stair climbing); **97139-Unlisted therapeutic procedure** (specify); **97150 Therapeutic procedure(s)**, group (2 or more individuals); **97750-Physical performance test or measurement** (e.g., musculoskeletal, functional capacity), with written report, each 15 minutes; **97535-Self care/home management training** (e.g., activities of daily living and compensatory training, meal preparation, safety procedures, and instructions in use of adaptive equipment), direct (one-on-one) contact by provider, each 15 minutes; **Physical therapy 97001 evaluation, 97002 Re-evaluation. Occupational therapy evaluation 97003, re-evaluation. 97004; Athlete training 97005; re-evaluation 97006**	Staff Initial
	Add total score here Maximum Score 40 pt. each form per activity
	See scale below or use own/facilities optional score system

20/ activity professional (Score 1-4)=1 (5-8) =2 (9-12) =3 (13-16) =4 (17-20) =5 If w/device add d if wish, ex: 1d, 2d, or If using 1-7 scale: (21-24) =6 (25-28) =7 40/clinician Score 1-8) =1 (9-16) =2 (17-24) =3 (25-32) =4 (33-40) =5 If w/device add d if wish, ex: 1d, 2d, or If using 1-7 scale: (41-48) =6 (49-56)

Aquatics
Socio-emotional Goals, Objectives, and Methods

SKILL	GOAL	OBJECTIVES SAMPLE	METHOD SAMPLE
Socialization/Community Integration	Increase social interactions, meaningful/fulfilling activities	-will interact with peers for pleasure, belonging needs, etc.; will engage in community integration experiences, use manners, social practices	Staff will take residents to swim center 1x a week and support/encourage them to socialize through community integration and being paired w/swimmers and group games
Team Playing/Sharing	Increase teamwork/sharing, meaningful/fulfilling activities	-will join in on a water sport game or water exercise with others and share, wait turn, support peers, show compassion, and patience to team members (listen, wait, make positive comments)	Staff will place a basketball floater in the pool and residents will be encouraged to play, share floats, form teams, strategize together, consider peers
Initiative and Motivation	Increase initiative and motivation/wellness, and quality of life	-will choose if they wish to swim or not, will choose if they wish to join in on team water game, will try a new swim technique	-Staff will support/encourage the resident to prepare to swim (change, shower first, go out to the pool in a timely fashion) for their own personal gains of activity -Staff will offer new techniques to motivate
Emotional Gratification	Increase emotional gratification/wellness, and quality of life	-will state that the swim class is a gratifying experience, or will show pleasure by smiling, laughing, deep focus on activity 1x a week	Staff will ask residents if they enjoyed the swim class and what they liked through verbal discussion, group discussions
Sense of Accomplishment	Increase feelings of self-worth, pride, productivity, dignity/wellness, and quality of life	-will look at the chart showing swimmers and personal bests, will use gestures to express pride in self, will talk about activity ability	A chart on the unit wall or a paper handed to the residents reflecting swim time, etc. will be available for residents to see their personal best/increased swim time
Self-esteem/self-identity	Increase self-esteem, feelings of belonging, dignity, self-worth, integrity, self-identity/wellness, and quality of life	-will state/communicate positive feelings about self and ability to swim, will join swim class to take an active role in health though exercising, will join the swim class based on own choices	-Staff will educate residents on the value of activity/exercise and encourage them to swim/exercise, -Staff will design a wall chart showing swimmers' names and personal swim time and endurance
Sensory Integration/Tolerating Stimulation	Increase sensory processing and enhance awareness of sensations and toleration/adaptation of sensory stimulations and demands	-will join in on exercise class, will listen and follow instructions, will use appropriate behavior for the setting, will wait turn, stand in line quietly; will quiet down when asked during swim class	Before swim class begins, staff will discuss the pool rules, appropriate behaviors, respect of property, safety, and respect of fellow swimmers while activity
Fostering Appropriate Behaviors	Increase social interaction, social opportunities and adjustment, safety, using appropriate behaviors during an activity for a calm environment/wellness, and quality of life	-will show adjustment to the smell of the pool, put hand or foot in the water, adjust to water/water temperature; will enter water and adjust to the pool temperature (2-4 min.) (read memo on temperatures)	-Staff will take residents to the pool and expose them to sensory stimulating experiences -Staff will support residents as they adjust to the stimulus one step at a time

TABLE 1.3

Recreational Objectives Observation Form
Aquatics - Socio-emotional Skills

PATIENT	Dependent (Totally dependent)	High Assistance (25+ ability)	Moderate Assist. (50+ ability)	Mild Assistance (75+ability)	Independent (Totally independent.)
SEE CODES BELOW USE OPTIONAL CODES IF APPROPRIATE	1	2	3	4	5
	3 cue/ 2-3 physical	2-3 cues/ 2 physical	2-3 cues/ 1 physical	1-2 cues	Encouragement

97530- Therapeutic activities or	SKILL	GOAL	OBJECTIVES ____times per ____	METHOD	OUTCOME DATE			
97537 Or 97535	SOCIALIZATION/ COMMUNITY INTEGRATION							
97537 Or 97535	TEAM PLAYING /SHARING							
97537 Or 97535	INITIATIVE AND MOTIVATION							
97537 Or 97535	EMOTIONAL GRATIFICATION							
97537 Or 97535	SENSE OF ACCOMPLISHMENT							
97537 Or 97535	SELF-ESTEEM/ SELF-IDENTITY							
97537 Or 97535	FOSTERING APPROPRIATE BEHAVIORS							
97533	SENSORY INTEGRATION/ TOLERATING							

97537-Community/work reintegration training (e.g., shopping, transportation, money management, avocational activities and/or work environment/modification analysis, work task analysis), direct (one-on-one) contact by provider, each 15 minutes; **97535-Self care/home management training** (e.g., activities of daily living and compensatory training, meal preparation, safety procedures, and instructions in use of adaptive equipment), direct (one-on-one) contact by provider, each 15 minutes; **97530-Therapeutic activities, direct (one-on-one)** patient contact by the provider (use of dynamic activities to improve functional performance), each 15 minutes; **97150-Therapeutic procedure(s), group (2 or more individuals); 97533-Sensory integration techniques** to enhance sensory processing and promote adaptive responses to environmental demands, direct (one-on-one) patient contact by the provider, each 15 minutes; **occupational therapy evaluation 97003, re-evaluation . 97004**	Staff Initial			
	Add total score here-Maximum Score 40 pt. each form per activity			
	See scale below or use own/facilities optional score system			

(Score 1-8)=1 (9-16) =2 (17-24) =3 (25-32) =4 (33-40) =5 If w/device add d if wish, ex: 1d, 2d, or If using 1-7 scale: (41-48) =6 (49-56)

Bowling /Table Bowling

Objectives and benefits

Cognitive Challenges: attention, memory, language, orientation, following patterns, keeping rhythm, perceptual awareness, and cognitive stimulation

Physical Needs: fine motor skills, gross motor skills, coordination, range of motion, flexibility, posture, balance, backward and forward movement, gait, following step patterns, circulation, cardio-vascular workout

Socio-emotional Needs: socialization, community integration, initiative and motivation, emotional gratification, sense of accomplishment, self-esteem, tolerating stimulation, fostering appropriate behaviors

Supplies: A tabletop bowling machine or bowling set. Be sure pins are light enough for the elderly to hit and knock over. Also keep in mind that the bowling pieces may need to be a soft material so the noise is not upsetting.

Time: 30 minutes

Staff/older adult ratio: 1:6 or as assessed per needs of individuals or group

Instructions: Set up bowling pins on a large table. Have them warm up for bowling by leading them in a sub maximal active warm-up first. This will gradually increase their body temperature, blood flow to the muscles, and synovial fluid to the joints. Then you may lead them in a three to five minute stretching exercise.

Bring each client up to the table for their turn. Help them pick up and slide the ball down the length of the table in an effort to knock down the pins. The score system is quite difficult; therefore the staff will generally have to keep count. In the case of the elderly, however, counting the number of fallen pins may be enough. If you have a resident who likes to keep score this can be very challenging, fun, and good for their math and cognitive skills.

The CDC recommends that older adults participate in moderate-intensity aerobic activity 3-5 days a week for at least 30 minutes. This will help older adults to increase endurance, strength, and balance. It is also recommended that older adults engage in activities that include stretching everyday and strength training activities 2-3 days per week. (CDC, NCCDPHP. Special focus: healthy aging. Chronic Disease Notes and Reports 1999; 12(3):10-11. Insert CDC recommendations obtained from aoa.hhs.gov 2005

* All older adults engaging in activities should have physician approval to engage in physical activities.

Bowling/Table Bowling
Cognitive Goals, Objectives, and Methods

SKILL	GOAL	OBJECTIVES SAMPLE	METHOD SAMPLE
Orientation	Show increased awareness of, time/ "timeframe," people, circumstances, and past experiences vs. present experiences, to engage in present-time activities, or for a reminiscing intended question	-will respond with correct answer to two choice questions Or yes/no, will follow rules, state where they are, time of day, present company of people on own and with the correct answer during bowling 1x a week	Staff will ask residents a series of questions to stimulate focus to the present setting Or past if a reminiscing exercise (Ex: "When have you bowled before? Where are we?")
Attention	Show increased attention span, task for function, and to engage in meaningful, recreational/fulfilling activities	-will make eye-contact with staff instructor, will read, listen, and follow bowling rules; will wait turn, stand at end of table/lane, initiate task 1x a week	Staff will address or stand in front of resident, make eye-contact, ask questions, or use others methods to get resident's attention/gauge attention
Memory	Show increased memory skills of recall, recognition, retention of information, working memory	-will repeat/retain how to swing ball back and roll, will repeat/recall how to roll the ball (or) will remember lesson at next class 1x a week	Staff will show steps on how to bowl, and ask residents to repeat the actions at present or future time (minutes, days, etc.)
Language	Show increased ability to communicate use of words, phrases, sentence structure, comprehension, interpretation	-will be asked a question and answer yes/no, will interact h peers and staff, will interpret instructor's request and follow (for interpretation skills) during bowling 1x a week	Staff will ask questions to stimulate a communication (Ex: "Tell me about your experience bowling.") Or for Interpretation/Lang. skills (Ex: "Hand me your ball.")
Cognitive Stimulation (awareness, seeks information in)	Increased stimulus/exposure for visual/ motor memory, cognitive experiences/awareness and brain stimulation to enhance (function, pragmatics, neuron-plasticity)	-will interact with peers, will listen to suggestions on strategies to knock down pins, will listen/seek cognitive stimulation, will engage in a game of bowling, will accept challenge of input information and engage/interact in bowling activity	Staff will set up a bowling game and talk about ways to hit all the pins to stimulate visual/motor memory, thinking, and cognitive awareness
Perceptual Awareness	Show increased abilities of depth perception, visual-spatial awareness, and acuity (for discrimination, comparison, and categorizing), safety	-will stay in own lane, will stay within own space next to others, will visually strategize path of ball/dimensions	-Staff will instruct the residents on where they need to stay in their lanes, area -Will use bowling game as a way to increase visual acuity, visual-spatial abilities, etc.
Problem-solving (goes beyond thinking/stimulus and initiates thinking process)	Increase problem-solving ability, processing of information, thinking, reasoning, and use of good judgment and decision-making	-will roll/push ball with two hands stretch, will swing arm and straighten to roll ball down lane, will use critical-thinking on best direction to roll/hit pins to knock them down	Staff will show the resident the step-by-step actions to bowl and possibilities to hit the ball, and have residents attempt to knock down all the pins
Complete a Task	Increase ability to complete a task	will recall/retain and sort/gather information, problem-solve, and complete the bowling activity or game, will follow through on steps of bowling	Staff will show the resident the step-by-step actions to bowl, encourage, and make use of adaptive devices, if needed, and supply necessary materials and support

TABLE 2.1

Recreational Objectives Observation Form
Bowling/Table Bowling - Cognitive skills

PATIENT	Dependent (Totally dependent)	High Assistance (25+ ability)	Moderate Assist. (50+ ability)	Mild Assistance (75+ability)	Independent (Totally independent)
SEE CODES BELOW USE OPTIONAL CODES IF APPROPRIATE	1	2	3	4	5
	3 cue/ 2-3 physical	2-3 cues/ 2 physical	2-3 cues/ 1 physical	1-2 cues	Encouragement

97530- Therapeutic activities or	SKILL	GOAL	OBJECTIVES ____times per ____	METHOD	OUTCOME DATE			
97532 Cognitive skills	ORIENTATION							
97532 Cognitive skills	ATTENTION							
97532 Cognitive skills	MEMORY							
97532 Cognitive skills	PROBLEM-SOLVING							
97532 Cognitive skills	COMPLETE A TASK							
97139 Speech Therapy	LANGUAGE							
97533	SENSORY STIMULATION/ COGNITIVE STIMULATION							
97532	PERCEPTUAL AWARENESS							

97532-Development of cognitive skills to improve attention, memory, problem-solving, includes compensatory training and/or sensory integrative activities, direct (one-on-one) patient contact by the provider, each 15 minutes; **97530-Therapeutic activities**, direct (one-on-one) patient contact by the provider (use of dynamic activities to improve functional performance), each 15 minutes; **97533-Sensory integration techniques** to enhance sensory processing and promote adaptive responses to environmental demands, direct (one-on-one) patient contact by the provider, each 15 minutes; **97150-Therapeutic procedure(s)**, group (2 or more individuals); **97139-Unlisted therapeutic procedure** (specify) minutes; **97003- occupational therapy evaluation**; **97004- re-evaluation**	Staff Initial				
	Add total score here -Maximum Score 40 pt. each form per activity				
	See scale below or use own/facilities optional score system				

(Score 1-8)=1 (9-16) =2 (17-24) =3 (25-32) =4 (33-40) =5 If w/device add d if wish, ex: 1d, 2d, or If using 1-7 scale: (41-48) =6 (49-56)

Bowling/Table Bowling
Physical Goals, Objectives, and Methods

SKILL	GOAL	OBJECTIVES SAMPLE	METHOD SAMPLE
Fine motor skills	Increase fine motor skills, including: using fingers, toes, hand-eye coordination, and dexterity	-will place fingers in ball, or pick up small ball, or use hands to push ball _____ time(s) this week	Staff will give residents instructions on the steps to bowl, including use of the fine motor skills
Gross motor skills	Increase large motor skills	-will bend, stretch, and do bowling movements/mechanics _____ time(s) this week	Staff will give residents instructions, and residents will be involved in a bowling activity using large motor skills of bending, lifting, turning, etc.
Perceptual speed and motor function	Increase speed and motor ability for function, safety, meaningful/fulfilling activities	-will react and throw ball down lane in coordinated movement and speed (within one minute), will join in on a bowling race game (with Dr. approval)	Staff will encourage residents to increase pace of actions while bowling, sliding bowl down the aisle by decreasing time between standing to bowl and release of the ball
Following step patterns/backwards forward movement	Increase strength, balance, endurance, meaningful/fulfilling activities	-will walk forward to table, will turn, will take backwards and forwards steps as is done for bowling; will walk backwards, forwards, turn, move all directions	Staff will show resident the mechanics of bowling which require walking forward/backwards, then forward and rolling the ball
For clinician/Dr. approved use only	For clinician/Dr. approved use only	-will lift arms, legs, turn trunk, bend (to capacity - set by Dr./clinician), will extend and flex (to capacity - set by clinician)	Staff will perform or give residents instructions on full swing of arms for bowling mechanics (if approved by Dr./clinician)
Balance and Posture (approved by Dr. and capacity tests)	Increase balance and improve body alignment and flexibility	-when ready to bowl, will stand straight using proper body alignment/posture as they stand to bowl 2-3 min	Staff will show residents proper posture and ask them to hold body in straight alignment (with device/support if needed)
Gait/Following Step patterns/ Backwards/Forward movement	Increase strength, balance, endurance, meaningful/fulfilling activities	-will stand up, without losing balance, and walk up to the lane at a safe pace (approved by Dr. and capacity tests), If approved, clinical specialist: _____ft. ______________________	-Staff will have residents walk to and from lane, etc. (with device/support if needed) -Staff will show proper standing for bowling including proper balance, steps, and holding body in alignment
Cardio-vascular Workout*	Increase circulation, blood flow, stamina	-will bowl at a safe pace (approved by Dr. and capacity tests), If approved, clinical specialist: ______________________	Staff will have residents do bowling activity (according to ability and approved amount of exercise)

TABLE 2.2

Recreational Objectives Observation Form
Bowling/Table Bowling- Physical Skills

PATIENT		Dependent (Totally dependent)	High Assistance (25+ ability)	Moderate Assist. (50+ ability)	Mild Assistance (75+ability)	Independent (Totally independent.)			
SEE CODES BELOW		1	2	3	4	5			
USE OPTIONAL CODES IF APPROPRIATE		3 cue/ 2-3 physical	2-3 cues/ 2 physical	2-3 cues/ 1 physical	1-2 cues	Encouragement			
97530- Therapeutic activities or	**SKILL**	**GOAL**	**OBJECTIVES** ____times per ____		**METHOD**	**OUTCOME DATE**			
97530 Therapeutic Activity	FINE MOTOR SKILLS								
97110/ 97530	GROSS MOTOR SKILLS								
97110/ 97530/ If under cognitive code 97532	PERCEPTUAL SPEED/ MOTOR FUNCTION								
97530 or Gait training 97116-	STEP PATTERNS								
		Licensed/ Clinician	Dr. approved use only		Licensed/ Clinician				
97110	RANGE OF MOTION								
97112	POSTURE AND BALANCE								
97110 Or Gait training 97116-	GAIT (INCLUDES STAIR CLIMBING)								
97110	CARDIO-VASCULAR WORKOUT*								

97110-Therapeutic procedure, one or more areas, each 15 minutes; therapeutic exercises to develop strength and endurance, range of motion, and flexibility; 97112-Neuromuscular reeducation of movement, balance, coordination, kinesthetic sense, posture, and proprioception; **97113-Aquatic therapy** with therapeutic exercises; **97116-Gait training** (includes stair climbing); **97139-Unlisted therapeutic procedure** (specify); **97150 Therapeutic procedure(s)**, group (2 or more individuals); **97750-Physical performance test or measurement** (e.g., musculoskeletal, functional capacity), with written report, each 15 minutes; **97535-Self care/home management training** (e.g., activities of daily living and compensatory training, meal preparation, safety procedures, and instructions in use of adaptive equipment), direct (one-on-one) contact by provider, each 15 minutes; **Physical therapy 97001 evaluation, 97002 Re-evaluation. occupational therapy evaluation 97003, re-evaluation. 97004; Athlete training 97005; re-evaluation 97006**	Staff Initial				
	Add total score here Maximum Score 40 pt. each form per activity				
	See scale below or use own/facilities optional score system				

Score 1-8) =1 (9-16) =2 (17-24) =3 (25-32) =4 (33-40) =5 If w/device add d if wish, ex: 1d, 2d, or If using 1-7 scale: (41-48) =6 (49-56)

Bowling/Table Bowling
Socio-emotional Goals, Objectives, and Methods

SKILL	GOAL	OBJECTIVES SAMPLE	METHOD SAMPLE
Socialization/Community Integration	Increase social interactions, meaningful/fulfilling activities	-will interact with peers for pleasure, belonging needs, etc. (for social skills), will use manners/social practices (for community adaptation), will put coin in bus pay slot while on bus trip for bowling alley	Staff will take residents to a bowling center/activity 1x week and support/encourage residents to socialize through community integration and being paired w/other bowlers/group games
Team Playing/Sharing	Increase teamwork/sharing, meaningful/fulfilling activities	-will join in on game with others and share, wait turn, support peers during activity	Staff will set up bowling table or take residents to a bowling alley, and residents will be encouraged to play, share, form teams, strategize together
Initiative and Motivation	Increase initiative and motivation/wellness, and quality of life	-will choose if they wish to bowl or not, or will choose if they wish to join in on team game; will try a new bowling technique, will do all bowling moves on own or with assistance, will increase amount of bowling games after stating own goal	-Staff will support/encourage the resident to pick out a correct pair of bowling shoes (if at bowling center), stand up when it is there turn to bowl, etc in a timely fashion, for their own personal gains of bowling -Staff will offer new techniques to motivate while bowling
Emotional Gratification	Increase emotional gratification/wellness, and quality of life	-will state that bowling is a gratifying experience or will show pleasure by smiling, laughing, deep focus	Staff will ask residents if they enjoyed bowling and what they liked through verbal discussion, group discussions
Sense of Accomplishment	Increase feelings of self-worth, pride, productivity, dignity/wellness, and quality of life	-will use gestures to express pride in self, will talk about their accomplishments of bowling, hang award on door	A chart on the unit wall or a paper handed to the residents reflecting bowling scores, etc. will be available for residents to see their personal best/increased bowling score.
Self-esteem/self-identity	Increase self-esteem, feelings of belonging, dignity, self-worth, integrity, self-identity/wellness, and quality of life	-will state/communicate positive feelings ability to bowl, will join bowling class to take an active role in health though exercising, will join the bowling activity based on own choices	-Staff will educate residents on the value of bowling/exercise and encourage them to bowl/exercise -Staff will design a wall chart showing bowlers' names and personal bowling scores
Sensory Integration/Tolerating Stimulation	Increase sensory processing and enhance awareness of sensations and toleration/adaptation of sensory stimulations and demands	-will adjust to the sounds of center, bowling pins dropping, other noises, lights, and peers during activity; will show adjustment to stimulus by staying in area with increased timing _____ time(s) this week	-Staff will take residents to the bowling alley/or given a bowling activity and exposed to sensory stimulating experiences -Staff will support resident as they adjust to the stimulus one step at a time
Fostering Appropriate Behaviors	Increase social interaction, social opportunities and adjustment, safety, using appropriate behaviors during an activity for a calm environment/wellness, and quality of life	-will join in on bowling class, listen, follow instructions, use appropriate behavior for the setting; will wait turn, stand in line quietly; will quiet down	Before bowling activity begins, staff will discuss the rules, appropriate behaviors, respect of property, safety, and respect of fellow bowlers

TABLE 2.3

Recreational Objectives Observation Form
Bowling/Table Bowling- Socio-emotional Skills

PATIENT	Dependent (Totally dependent)	High Assistance (25+ ability)	Moderate Assist. (50+ ability)	Mild Assistance (75+ability)	Independent (Totally independent.)
SEE CODES BELOW USE OPTIONAL CODES IF APPROPRIATE	1	2	3	4	5
	3 cue/ 2-3 physical	2-3 cues/ 2 physical	2-3 cues/ 1 physical	1-2 cues	Encouragement

97530-Therapeutic activities or	SKILL	GOAL	OBJECTIVES ____times per ____	METHOD	OUTCOME DATE			
97537 Or 97535	SOCIALIZATION/ COMMUNITY INTEGRATION							
97537 Or 97535	TEAM PLAYING /SHARING							
97537 Or 97535	INITIATIVE AND MOTIVATION							
97537 Or 97535	EMOTIONAL GRATIFICATION							
97537 Or 97535	SENSE OF ACCOMPLISHMENT							
97537 Or 97535	SELF-ESTEEM/ SELF-IDENTITY							
97537 Or 97535	FOSTERING APPROPRIATE BEHAVIORS							
97533	SENSORY INTEGRATION/ TOLERATING							

97537-Community/work reintegration training (e.g., shopping, transportation, money management, avocational activities and/or work environment/modification analysis, work task analysis), direct (one-on-one) contact by provider, each 15 minutes; **97535-Self care/home management training** (e.g., activities of daily living and compensatory training, meal preparation, safety procedures, and instructions in use of adaptive equipment), direct (one-on-one) contact by provider, each 15 minutes; **97530-Therapeutic activities, direct (one-on-one)** patient contact by the provider (use of dynamic activities to improve functional performance), each 15 minutes; **97150-Therapeutic procedure(s), group (2 or more individuals); 97533-Sensory integration techniques** to enhance sensory processing and promote adaptive responses to environmental demands, direct (one-on-one) patient contact by the provider, each 15 minutes; **occupational therapy evaluation 97003, re-evaluation . 97004**	Staff Initial				
	Add total score here-Maximum Score 40 pt. each form per activity				
	See scale below or use own/facilities optional score system				

(Score 1-8)=1 (9-16) =2 (17-24) =3 (25-32) =4 (33-40) =5 If w/device add d if wish, ex: 1d, 2d, or If using 1-7 scale: (41-48) =6 (49-56)

Dancing

Objectives and benefits

Cognitive Challenges: attention, memory, language, orientation, following patterns, keeping rhythm, perceptual awareness, and cognitive stimulation

Physical Needs: fine motor skills, gross motor skills, coordination, range of motion, flexibility, posture, balance, backward and forward movement, gait, following step patterns, circulation, cardio-vascular workout

Socio-emotional Needs: socialization, community integration, initiative and motivation, emotional gratification, sense of accomplishment, self-esteem, tolerating stimulation, fostering appropriate behaviors, relaxation, solace and healing

Supplies: Tape player, keyboard, movie, musical instruments, radio

Time: 30 minutes

Staff/older adult ratio: 1:1 or as assessed per needs of individuals or group. Also keep in mind the amount of space available for a safe dancing area.

Instructions: Have older adults warm up for dancing by leading them in a sub maximal active warm-up first. This will gradually increase their body temperature, blood flow to the muscles, and synovial fluid to the joints. Then you may lead them in a three to five minute stretching exercise.

Have older adults join in a circle or stand together in a line. Put on the music. You may choose the music or allow them to choose their own music. It could be based on a theme for example holiday or country western. If you are doing a line dance it would be great to have a client or staff member who knows some dance moves. Start off the dance. Help those who can dance but need additional help. If there are older adults in wheel chairs, encourage them to do moves from their chairs, or, if they are able, offer them assistance in standing. Encourage free movement as well as following directions for a line dance.

It is extremely crucial to watch older adults at all times. Residents should already have a flow sheet on their individual abilities on balance and gait. With their needs in mind, watch the older adult's ability to stand and dance. Even those who have no regular balance trouble can fall. For safety purposes, be sure to have plenty of staff available to catch older adults losing their balance. If there are extra chairs you can offer older adults one to hold onto as they dance, but do not let them rely on a chair for full support. Once safety has been assured, let them enjoy themselves in dance creativity.

The CDC recommends that older adults participate in moderate-intensity aerobic activity 3-5 days a week for at least 30 minutes. This will help older adults to increase endurance, strength, and balance. It is also recommended that older adults engage in activities that include stretching everyday and strength training activities 2-3 days per week. (CDC, NCCDPHP. Special focus: healthy aging. Chronic Disease Notes and Reports 1999; 12(3):10-11. Insert CDC recommendations obtained from aoa.hhs.gov 2005

* All older adults engaging in activities should have physician approval to engage in physical activities.

Dancing
Cognitive Goals, Objectives and Methods

SKILL	GOAL	OBJECTIVES SAMPLE	METHOD SAMPLE
Orientation	Show increased awareness of, time/"timeframe," people, circumstances, and past experiences vs. present experiences, to engage in present-time activities, or for a reminiscing intended question	-will respond with correct answer to two choice questions, will state where they are, time of day, present company of people on own and with the correct answer	The resident will be asked a series of questions to stimulate focus to the present setting Or past if reminiscing exercise (Ex: "What are your favorite dances? What where the favorite dances in your twenties? Who did you dance with? Who is your dance partner right now?")
Attention	Show increased attention span, task for function, and to engage in meaningful, recreational/fulfilling activities	-will make eye-contact with dance instructor and staff for _____ sec(s), will verbalize with staff and instructor, will read/listen to dance steps and do the action as stated	Staff will address resident, make eye-contact, ask questions, or use others forms to get resident's attention/gauge attention (Ex: "Can you tell me what dance we will be doing?")
Memory	Show increased memory skills of recall, recognition, retention of information, working memory	-will repeat/recall how to do the dance moves, will repeat/recall how to do the free style (3 minutes/10 min. later), will remember lesson at next class	-Staff will show steps on how to dance, and ask residents to repeat the actions 3 minutes later -Staff will ask residents to bring sneakers to dance class and see if they remember
Language	Show increased ability to communicate use of words, phrases, ntence structure, comprehension, interpretation	-will be asked a question and answer yes/no, or will interact with peers/staff, will interpret instructor's request and follow	Staff will ask questions to stimulate a communication k: "Tell me about your dance experiences.") Or for Interpretation/Lang. skills (Ex: "Bring your sneakers to nce class today.")
Cognitive Stimulation (awareness, seeks information in)	Increased stimulus/exposure for visual/ motor memory, cognitive experiences/awarenes s and brain stimulation to enhance (function, pragmatics, neuroplasticity)	-will interact with peers, will engage in a dance routine, will listen/seek cognitive stimulation, will accept challenge of input information and engage/interact in dancing	-Staff will set up a dance routine and ask residents to dress up in a period outfit using ingenuity -Staff will show the resident the step-by-step actions to dance a particular dance
Perceptual Awareness	Show increased abilities of depth perception, visio-spatical awareness, and acuity (for discrimination, comparison, and categorizing), safety	-will stay within own space next to others, will maneuver around the room successfully (when appropriate)	Staff will instruct the residents on where they need to stay in their lanes, dance area, spatial relation to peers
Problem-solving (goes beyond thinking/stimulus and initiates thinking process)	Increase problem-solving ability, processing of information, thinking, reasoning, and use of good judgment and decision-making	-will make a creative outfit for dance party, will follow rhythm of dance workout and timing, will do synchronized dance or movements when asked, will do the dance steps in order sequence	-Staff will line residents up for synchronized dance with peers using a music tape -Staff will talk about/show dance moves and offer the residents stimulating dances for processing info., step judgments etc
Complete a Task	Increase ability to complete a task	will recall/retain and sort/gather information, problem-solve, and complete activity	-Staff will explain the procedure/agenda regarding dancing, and answer questions regarding understanding of required steps -Staff will instruct, encourage, make use of adaptive devices, if needed, and supply necessary materials and support

TABLE 3.1

Recreational Objectives Observation Form
Dancing - Cognitive skills

PATIENT		Dependent (Totally dependent)	High Assistance (25+ ability)	Moderate Assist. (50+ ability)	Mild Assistance (75+ability)	Independent (Totally independent)			
SEE CODES BELOW USE OPTIONAL CODES IF APPROPRIATE		1	2	3	4	5			
		3 cue/ 2-3 physical	2-3 cues/ 2 physical	2-3 cues/ 1 physical	1-2 cues	Encouragement			
97530- Therapeutic activities or	**SKILL**	**GOAL**	**OBJECTIVES** ____times per ____		**METHOD**	**OUTCOME DATE**			
97532 Cognitive skills	ORIENTATION								
97532 Cognitive skills	ATTENTION								
97532 Cognitive skills	MEMORY								
97532 Cognitive skills	PROBLEM-SOLVING								
97532 Cognitive skills	COMPLETE A TASK								
97139 Speech Therapy 97532 Cognitive skills	LANGUAGE								
97533	SENSORY STIMULATION/ COGNITIVE STIMULATION								
97532	PERCEPTUAL AWARENESS								

97532-Development of cognitive skills to improve attention, memory, problem-solving, includes compensatory training and/or sensory integrative activities, direct (one-on-one) patient contact by the provider, each 15 minutes; **97530-Therapeutic activities**, direct (one-on-one) patient contact by the provider (use of dynamic activities to improve functional performance), each 15 minutes; **97533-Sensory integration techniques** to enhance sensory processing and promote adaptive responses to environmental demands, direct (one-on-one) patient contact by the provider, each 15 minutes; **97150-Therapeutic procedure(s)**, group (2 or more individuals); **97139-Unlisted therapeutic procedure** (specify) minutes; **97003- occupational therapy evaluation**; **97004- re-evaluation**	Staff Initial				
	Add total score here -Maximum Score 40 pt. each form per activity				
	See scale below or use own/facilities optional score system				

(Score 1-8)=1 (9-16) =2 (17-24) =3 (25-32) =4 (33-40) =5 If w/device add d if wish, ex: 1d, 2d, or If using 1-7 scale: (41-48) =6 (49-56)

Dancing
Physical Goals, Objectives, and Methods

SKILL	GOAL	OBJECTIVES SAMPLE	METHOD SAMPLE
FINE MOTOR SKILLS	Increase fine motor skills, including: using fingers, toes, hand-eye coordination, and dexterity	-will clap, snap, and shake fingers	Staff will give music along with instructions on the steps to a particular dance, and include small motor abilities
GROSS MOTOR SKILLS	Increase large motor skills	-will bend, stretch, turn and do dance movements	Staff will give residents music along with instructions on the steps to a particular dance
PERCEPTUAL SPEED AND MOTOR FUNCTION	Increase speed and motor ability for function, safety, meaningful/ fulfilling activities	-will do a slow style dance, will do a moderate style dance, will do a fast-paced dance routine game (with Dr. approval)	Staff will introduce music with faster and faster beats and movements to increase perceptual speed and motor skills
FOLLOWING STEP PATTERNS/ BACKWARDS FORWARD MOVEMENT	Increase strength, balance, endurance, meaningful/fulfilling activities	-will walk forward during dance, will turn, change direction of path; will walk backwards, will walk backwards and forwards, will walk backwards, forwards, turn, move all directions	Staff will ask residents to dance forwards/backwards and turn (with support device if needed) while listening to music, and do these actions during dance
FOR CLINICIAN/ DR. APPROVED USE ONLY	For clinician/Dr. approved use only	-will lift arms, legs, trunk (to capacity - set by Dr./clinician), will extend and flex (to capacity - set by clinician)	Staff will instruct residents to do exercises that include flexing, extending muscles
BALANCE AND POSTURE (approved by Dr. and capacity tests)	Increase balance and improve body alignment and flexibility	-will hold on to a railing and show proper posture for 3 min., will stand to do dance moves using proper alignment/posture	While dancing, staff will show residents proper posture and ask residents to hold body in straight alignment/posture for at 3 minutes (then increase)
GAIT/ FOLLOWING STEP PATTERNS/ BACKWARDS/ FORWARD MOVEMENT	Increase strength, balance, endurance, meaningful/fulfilling activities	-will stand up, without losing balance, and walk at a safe pace (approved by Dr. and capacity tests), If approved, clinical specialist: _____ ft. ______________________________	Staff will show residents the proper posture / balance and gait for dance steps, and have them hold body in straight alignment/posture (may hold on to railing for safety or use device if needed) (with Dr. approval)
CARDIO-VASCULAR WORKOUT*	Increase circulation, blood flow, stamina	-will dance at a safe pace (approved by Dr. and capacity tests), If approved, clinical specialist: ______________________________	Staff will have residents do dance routine (according to ability and approved amount of dancing)

TABLE 3.2

Recreational Objectives Observation Form

Dancing- Physical Skills

PATIENT		Dependent (Totally dependent)	High Assistance (25+ ability)	Moderate Assist. (50+ ability)	Mild Assistance (75+ability)	Independent (Totally independent.)
SEE CODES BELOW USE OPTIONAL CODES IF APPROPRIATE		1	2	3	4	5
		3 cue/ 2-3 physical	2-3 cues/ 2 physical	2-3 cues/ 1 physical	1-2 cues	Encouragement
97530- Therapeutic activities or	**SKILL**	**GOAL**	**OBJECTIVES** ____times per ____		**METHOD**	**OUTCOME DATE**
97530 Therapeutic Activity	FINE MOTOR SKILLS					
97110/ 97530	GROSS MOTOR SKILLS					
97110/ 97530/ If under cognitive code 97532	PERCEPTUAL SPEED/ MOTOR FUNCTION					
97530 or Gait training971 16-	STEP PATTERNS					
		Licensed/ Clinician	Dr. approved use only		Licensed/ Clinician	
97110	RANGE OF MOTION					
97112	POSTURE AND BALANCE					
97110 Or Gait training 97116-	GAIT (INCLUDES STAIR CLIMBING)					
97110	CARDIO-VASCULAR WORKOUT*					

97110-Therapeutic procedure, one or more areas, each 15 minutes; therapeutic exercises to develop strength and endurance, range of motion, and flexibility; 97112-Neuromuscular reeducation of movement, balance, coordination, kinesthetic sense, posture, and proprioception; **97113-Aquatic therapy** with therapeutic exercises; **97116-Gait training** (includes stair climbing); **97139-Unlisted therapeutic procedure** (specify); **97150 Therapeutic procedure(s)**, group (2 or more individuals); **97750-Physical performance test or measurement** (e.g., musculoskeletal, functional capacity), with written report, each 15 minutes; **97535-Self care/home management training** (e.g., activities of daily living and compensatory training, meal preparation, safety procedures, and instructions in use of adaptive equipment), direct (one-on-one) contact by provider, each 15 minutes; **Physical therapy 97001 evaluation, 97002 Re-evaluation. occupational therapy evaluation 97003, re-evaluation. 97004; Athlete training 97005; re-evaluation 97006**

Staff Initial	
Add total score here Maximum Score 40 pt. each form per activity	
See scale below or use own/facilities optional score system	

Score 1-8) =1 (9-16) =2 (17-24) =3 (25-32) =4 (33-40) =5 If w/device add d if wish, ex: 1d, 2d, or If using 1-7 scale: (41-48) =6 (49-56) Current Procedural Terminology © 2005 American Medical Association. All rights reserved. Recreational Objectives Observational form © 2005. All rights reserved. Patent pending.

Dancing
Socio-emotional Goals, Objectives, and Methods

SKILL	GOAL	OBJECTIVES SAMPLE	METHOD SAMPLE
SOCIALIZATION/COMMUNITY INTEGRATION	Increase social interactions, meaningful/fulfilling activities	-will interact with peers, will engage in community integration experiences (for social skills), will use manners, social practices (for community adaptation), will attend a ball.	Staff will take residents to dance center or do dancing activity and support/encourage residents to socialize through community integration and being paired w/partners or line dancers
TEAM PLAYING/SHARING	Increase teamwork/sharing, meaningful/fulfilling activities	-will join in on a dance class with others and share, wait turn, support peers _____ time(s) this week.	Staff will encourage and support residents to dance, form teams, strategize, work together to choose dances, etc. -Residents will support and encourage each other while dancing
INITIATIVE AND MOTIVATION	Increase initiative and motivation/wellness, and quality of life	-will choose if they wish to dance, will choose if they wish to join in on partner/group/line dance; will try a new dance technique, will do all swim moves on own, will increase amount of steps to a dance after stating own goal	Staff will support/encourage the resident to prepare for dance class, go out to the dance activity in a timely fashion for their own personal gains of dancing -Staff will offer new dance techniques to motivate
EMOTIONAL GRATIFICATION	Increase emotional gratification/wellness, and quality of life	-will state that the dance class is a gratifying experience, or will show pleasure by smiling, laughing, deep focus on dancing	Staff will ask residents if they enjoyed the dance class and what they liked through verbal discussion, group discussions
SENSE OF ACCOMPLISHMENT	Increase feelings of self-worth, pride, productivity, dignity/wellness, and quality of life	-will use gestures to express pride in self, will talk about their accomplishments of being a good dancer	Staff will hang up a chart on the unit wall or hand residents a paper that reflects dance team awards, residents' personal best, theme dances, costumes, etc. during dances
SELF-ESTEEM/ SELF-IDENTITY	Increase self-esteem, feelings of belonging, dignity, self-worth, integrity, self-identity/wellness, and quality of life	-will state/communicate positive feelings about self and ability to dance, will join dance class to take an active role in health though exercising, will join the dance class based on own choices	-Staff will educate residents on the value of dance/exercise and encourage them to dance -Staff will design a wall chart showing best team dance (be sure to acknowledge all dancers) -Staff will encourage cultural dances to be shared
SENSORY INTEGRATION/TOLERATING STIMULATION	Increase sensory processing and enhance awareness of sensations and toleration/adaptation of sensory stimulations and demands	-will adjust to the music and others dancing, will tolerate noise, movements of others	-Staff will take residents to a dance activity and expose them to sensory stimulating experiences -Staff will support residents as they adjust to the stimulus, one step at a time
FOSTERING APPROPRIATE BEHAVIORS	Increase social interaction, social opportunities and adjustment, safety, using appropriate behaviors during an activity for a calm environment/wellness, and quality of life	-will join in on dance class, will listen and follow instructions, use appropriate behavior for the setting, will wait turn, stand in line quietly, wait for music, will quiet down when asked	Before dance class begins, staff will discuss the activity rules, appropriate behaviors, respect of property, safety, and respect of fellow dancers while dancing

TABLE 3.3

Recreational Objectives Observation Form
Dancing- Socio-emotional Skills

PATIENT		Dependent (Totally dependent)	High Assistance (25+ ability)	Moderate Assist. (50+ ability)	Mild Assistance (75+ability)	Independent (Totally independent.)			
SEE CODES BELOW USE OPTIONAL CODES IF APPROPRIATE		1	2	3	4	5			
		3 cue/ 2-3 physical	2-3 cues/ 2 physical	2-3 cues/ 1 physical	1-2 cues	Encouragement			
97530- Therapeutic activities or	SKILL	GOAL	OBJECTIVES ____times per ____		METHOD	OUTCOME DATE			
97537 Or 97535	SOCIALIZATION/ COMMUNITY INTEGRATION								
97537 Or 97535	TEAM PLAYING /SHARING								
97537 Or 97535	INITIATIVE AND MOTIVATION								
97537 Or 97535	EMOTIONAL GRATIFICATION								
97537 Or 97535	SENSE OF ACCOMPLISHM ENT								
97537 Or 97535	SELF-ESTEEM/ SELF-IDENTITY								
97537 Or 97535	FOSTERING APPROPRIATE BEHAVIORS								
97533	SENSORY INTEGRATION/ TOLERATING								

97537-Community/work reintegration training (e.g., shopping, transportation, money management, avocational activities and/or work environment/modification analysis, work task analysis), direct (one-on-one) contact by provider, each 15 minutes; **97535-Self care/home management training** (e.g., activities of daily living and compensatory training, meal preparation, safety procedures, and instructions in use of adaptive equipment), direct (one-on-one) contact by provider, each 15 minutes; **97530-Therapeutic activities, direct (one-on-one)** patient contact by the provider (use of dynamic activities to improve functional performance), each 15 minutes; **97150-Therapeutic procedure(s), group (2 or more individuals)**; **97533-Sensory integration techniques** to enhance sensory processing and promote adaptive responses to environmental demands, direct (one-on-one) patient contact by the provider, each 15 minutes; **occupational therapy evaluation 97003, re-evaluation . 97004**	Staff Initial				
	Add total score here-Maximum Score 40 pt. each form per activity				
	See scale below or use own/facilities optional score system				

(Score 1-8)=1 (9-16) =2 (17-24) =3 (25-32) =4 (33-40) =5 If w/device add d if wish, ex: 1d, 2d, or If using 1-7 scale: (41-48) =6 (49-56)

Exercise and Weight Lifting

Objectives and benefits

***Cognitive Challenges**:* attention, memory, language, orientation, following patterns, keeping rhythm, perceptual awareness, and cognitive stimulation

***Physical Needs**:* fine motor skills, gross motor skills, coordination, range of motion, flexibility, posture, balance, backward and forward movement, gait, following step patterns, circulation, cardio-vascular workout

Socio-emotional Needs: socialization, community integration, initiative and motivation, emotional gratification, sense of accomplishment, self-esteem, tolerating stimulation, fostering appropriate behaviors

Supplies: Weights for weight-lifting, exercise tapes, a room with floor mats or carpet.

Time: 10–30 minutes as capable and prescribed as a suitable workout time.

Staff/older adult ratio: 1:6 or as assessed per needs of individuals or group.

Instructions: Have older adults join together for an exercise class. Have them warm up for exercising by leading them in them in a sub maximal active warm-up first. This will gradually increase their body temperature, blood flow to the muscles, and synovial fluid to the joints. Then you may lead them in a three to five minute stretching exercise. Have a staff member show the older adults the exercise moves. Have them repeat and follow the exercise routine. You can use weights or small dumbbells to enhance exercise activities. You can also introduce weight lifting as the next level of strengthening in a progressive exercise program.

The CDC recommends that older adults participate in moderate-intensity aerobic activity 3-5 days a week for at least 30 minutes. This will help older adults to increase endurance, strength, and balance. It is also recommended that older adults engage in activities that include stretching everyday and strength training activities 2-3 days per week. (CDC, NCCDPHP. Special focus: healthy aging. Chronic Disease Notes and Reports 1999; 12(3):10-11. Insert CDC recommendations obtained from aoa.hhs.gov 2005

* All older adults engaging in activities should have physician approval to engage in physical activities.

Exercise and Weight Lifting
Cognitive Goals, Objectives, and Methods

SKILL	GOAL	OBJECTIVES SAMPLE	METHOD SAMPLE
ORIENTATION	Show increased awareness of, time/"timeframe," people, circumstances, and past experiences vs. present experiences, to engage in present-time activities, or for a reminiscing intended question	-will respond with correct answer to two choice questions Or yes/no answer, will state where they are, time of day, present company of people on own and with the correct answer	Staff will ask resident a series of questions to stimulate focus to the present setting Or past if reminiscing exercise (Ex: "Where are you in the exercise room, the YWCA or at home?")
ATTENTION	Show increased attention span, task for function, and to engage in meaningful, recreational/fulfilling activities	-will make eye-contact with instructor for _____ sec(s), will verbalize with staff and instructor, will read/listen to exercise room rules, will say yes/no to show understand	Staff will address, instruct, or stand in front of resident, make eye-contact, ask questions or use others forms to get resident's attention/gauge attention
MEMORY	Show increased memory skills of recall, recognition, retention of information, working memory	-will repeat/recall how to do push ups, will repeat/recall how to do side kicks, will remember lesson at next class	Staff will show steps on how to do the exercise, and ask residents to repeat the actions after an increased amount of time
LANGUAGE	Show increased ability to communicate use of words, phrases, sentence structure, comprehension, interpretation	-will be asked a question and answer yes/no, will be asked what favorite exercise is and reply on own or with two choice method, will interact with peers and staff; will interpret instructor's request and follow	Staff will ask questions to stimulate communication (Ex: "What kinds of exercise did you do?") Or for Interpretation/Lang. skills (Ex: "Let me see you do a side kick, etc.")
COGNITIVE STIMULATION (awareness, seeks information in)	Increased stimulus/exposure for visual/ motor memory, cognitive experiences/awareness and brain stimulation to enhance (function, pragmatics, neuroplasticity)	-will look around the room, will interact with peers while doing an exercise workout, will listen/seek cognitive stimulation, will accept challenge of input information and engage/interact in dancing	Staff will offer exercises to stimulate motor memory functions
PERCEPTUAL AWARENESS	Show increased abilities of depth perception, visio-spatical awareness, and acuity (for discrimination, comparison, and categorizing), safety	-will stay within own space next to others, will maneuver around room, will put items away in proper containers in associated area, will play basketball and hit the target	-Staff will instruct the residents on where they need to stay in their area of exercise mat -Staff may use equipment (if safe ability) -Staff may use punching bags to help with vision concerns
PROBLEM-SOLVING (goes beyond thinking/stimulus and initiates thinking process)	Increase problem-solving ability, processing of information, thinking, reasoning, and use of good judgment and decision-making	-will follow rhythm of workout, will do synchronized workouts, will repeat the rhythm movements when asked to, will stretch, bend, and move arms, legs, etc.; will use light weights and do a set as instructed	Staff will direct the residents in an exercise using a series (Ex: arm lifts and saying 1,2,3 lift, for following rhythms of exercise workout and timing)
COMPLETE A TASK	Increase ability to complete a task	will recall/retain and sort/gather information, problem-solve, and complete activity	Staff will show the resident the step-by-step actions of the exercise, and ask resident to repeat the steps until all the steps have been done

TABLE 4.1

Recreational Objectives Observation Form
Exercise and Weight Lifting - Cognitive skills

PATIENT		Dependent (Totally dependent)	High Assistance (25+ ability)	Moderate Assist. (50+ ability)	Mild Assistance (75+ability)	Independent (Totally independent)			
SEE CODES BELOW USE OPTIONAL CODES IF APPROPRIATE		1	2	3	4	5			
		3 cue/ 2-3 physical	2-3 cues/ 2 physical	2-3 cues/ 1 physical	1-2 cues	Encouragement			
97530-Therapeutic activities or	**SKILL**	**GOAL**	**OBJECTIVES** ____times per ____		**METHOD**	**OUTCOME DATE**			
97532 Cognitive skills	ORIENTATION								
97532 Cognitive skills	ATTENTION								
97532 Cognitive skills	MEMORY								
97532 Cognitive skills	PROBLEM-SOLVING								
97532 Cognitive skills	COMPLETE A TASK								
97139 Speech Therapy 97532 Cognitive skills	LANGUAGE								
97533	SENSORY STIMULATION/ COGNITIVE STIMULATION								
97532	PERCEPTUAL AWARENESS								

97532-Development of cognitive skills to improve attention, memory, problem-solving, includes compensatory training and/or sensory integrative activities, direct (one-on-one) patient contact by the provider, each 15 minutes; **97530-Therapeutic activities**, direct (one-on-one) patient contact by the provider (use of dynamic activities to improve functional performance), each 15 minutes; **97533-Sensory integration techniques** to enhance sensory processing and promote adaptive responses to environmental demands, direct (one-on-one) patient contact by the provider, each 15 minutes; **97150-Therapeutic procedure(s)**, group (2 or more individuals); **97139-Unlisted therapeutic procedure** (specify) minutes; **97003- occupational therapy evaluation**; **97004- re-evaluation**	Staff Initial				
	Add total score here -Maximum Score 40 pt. each form per activity				
	See scale below or use own/facilities optional score system				

(Score 1-8)=1 (9-16) =2 (17-24) =3 (25-32) =4 (33-40) =5 If w/device add d if wish, ex: 1d, 2d, or If using 1-7 scale: (41-48) =6 (49-56)

Exercise and Weight Lifting
Physical Goals, Objectives, and Methods

SKILL	GOAL	OBJECTIVES SAMPLE	METHOD SAMPLE
FINE MOTOR SKILLS	Increase fine motor skills, including: using fingers, toes, hand-eye coordination, and dexterity	-will use hands, fingers, toes in extension/flexion, will pick up small weights	Staff will give residents instructions, and residents will be involved in an exercise workout which includes small motor skills (lifting fingers, hands)
GROSS MOTOR SKILLS	Increase large motor skills	-will bend, stretch, and do movements during workout, involving large motor skills (legs, arms, trunk)	Staff will give residents instructions, and residents will be involved in an exercise workout, which includes large motor skills (lifting legs, arms, etc.) (Ex: do 10 sidekicks)
PERCEPTUAL SPEED AND MOTOR FUNCTION	Increase speed and motor ability for function, safety, meaningful/fulfilling activities	-will do movement 3-5 min., will do movement 5-10 min., etc.; will increase own time, will join in on a race game (with Dr. approval)	-Staff will direct residents in an exercise workout involving movement and reaction time -Staff will increase the exercise speed as resident's ability allows (dry approved or safe) (Ex: touch nose 10 x by bending elbow and touching nose)
FOLLOWING STEP PATTERNS/ BACKWARDS FORWARD MOVEMENT	Increase strength, balance, endurance, meaningful/fulfilling activities	-will walk forward, will turn, will walk backwards, will walk backwards and forwards, will walk backwards, forwards, and turn all directions	Staff will ask residents to walk forwards/ backwards and turn during (support device if needed) exercise routine
FOR CLINICIAN/ DR. APPROVED USE ONLY	For clinician/Dr. approved use only	-will lift arms, legs (to capacity - set by Dr./clinician), will extend and flex (to capacity - set by clinician)	Staff will instruct resident to do exercises that include flexing, extending muscles (with Dr. approval)
BALANCE AND POSTURE (approved by Dr. and capacity tests)	Increase balance and improve body alignment and flexibility	-will sit in chair and maintain posture, will stand using adequate posture	Staff will show residents proper posture and how to hold body in straight alignment/posture
GAIT/ FOLLOWING STEP PATTERNS/ BACKWARDS/ FORWARD MOVEMENT	Increase strength, balance, endurance, meaningful/fulfilling activities	-will stand up without losing balance and walk a safe pace (approved by Dr. and capacity tests) If approved clinical specialist: _____ ft. ______________________________	Staff will show residents proper stance/alignment to increase balance by standing still, building strength in lower legs (Dr./clinician approved) (support if needed)
CARDIO-VASCULAR WORKOUT*	Increase circulation, blood flow, stamina	-will exercise at a safe pace (approved by Dr. and capacity tests), If approved clinical specialist: _______________ ____________________________	Staff will offer residents an exercise class/workout according to ability and Dr./clinician approved amount of exercise

TABLE 4.2

Recreational Objectives Observation Form
Exercising and Weight Lifting- Physical Skills

PATIENT		Dependent (Totally dependent)	High Assistance (25+ ability)	Moderate Assist. (50+ ability)	Mild Assistance (75+ability)	Independent (Totally independent.)
SEE CODES BELOW		1	2	3	4	5
USE OPTIONAL CODES IF APPROPRIATE		3 cue/ 2-3 physical	2-3 cues/ 2 physical	2-3 cues/ 1 physical	1-2 cues	Encouragement
97530- Therapeutic activities or	**SKILL**	**GOAL**	**OBJECTIVES** ____times per ____		**METHOD**	**OUTCOME DATE**
97530 Therapeutic Activity	FINE MOTOR SKILLS					
97110/ 97530	GROSS MOTOR SKILLS					
97110/ 97530/ If under cognitive code 97532	PERCEPTUAL SPEED/ MOTOR FUNCTION					
97530 or Gait training 97116-	STEP PATTERNS					
		Licensed/ Clinician	Dr. approved use only		Licensed/ Clinician	
97110	RANGE OF MOTION					
97112	POSTURE AND BALANCE					
97110 Or Gait training 97116-	GAIT (INCLUDES STAIR CLIMBING)					
97110	CARDIO-VASCULAR WORKOUT*					

97110-Therapeutic procedure, one or more areas, each 15 minutes; therapeutic exercises to develop strength and endurance, range of motion, and flexibility; 97112-Neuromuscular reeducation of movement, balance, coordination, kinesthetic sense, posture, and proprioception; **97113-Aquatic therapy** with therapeutic exercises; **97116-Gait training** (includes stair climbing); **97139-Unlisted therapeutic procedure** (specify); **97150 Therapeutic procedure(s)**, group (2 or more individuals); **97750-Physical performance test or measurement** (e.g., musculoskeletal, functional capacity), with written report, each 15 minutes; **97535-Self care/home management training** (e.g., activities of daily living and compensatory training, meal preparation, safety procedures, and instructions in use of adaptive equipment), direct (one-on-one) contact by provider, each 15 minutes; **Physical therapy 97001 evaluation, 97002 Re-evaluation. occupational therapy evaluation 97003, re-evaluation. 97004; Athlete training 97005; re-evaluation 97006**	Staff Initial Add total score here Maximum Score 40 pt. each form per activity See scale below or use own/facilities optional score system

Score 1-8) =1 (9-16) =2 (17-24) =3 (25-32) =4 (33-40) =5 If w/device add d if wish, ex: 1d, 2d, or If using 1-7 scale: (41-48) =6 (49-56) Current Procedural Terminology © 2005 American Medical Association. All rights reserved. Recreational Objectives Observational forms © 2005. All rights reserved. Patent pending.

Exercise and Weight Lifting
Socio-emotional Goals, Objectives, and Methods

SKILL	GOAL	OBJECTIVES SAMPLE	METHOD SAMPLE
Socialization/Community Integration	Increase social interactions, meaningful/fulfilling activities	-will interact with peers, will engage in community integration experiences (for social skills), will use manners, social practices (for community adaptation), will attend the "YMCA", etc.	Staff will take residents to a center or implement an exercise routine to support and encourage socialization through community integration and being paired w/partners and teams
Team Playing/Sharing	Increase teamwork/sharing, meaningful/fulfilling activities	-will join in on a sport game, or exercise with others and share, wait turn, support peers	Staff will encourage residents to share equipment, strategize, work as a team, include all members
Initiative and Motivation	Increase initiative and motivation/wellness, and quality of life	-will choose if they wish to exercise, will choose if they wish to join in on team game/workout, will try a new technique, game; will do all moves on own (or with assistance), but own imitative; will increase amount of exercise after stating goal	Staff will support and encourage the resident to prepare to exercise by changing or putting on sneakers. etc. in a timely fashion for their own personal gains of exercising -Staff will offer new exercise routines to motivate
Emotional Gratification	Increase emotional gratification/wellness, and quality of life	-will state that the class is a gratifying experience, or will show pleasure by smiling, laughing, deep focus on exercise workout	Staff will ask resident if they enjoyed the exercise class to stimulate communication of emotional well-being
Sense of Accomplishment	Increase feelings of self-worth, pride, productivity, dignity/wellness, and quality of life	-will use gestures to express pride in self, will talk about their accomplishments of exercise, amount of weights they can lift, pace, etc. during lunch time	Staff will place a chart on the unit wall or hand out a paper to the residents that reflects "steps to success exercise program" and residents' accomplishments
Self-esteem/self-identity	Increase self-esteem, feelings of belonging, dignity, self-worth, integrity, self-identity/wellness, and quality of life	-will state/communicate positive feelings about self and ability to do exercises, will join class to take an active role in health though exercising, will join the swim class based on own choices	Staff will educate residents on the value of exercise and will encourage them to exercise -Staff will design a wall chart showing swimmers names and personal swim time and endurance
Sensory Integration/Tolerating Stimulation	Increase sensory processing and enhance awareness of sensations and toleration/adaptation of sensory stimulations and demands	-will adjust to noises (sounds of equipment, peers), and vibration of machines	-Staff will have residents join in on exercises and be exposed to sensory experiences -Staff will support residents as they adjust to the stimulus one step at a time
Fostering Appropriate Behaviors	Increase social interaction, social opportunities and adjustment, safety, using appropriate behaviors during an activity for a calm environment/wellness, and quality of life	-will join in on exercise class, listen, and follow instructions, use appropriate behavior for the setting; will wait turn, stand in line quietly; will quiet down when asked	Before exercise class, staff will discuss the gym rules, appropriate behaviors, respect of property, safety, and respect of peers and staff

Table 4.3

Recreational Objectives Observation Form
Exercise and Weight Lifting Socio-emotional Skills

PATIENT		Dependent (Totally dependent)	High Assistance (25+ ability)	Moderate Assist. (50+ ability)	Mild Assistance (75+ability)	Independent (Totally independent.)
SEE CODES BELOW USE OPTIONAL CODES IF APPROPRIATE		1	2	3	4	5
		3 cue/ 2-3 physical	2-3 cues/ 2 physical	2-3 cues/ 1 physical	1-2 cues	Encouragement
97530- Therapeutic activities or	**SKILL**	**GOAL**	**OBJECTIVES** ____times per ____		**METHOD**	**OUTCOME DATE**
97537 Or 97535	SOCIALIZATION/ COMMUNITY INTEGRATION					
97537 Or 97535	TEAM PLAYING /SHARING					
97537 Or 97535	INITIATIVE AND MOTIVATION					
97537 Or 97535	EMOTIONAL GRATIFICATION					
97537 Or 97535	SENSE OF ACCOMPLISHM ENT					
97537 Or 97535	SELF-ESTEEM/ SELF-IDENTITY					
97537 Or 97535	FOSTERING APPROPRIATE BEHAVIORS					
97533	SENSORY INTEGRATION/ TOLERATING					

97537-Community/work reintegration training (e.g., shopping, transportation, money management, avocational activities and/or work environment/modification analysis, work task analysis), direct (one-on-one) contact by provider, each 15 minutes; **97535-Self care/home management training** (e.g., activities of daily living and compensatory training, meal preparation, safety procedures, and instructions in use of adaptive equipment), direct (one-on-one) contact by provider, each 15 minutes; **97530-Therapeutic activities, direct (one-on-one)** patient contact by the provider (use of dynamic activities to improve functional performance), each 15 minutes; **97150-Therapeutic procedure(s), group (2 or more individuals); 97533-Sensory integration techniques** to enhance sensory processing and promote adaptive responses to environmental demands, direct (one-on-one) patient contact by the provider, each 15 minutes; **occupational therapy evaluation 97003, re-evaluation . 97004**	Staff Initial Add total score here-Maximum Score 40 pt. each form per activity See scale below or use own/facilities optional score system

(Score 1-8)=1 (9-16) =2 (17-24) =3 (25-32) =4 (33-40) =5 If w/device add d if wish, ex: 1d, 2d, or If using 1-7 scale: (41-48) =6 (49-56) Current Procedural Terminology © 2005 American Medical Association. All rights reserved. Recreational Objectives Observational form © 2005. All rights reserved. Patent pending.

Golf /Miniature Golf

Objectives and benefits

Cognitive Challenges: attention, memory, language, orientation, following patterns, keeping rhythm, perceptual awareness, and cognitive stimulation

Physical Needs: fine motor skills, gross motor skills, coordination, range of motion, flexibility, posture, balance, backward and forward movement, gait, following step patterns, circulation, cardio-vascular workout

Socio-emotional Needs: socialization, community integration, initiative and motivation, emotional gratification, sense of accomplishment, self-esteem, tolerating stimulation, fostering appropriate behaviors

Supplies: Availability of golfing range, miniature golf center

Time: 20–30 minutes

Staff/older adult ratio: 1:2 or as assessed per needs of individuals or group

Instructions: Have them warm up for activity by leading them in a sub maximal active warm-up first. This will gradually increase their body temperature, blood flow to the muscles, and synovial fluid to the joints. You may then lead them in a three to five minute stretching exercise.

The activity could be done as a leisure activity that allows older adults to play golf at their own pace, with peers for casual play or with the help of a golf instructor.

Golf can be played with a simple "course" on the unit, at a miniature golf center or on an actual golfing range. Equipment can range from simple golf club and cup/net and a ball on unit, with challenges on a small mini-course or true golf on a range. Have the resident swing the club and attempt to sink the ball in the hole. Increase challenge of ball going up hills, around the course etc.

Due to medications or falling potential, older adults should be supervised very carefully. Older adults with restrictions may be able to use special equipment available for the use of the physically challenged. It might be helpful to ask the facility what they have available to support those with limited ability to join in on golf activities.

Golfing is an activity many older adults wish to continue to engage in when they have reached retirement age. When issues such as cognitive diseases/Alzheimer's disease are of concern, special supportive environments or precautions may be put in place to allow the older adult to still engage in this pleasurable activity and gain benefits in physical, cognitive and socio-emotional well-being. In the case of residents who are capable of full physical abilities and approval by a doctor, Pilates have become very popular among golf players. Pilates can help the golf player to maintain better focus, movement control, flexibility, and stance when swinging. Pilate's instructors now offer Pilate golf clinics. Please see the Pilates chart in the special considerations section.

The CDC recommends that older adults participate in moderate-intensity aerobic activity 3-5 days a week for at least 30 minutes. This will help older adults to increase endurance, strength, and balance. It is also recommended that older adults engage in activities that include stretching everyday and strength training activities 2-3 days per week. (CDC, NCCDPHP. Special focus: healthy aging. Chronic Disease Notes and Reports 1999; 12(3):10-11. Insert CDC recommendations obtained from aoa.hhs.gov 2005

* All older adults engaging in activities should have physician approval to engage in physical activities.

Golf/Miniature Golf
Cognitive Goals, Objectives, and Methods

SKILL	GOAL	OBJECTIVES SAMPLE	METHOD SAMPLE
ORIENTATION	Show increased awareness of, time/"timeframe," people, circumstances, and past experiences vs. present experiences, to engage in present-time activities, or for a reminiscing intended question	-will respond with correct answer to two choice questions (Ex: "Are you at the mall or at the sports center?") Or yes/no answer, will state where they are, time of day, present company of people on own and with the correct answer	Staff will ask residents a series of questions to stimulate focus to the present setting, Or past if reminiscing exercise (Ex: "When have you played volleyball before? Where are we?")
ATTENTION	Show increased attention span, task for function, and to engage in meaningful, recreational/fulfilling activities	-will make eye-contact with instructor for _____ sec(s), will verbalize with staff, will read/listen to rules, will say yes/no to show understand	Staff will address or stand in front of resident, make eye-contact, ask questions, or use others methods to get resident's attention/gauge attention
MEMORY	Show increased memory skills of recall, recognition, retention of information, working memory	-will repeat/recall and retain rules, will repeat /recall how to throw and hit the ball, will remember lesson at next class	Staff will show steps on how to play the game and ask residents to repeat the actions
LANGUAGE	Show increased ability to communicate use of words, phrases, sentence structure, comprehension, interpretation	-will be asked a question and answer yes/no to a two choice question; will interact with peers and staff, will interpret instructor's request and follow directions	Staff will ask questions to stimulate a communication (Ex: "Do you want to golf?") Or Interpretation/Lang. skills (Ex: "Hand me the golf club.")
COGNITIVE STIMULATION (awareness, seeks information in)	Increased stimulus/exposure for visual/ motor memory, cognitive experiences/awareness and brain stimulation to enhance (function, pragmatics, neuro-plasticity)	-will listen/seek cognitive stimulation, will accept challenge of input information and engage/interact in game	Staff will set up a game and introduce residents to stimulation experiences
PERCEPTUAL AWARENESS	Show increased abilities of depth perception, visual-spatial awareness, and acuity (for discrimination, comparison, and categorizing), safety	-will gauge distance to hole). will stay within own space next to others, will maneuver around peers, net	-Staff will instruct the residents on where they need to stay in their area -Staff will use the game to help residents understand/practice/ increase depth perception skills
PROBLEM-SOLVING (goes beyond thinking/ stimulus and initiates thinking process)	Increase problem-solving ability, processing of information, thinking, reasoning, and use of good judgment and decision-making	-will use good judgment of speed and motor coordination, movement or strength and distance to hit club/ to hole; will consider dimensions, force of arm strength to aim/swing; will consider strategies to hit the ball	-Staff will direct the residents on using a series of techniques for golf -Staff will answer questions regarding understanding of steps and offer the residents challenging strategies for processing info, step judgments -Staff will have residents attempt to hit the ball, considering dimensions, strategies
COMPLETE A TASK	Increase ability to complete a task		

TABLE 5.1

Recreational Objectives Observation Form
Golf/Miniature Golf Cognitive skills

PATIENT	Dependent (Totally dependent)	High Assistance (25+ ability)	Moderate Assist. (50+ ability)	Mild Assistance (75+ability)	Independent (Totally independent)
SEE CODES BELOW USE OPTIONAL CODES IF APPROPRIATE	1	2	3	4	5
	3 cue/ 2-3 physical	2-3 cues/ 2 physical	2-3 cues/ 1 physical	1-2 cues	Encouragement

97530-Therapeutic activities or	SKILL	GOAL	OBJECTIVES ____times per ____	METHOD	OUTCOME DATE			
97532 Cognitive skills	ORIENTATION							
97532 Cognitive skills	ATTENTION							
97532 Cognitive skills	MEMORY							
97532 Cognitive skills	PROBLEM-SOLVING							
97532 Cognitive skills	COMPLETE A TASK							
97139 Speech Therapy 97532 Cognitive skills	LANGUAGE							
97533	SENSORY STIMULATION/ COGNITIVE STIMULATION							
97532	PERCEPTUAL AWARENESS							

97532-Development of cognitive skills to improve attention, memory, problem-solving, includes compensatory training and/or sensory integrative activities, direct (one-on-one) patient contact by the provider, each 15 minutes; **97530-Therapeutic activities**, direct (one-on-one) patient contact by the provider (use of dynamic activities to improve functional performance), each 15 minutes**; 97533-Sensory integration techniques** to enhance sensory processing and promote adaptive responses to environmental demands, direct (one-on-one) patient contact by the provider, each 15 minutes; **97150-Therapeutic procedure(s)**, group (2 or more individuals); **97139-Unlisted therapeutic procedure** (specify) minutes; **97003- occupational therapy evaluation**; **97004- re-evaluation**	Staff Initial				
	Add total score here -Maximum Score 40 pt. each form per activity				
	See scale below or use own/facilities optional score system				

(Score 1-8)=1 (9-16) =2 (17-24) =3 (25-32) =4 (33-40) =5 If w/device add d if wish, ex: 1d, 2d, or If using 1-7 scale: (41-48) =6 (49-56)

Golf/Miniature Golf
Physical Goals, Objectives, and Methods

SKILL	GOAL	OBJECTIVES SAMPLE	METHOD SAMPLE
FINE MOTOR SKILLS	Increase fine motor skills, including: using fingers, toes, hand-eye coordination, and dexterity	-will use club/hands to hit the ball, will pick up ball	Staff will give instructions, and residents will be involved in a game that requires small motor skills
GROSS MOTOR SKILLS	Increase large motor skills	-will bend, stretch, jump, hit the ball (may also do from chair)	Staff will give instructions, and residents will be involved in a volleyball game that requires large motor skills
PERCEPTUAL SPEED AND MOTOR FUNCTION	Increase speed and motor ability for function, safety, meaningful/fulfilling activities	-will increase acuity and hit the ball faster (with Dr. approval)	-Staff will give residents instructions on how to play the game -Staff will use varied types of game equipment (balloon or ball) to support resident's ability to hit the ball.
FOLLOWING STEP PATTERNS/ BACKWARDS FORWARD MOVEMENT	Increase strength, balance, endurance, meaningful/fulfilling activities	-will stand/sit and swing club to make contact with the ball	Staff will ask residents to walk forwards/backwards and turn during the game while hitting the ball (support device if needed), or can be done sitting in a chair
FOR CLINICIAN/ DR. APPROVED USE ONLY	For clinician/Dr. approved use only	-will lift arms, legs, bend, reach (to capacity - set by Dr./clinician), will extend and flex (to capacity - set by clinician)	Staff/clinician will instruct residents to do exercises that include flexing, extending muscles
BALANCE AND POSTURE (approved by Dr. and capacity tests)	Increase balance and improve body alignment and flexibility	-will maintain posture, will stand and maintain posture	Staff will remind residents of proper posture and ask residents to hold body in straight alignment/ posture
GAIT/ FOLLOWING STEP PATTERNS/ BACKWARDS/ FORWARD MOVEMENT	Increase strength, balance, endurance, meaningful/fulfilling activities	-will stand up without losing balance and walk a safe pace (approved by Dr. and capacity tests), If approved clinical specialist: ____ ft. ________________________________	Staff will call residents to the activity and have them walk to activity (w/device if needed) to work on leg strength (if approved by clinician etc.)
CARDIO-VASCULAR WORKOUT*	Increase circulation, blood flow, stamina	-will play the game at a safe pace (approved by Dr. and capacity tests), If approved clinical specialist: ________________________________	Staff/clinician will have residents play game (according to doctor approved ability and approved amount of exercise)

TABLE 5.2

Recreational Objectives Observation Form
Golf/Miniature Golf -Physical Skills

PATIENT	Dependent (Totally dependent)	High Assistance (25+ ability)	Moderate Assist. (50+ ability)	Mild Assistance (75+ability)	Independent (Totally independent.)
SEE CODES BELOW USE OPTIONAL CODES IF APPROPRIATE	1	2	3	4	5
	3 cue/ 2-3 physical	2-3 cues/ 2 physical	2-3 cues/ 1 physical	1-2 cues	Encouragement

97530- Therapeutic activities or	SKILL	GOAL	OBJECTIVES ____times per ____	METHOD	OUTCOME DATE			
97530 Therapeutic Activity	FINE MOTOR SKILLS							
97110/ 97530	GROSS MOTOR SKILLS							
97110/ 97530/ If under cognitive code 97532	PERCEPTUAL SPEED/ MOTOR FUNCTION							
97530 or Gait training 97116-	STEP PATTERNS							
		Licensed/ Clinician	Dr. approved use only	Licensed/ Clinician				
97110	RANGE OF MOTION							
97112	POSTURE AND BALANCE							
97110 Or Gait training 97116-	GAIT (INCLUDES STAIR CLIMBING)							
97110	CARDIO-VASCULAR WORKOUT*							

97110-Therapeutic procedure, one or more areas, each 15 minutes; therapeutic exercises to develop strength and endurance, range of motion, and flexibility; 97112-Neuromuscular reeducation of movement, balance, coordination, kinesthetic sense, posture, and proprioception; **97113-Aquatic therapy** with therapeutic exercises; **97116-Gait training** (includes stair climbing); **97139-Unlisted therapeutic procedure** (specify); **97150 Therapeutic procedure(s)**, group (2 or more individuals); **97750-Physical performance test or measurement** (e.g., musculoskeletal, functional capacity), with written report, each 15 minutes; **97535-Self care/home management training** (e.g., activities of daily living and compensatory training, meal preparation, safety procedures, and instructions in use of adaptive equipment), direct (one-on-one) contact by provider, each 15 minutes; **Physical therapy 97001 evaluation, 97002 Re-evaluation. occupational therapy evaluation 97003, re-evaluation. 97004; Athlete training 97005; re-evaluation 97006**	Staff Initial			
	Add total score here Maximum Score 40 pt. each form per activity			
	See scale below or use own/facilities optional score system			

Score 1-8) =1 (9-16) =2 (17-24) =3 (25-32) =4 (33-40) =5 If w/device add d if wish, ex: 1d, 2d, or If using 1-7 scale: (41-48) =6 (49-56) Current Procedural Terminology © 2005 American Medical Association. All rights reserved. Recreational Objectives Observational forms © 2005. All rights reserved. Patent pending.

Golf/Miniature Golf
Socio-emotional Goals, Objectives and Methods

Skill	Goal	Objectives Sample	Method Sample
Socialization/Community Integration	Increase social interactions, meaningful/fulfilling activities	-will interact with peers, will engage in community integration experiences (for social skills), will use manners, social practices	Staff will engage residents in a sport and support/encourage residents to socialize through community integration and being paired w/group for games
Team Playing/Sharing	Increase teamwork/sharing, meaningful/fulfilling activities	-will join in on the game with others and share, wait turn, support peers	Staff will encourage residents to play, form teams, strategize together, include all members in play
Initiative and Motivation	Increase initiative and motivation/wellness, and quality of life	-will choose if they wish to play or not, will try a new technique, will initiate playing on own (or with assistance), will increase amount of practice after stating own goal	-Staff will support and encourage the residents to prepare/join activities for their own personal gains -Staff will offer new techniques to motivate resident's interests and desires
Emotional Gratification	Increase emotional gratification/wellness, and quality of life	-will state that the game was a gratifying experience or will show pleasure by smiling, laughing, deep focus, and involvement during the game	Staff will ask residents if they enjoyed golfing and what they liked through the use of verbal discussion, group discussions or as observed
Sense of Accomplishment	Increase feelings of self-worth, pride, productivity, dignity/wellness, and quality of life	-will use gestures to express pride in self , will talk about their accomplishments while playing he game	Staff will place a chart on the unit wall or hand a paper to the residents that reflect the team scores, the charts/paper etc. will be available for residents to see their personal best
Self-esteem/self-identity	Increase self-esteem, feelings of belonging, dignity, self-worth, integrity, self-identity/wellness, and quality of life	-will state/communicate positive feelings about self and ability to play, will join game to take an active role in health though exercising, will join the game based on own choices	Staff will educate residents on the value of exercise and will encourage residents to join sports games
Fostering Appropriate Behaviors	Increase social interaction, social opportunities and adjustment, safety, using appropriate behaviors during an activity for a calm environment/wellness, and quality of life	-will adjust to the noises, other's movements, surroundings, etc.	-Staff will engage residents in sports to expose residents to sensory stimulating experiences -Staff will support residents as they adjust to the stimulus one step at a time
Sensory Integration/Tolerating Stimulation	Increase sensory processing and enhance awareness of sensations and toleration/adaptation of sensory stimulations and demands	-will join in on golf lesson, listen and follow instructions, use appropriate behavior for the setting; will wait turn, stand in line quietly; will quiet down when asked	Before class begins, staff will discuss the rules, appropriate behaviors, respect of property, safety, and respect of fellow team players

TABLE 5.3

Recreational Objectives Observation Form
Golf/Miniature Golf - Socio-emotional Skills

PATIENT	Dependent (Totally dependent)	High Assistance (25+ ability)	Moderate Assist. (50+ ability)	Mild Assistance (75+ability)	Independent (Totally independent.)
SEE CODES BELOW USE OPTIONAL CODES IF APPROPRIATE	1	2	3	4	5
	3 cue/ 2-3 physical	2-3 cues/ 2 physical	2-3 cues/ 1 physical	1-2 cues	Encouragement

97530-Therapeutic activities or	SKILL	GOAL	OBJECTIVES ____times per ____	METHOD	OUTCOME DATE			
97537 Or 97535	SOCIALIZATION/ COMMUNITY INTEGRATION							
97537 Or 97535	TEAM PLAYING /SHARING							
97537 Or 97535	INITIATIVE AND MOTIVATION							
97537 Or 97535	EMOTIONAL GRATIFICATION							
97537 Or 97535	SENSE OF ACCOMPLISHM ENT							
97537 Or 97535	SELF-ESTEEM/ SELF-IDENTITY							
97537 Or 97535	FOSTERING APPROPRIATE BEHAVIORS							
97533	SENSORY INTEGRATION/ TOLERATING							

97537-Community/work reintegration training (e.g., shopping, transportation, money management, avocational activities and/or work environment/modification analysis, work task analysis), direct (one-on-one) contact by provider, each 15 minutes; **97535-Self care/home management training** (e.g., activities of daily living and compensatory training, meal preparation, safety procedures, and instructions in use of adaptive equipment), direct (one-on-one) contact by provider, each 15 minutes; **97530-Therapeutic activities, direct (one-on-one)** patient contact by the provider (use of dynamic activities to improve functional performance), each 15 minutes; **97150-Therapeutic procedure(s), group (2 or more individuals); 97533-Sensory integration techniques** to enhance sensory processing and promote adaptive responses to environmental demands, direct (one-on-one) patient contact by the provider, each 15 minutes; **occupational therapy evaluation 97003, re-evaluation . 97004**	Staff Initial				
	Add total score here-Maximum Score 40 pt. each form per activity				
	See scale below or use own/facilities optional score system				

(Score 1-8)=1 (9-16) =2 (17-24) =3 (25-32) =4 (33-40) =5 If w/device add d if wish, ex: 1d, 2d, or If using 1-7 scale: (41-48) =6 (49-56) Current Procedural Terminology © 2005 American Medical Association. All rights reserved. Recreational Objectives Observational form © 2005. All rights reserved. Patent pending.

Ring Toss/Tic-Tac-Toe/Horseshoes

Objectives and benefits

Cognitive Challenges: attention, memory, language, orientation, following patterns, keeping rhythm, perceptual awareness, and cognitive stimulation

Physical Needs: fine motor skills, gross motor skills, coordination, range of motion, flexibility, posture, balance, backward and forward movement, gait, following step patterns, circulation, cardio-vascular workout

Socio-emotional Needs: socialization, community integration, initiative and motivation, emotional gratification, sense of accomplishment, self-esteem, tolerating stimulation, fostering appropriate behaviors

Supplies: A ring toss game, a tic-tac-toe game board that sits on the floor, an indoor/outdoor horseshoe set, a sand bag toss with board.

Time: 30 minutes.

Staff/older adult ratio: 1:10 or as assessed per needs of individuals or group. The need of assistance will be crucial for those with restricted use of arms. Those who are blind or sight-limited should be encouraged to play. They can be guided by being told the distances and directions of the games. It can be quite a challenge and yet very rewarding and fun.

Instructions: Have them warm up for the activity by leading them in them in a sub maximal active warm-up first. This will gradually increase their body temperature, blood flow to the muscles, and synovial fluid to the joints. Then you may lead them in a three to five minute stretching exercise. Have residents lined up a distance where they are capable of mastering the toss and range of hand-eye coordination. Give them three tosses. You may then take scores and have a prize for the top thrower of the day, or just play for fun. You can move the ring toss/etc. a bit further away as the game continues. It is always a challenge to find enough gross motor skills activities in an adult care population, so this game is certainly worth adapting. Have fun!

The CDC recommends that older adults participate in moderate-intensity aerobic activity 3-5 days a week for at least 30 minutes. This will help older adults to increase endurance, strength, and balance. It is also recommended that older adults engage in activities that include stretching everyday and strength training activities 2-3 days per week. (CDC, NCCDPHP. Special focus: healthy aging. Chronic Disease Notes and Reports 1999; 12(3):10-11. Insert CDC recommendations obtained from aoa.hhs.gov 2005

* All older adults engaging in activities should have physician approval to engage in physical activities.

Ring Toss/ Tic Tac Toe Horseshoes
Cognitive Goals, Objectives, and Methods

Skill	Goal	Objectives Sample	Method Sample
Orientation	Show increased awareness of, time/"timeframe," people, circumstances, and past experiences vs. present experiences, to engage in present-time activities, or for a reminiscing intended question	-will respond with correct answer to two choice questions Or yes/no answer about time, place, etc.; will state where they are, time of day, present company of people on own and with the correct answer	Staff will ask residents a series of questions to stimulate focus to the present setting Or past if reminiscing exercise (Ex: "Have you played this game before? Where are we?")
Attention	Show increased attention span, task for function, and to engage in meaningful, recreational/fulfilling activities	-will make eye-contact with staff instructor for _____ sec., will verbalize with staff and instructor, will read/listen to rule, will say yes/no to show they understand or will do action	Staff will address or stand in front of resident, make eye-contact, ask questions, or use others methods to get resident's attention/gauge attention
Memory	Show increased memory skills of recall, recognition, retention of information, working memory	-will repeat/recall/retain, will play the game, will repeat/recall how to toss the ring	Staff will show steps on how to play the game and repeat the actions, and have residents repeat action again when asked
Language	Show increased ability to communicate use of words, phrases, sentence structure, comprehension, interpretation	-will be asked a question and answer yes/no, will interact with peers and staff, will interpret instructor's request and follow	Staff will ask questions to stimulate a communication for Interpretation/Lang. skills (Ex: "Hand me your horseshoes.")
Cognitive Stimulation (awareness, seeks information in)	Increased stimulus/exposure for visual/ motor memory, cognitive experiences/awareness and brain stimulation to enhance (function, pragmatics, neuroplasticity)	-will listen/seek cognitive stimulation, will accept challenge of input information and engage/interact in game	-Staff will instruct the residents on where they need to stay in their area -Staff will show the resident the step-by-step actions on how to do the game
Perceptual Awareness	Show increased abilities of depth perception, visio-spatical awareness, and acuity (for discrimination, comparison, and categorizing), safety	-will stay in own lanes, will stay within own space next to others, will put items away in proper containers associated with proper areas	-Staff will direct the residents on using a series of techniques for horseshoes, etc. -Staff will answer questions regarding understanding of steps, and offer the residents challenging strategies for processing info., step judgments
Problem-solving (goes beyond thinking/stimulus and initiates thinking process)	Increase problem-solving ability, processing of information, thinking, reasoning, and use of good judgment and decision-making	will use good judgment of speed and motor coordination, will consider dimensions, force of arm strength to aim/toss, will stretch, step, aim, and toss item as required	-Staff will explain the procedure/agenda regarding exercise -Staff will instruct, encourage, make use of adaptive devices if needed, and supply necessary materials and support
Complete a task	Increase ability to complete a task	-will recall/retain and sort/gather information, problem-solve, and complete activity	

TABLE 6.1

Recreational Objectives Observation Form
Ring Toss/Tic Tac Toe- Cognitive skills

PATIENT		Dependent (Totally dependent)	High Assistance (25+ ability)	Moderate Assist. (50+ ability)	Mild Assistance (75+ability)	Independent (Totally independent)			
SEE CODES BELOW USE OPTIONAL CODES IF APPROPRIATE		1	2	3	4	5			
		3 cue/ 2-3 physical	2-3 cues/ 2 physical	2-3 cues/ 1 physical	1-2 cues	Encouragement			
97530- Therapeutic activities or	**SKILL**	**GOAL**	**OBJECTIVES** ____times per ____		**METHOD**	**OUTCOME DATE**			
97532 Cognitive skills	ORIENTATION								
97532 Cognitive skills	ATTENTION								
97532 Cognitive skills	MEMORY								
97532 Cognitive skills	PROBLEM-SOLVING								
97532 Cognitive skills	COMPLETE A TASK								
97139 Speech Therapy 97532 Cognitive skills	LANGUAGE								
97533	SENSORY STIMULATION/ COGNITIVE STIMULATION								
97532	PERCEPTUAL AWARENESS								

97532-Development of cognitive skills to improve attention, memory, problem-solving, includes compensatory training and/or sensory integrative activities, direct (one-on-one) patient contact by the provider, each 15 minutes; **97530-Therapeutic activities**, direct (one-on-one) patient contact by the provider (use of dynamic activities to improve functional performance), each 15 minutes; **97533-Sensory integration techniques** to enhance sensory processing and promote adaptive responses to environmental demands, direct (one-on-one) patient contact by the provider, each 15 minutes; **97150-Therapeutic procedure(s)**, group (2 or more individuals); **97139-Unlisted therapeutic procedure** (specify) minutes; **97003- occupational therapy evaluation**; **97004- re-evaluation**	Staff Initial				
	Add total score here -Maximum Score 40 pt. each form per activity				
	See scale below or use own/facilities optional score system				

(Score 1-8)=1 (9-16) =2 (17-24) =3 (25-32) =4 (33-40) =5 If w/device add d if wish, ex: 1d, 2d, or If using 1-7 scale: (41-48) =6 (49-56)

Ring Toss, Tic Tac Toe, Horseshoes
Physical Goals, Objectives, and Methods

Skill	Goal	Objectives Sample	Method Sample
Fine motor skills	Increase fine motor skills, including: using fingers, toes, hand-eye coordination, and dexterity	-will grab rings and sack, and toss	Staff will give residents instructions on the steps to play the game, including the use of small motor skills (fingers, hand-eye coordination, etc.)
Gross motor skills	Increase large motor skills	-will reach, bend, stretch, and toss	Staff will give residents instructions, and the residents will be involved in game, including the use of large motor (arms, legs, etc.)
Perceptual speed and motor function	Increase speed and motor ability for function, safety, meaningful/fulfilling activities	-will toss ball at increased rates	-While playing the game, staff will call 1,2,3 As game continues the staff -Staff will decrease amount of time between tosses, but wait until residents have mastered ability to throw at each level
Following step patterns/backwards forward movement	Increase strength, balance, endurance, meaningful/fulfilling activities	-will pick up the ring/sack, will aim the ring/sack at the ring stand and pole; will lean forwards and toss the ring at the pole	Staff will ask residents to walk forwards/backwards and turn and toss horseshoe (device support if needed)
For clinician/Dr. approved use only	For clinician/Dr. approved use only	-will lift arms, legs (to capacity - set by Dr./clinician), will extend and flex (to capacity - set by clinician)	Staff will guide and support residents as they do exercises that include flexing, extending muscles
Balance and Posture (approved by Dr. and capacity tests)	Increase balance and improve body alignment and flexibility	-will sit in chair and maintain posture, will stand using adequate posture during the game	Staff will remind residents to hold body in straight alignment/posture
Gait/Following Step patterns/ Backwards/Forward movement	Increase strength, balance, endurance, meaningful/fulfilling activities	-will stand up without losing balance and walk a safe pace (approved by Dr. and capacity tests), If approved, clinical specialist: _____	-Staff will encourage residents to walk, as a way to build up leg strength for balance and gait -Staff will increase balance by standing still (support if needed) as they pitch forward to toss the ball onto the pole
Cardio-vascular Workout*	Increase circulation, blood flow, stamina	-will play game at a safe pace (approved by Dr. and capacity tests), If approved clinical specialist: ________________________	Staff will support residents in a safe workout (according to ability and approved amount of activity)

Table 6.2

Recreational Objectives Observation Form
Ring Toss/ Tic Tac Toe- Physical Skills

Patient	Dependent (Totally dependent)	High Assistance (25+ ability)	Moderate Assist. (50+ ability)	Mild Assistance (75+ability)	Independent (Totally independent.)
SEE CODES BELOW	1	2	3	4	5
USE OPTIONAL CODES IF APPROPRIATE	3 cue/ 2-3 physical	2-3 cues/ 2 physical	2-3 cues/ 1 physical	1-2 cues	Encouragement

97530- Therapeutic activities or	**Skill**	**Goal**	**Objectives** ____times per ____	**Method**	**Outcome Date**			
97530 Therapeutic Activity	Fine Motor skills							
97110/ 97530	Gross Motor Skills							
97110/ 97530/ If under cognitive code 97532	Perceptual Speed/ Motor Function							
97530 or Gait training 97116-	Step Patterns							
		Licensed/ Clinician	Dr. approved use only	Licensed/ Clinician				
97110	Range of Motion							
97112	Posture and Balance							
97110 Or Gait training 97116-	Gait (includes stair climbing)							
97110	Cardio-vascular Workout*							

97110-Therapeutic procedure, one or more areas, each 15 minutes; therapeutic exercises to develop strength and endurance, range of motion, and flexibility; 97112-Neuromuscular reeducation of movement, balance, coordination, kinesthetic sense, posture, and proprioception; **97113-Aquatic therapy** with therapeutic exercises; **97116-Gait training** (includes stair climbing); **97139-Unlisted therapeutic procedure** (specify); **97150 Therapeutic procedure(s)**, group (2 or more individuals); **97750-Physical performance test or measurement** (e.g., musculoskeletal, functional capacity), with written report, each 15 minutes; **97535-Self care/home management training** (e.g., activities of daily living and compensatory training, meal preparation, safety procedures, and instructions in use of adaptive equipment), direct (one-on-one) contact by provider, each 15 minutes; **Physical therapy 97001 evaluation, 97002 Re-evaluation. occupational therapy evaluation 97003, re-evaluation. 97004; Athlete training 97005; re-evaluation 97006**

Staff Initial

Add total score here
Maximum Score 40 pt.
each form per activity

See scale below
or use own/facilities
optional score system

Score 1-8) =1 (9-16) =2 (17-24) =3 (25-32) =4 (33-40) =5 If w/device add d if wish, ex: 1d, 2d, or If using 1-7 scale: (41-48) =6 (49-56)

Ring Toss, Tic Tac Toe, Horseshoes
Socio-emotional Goals, Objectives and Methods

Skill	Goal	Objectives Sample	Method Sample
Socialization/Community Integration	Increase social interactions, meaningful/fulfilling activities	-will interact with peers, will engage in community integration experiences (for social skills), will use manners, social practices	Staff will engage residents in an activity and support/encourage residents to socialize through community integration and being paired w/group members to play a game
Team Playing/Sharing	Increase teamwork/sharing, meaningful/fulfilling activities	-will join in on a game, will exercise with others and share, wait turn, support peers	Staff will encourage residents to play, share games, form teams, strategize together
Initiative and Motivation	Increase initiative and motivation/wellness, and quality of life	-will choose if they wish to engage in game, will choose if they wish to join in on game, will try a new technique, will do all moves on own or with assistance, will increase amount of tosses after stating own goal	-Staff will support/encourage the resident to participate for the resident's own personal gains -Staff will offer new techniques/strategies to motivate
Emotional Gratification	Increase emotional gratification/wellness, and quality of life	-will state that the game was a gratifying experience, or will show pleasure by smiling, laughing, deep focus on the game	Staff will ask residents if they enjoyed the game and what they liked through verbal discussion, group discussions
Sense of Accomplishment	Increase feelings of self-worth, pride, productivity, dignity/wellness, and quality of life	-will use gestures to express pride in self, will talk about their accomplishments of using a good aim, score, etc.	Staff will give residents a paper showing their score for residents to be able to see their personal best/increased, etc.
Self-esteem/self-identity	Increase self-esteem, feelings of belonging, dignity, self-worth, integrity, self-identity/wellness, and quality of life	-will state/communicate positive feelings about self and ability to play, will join in on game, will take an active role in maintaining health though exercising, will join game based on own choices	Staff will educate residents on the value of playing games/exercise and encourage residents to exercise
Sensory Integration/Tolerating Stimulation	Increase sensory processing and enhance awareness of sensations and toleration/adaptation of sensory stimulations and demands	-will adjust to the commotion, peers; can tolerate suspense or pressure to toss the ball in front of others _____ time(s) this week	Staff will expose residents to sensory stimulating experiences and support residents as they adjust to the stimulus one step at a time
Fostering Appropriate Behaviors	Increase social interaction, social opportunities and adjustment, safety, using appropriate behaviors during an activity for a calm environment/wellness, and quality of life	-will join in on game, listen and follow instructions, use appropriate behavior for the setting; will wait turn, stand in line quietly; will quiet down when asked	Before activity begins, staff will discuss game rules, appropriate behaviors, respect of property, safety, and respect of fellow game players

TABLE 6.3

Recreational Objectives Observation Form
Ring Toss/Tic Tac Toe - Socio-emotional Skills

PATIENT	Dependent (Totally dependent)	High Assistance (25+ ability)	Moderate Assist. (50+ ability)	Mild Assistance (75+ability)	Independent (Totally independent.)
SEE CODES BELOW USE OPTIONAL CODES IF APPROPRIATE	1	2	3	4	5
	3 cue/ 2-3 physical	2-3 cues/ 2 physical	2-3 cues/ 1 physical	1-2 cues	Encouragement

97530- Therapeutic activities or	SKILL	GOAL	OBJECTIVES ____times per ____	METHOD	OUTCOME DATE			
97537 Or 97535	SOCIALIZATION/ COMMUNITY INTEGRATION							
97537 Or 97535	TEAM PLAYING /SHARING							
97537 Or 97535	INITIATIVE AND MOTIVATION							
97537 Or 97535	EMOTIONAL GRATIFICATION							
97537 Or 97535	SENSE OF ACCOMPLISHMENT							
97537 Or 97535	SELF-ESTEEM/ SELF-IDENTITY							
97537 Or 97535	FOSTERING APPROPRIATE BEHAVIORS							
97533	SENSORY INTEGRATION/ TOLERATING							

97537-Community/work reintegration training (e.g., shopping, transportation, money management, avocational activities and/or work environment/modification analysis, work task analysis), direct (one-on-one) contact by provider, each 15 minutes; **97535-Self care/home management training** (e.g., activities of daily living and compensatory training, meal preparation, safety procedures, and instructions in use of adaptive equipment), direct (one-on-one) contact by provider, each 15 minutes; **97530-Therapeutic activities, direct (one-on-one)** patient contact by the provider (use of dynamic activities to improve functional performance), each 15 minutes; **97150-Therapeutic procedure(s), group (2 or more individuals); 97533-Sensory integration techniques** to enhance sensory processing and promote adaptive responses to environmental demands, direct (one-on-one) patient contact by the provider, each 15 minutes; **occupational therapy evaluation 97003, re-evaluation . 97004**	Staff Initial				
	Add total score here-Maximum Score 40 pt. each form per activity				
	See scale below or use own/facilities optional score system				

(Score 1-8)=1 (9-16) =2 (17-24) =3 (25-32) =4 (33-40) =5 If w/device add d if wish, ex: 1d, 2d, or If using 1-7 scale: (41-48) =6 (49-56)

Tennis

Objectives and benefits

Cognitive Challenges*:* attention, memory, language, orientation, following patterns, keeping rhythm, perceptual awareness, and cognitive stimulation

Physical Needs*:* fine motor skills, gross motor skills, coordination, range of motion, flexibility, posture, balance, backward and forward movement, gait, following step patterns, circulation, cardio-vascular workout

Socio-emotional Needs: socialization, community integration, initiative and motivation, emotional gratification, sense of accomplishment, self-esteem, tolerating stimulation, fostering appropriate behaviors

Supplies: Availability of tennis court.

Time: 20–30 minutes.

Staff/older adult ratio: 1:2 or as assessed per needs of individuals or group.

Instructions: Have them warm up for activity by leading them in a sub maximal active warm-up first. This will gradually increase their body temperature, blood flow to the muscles, and synovial fluid to the joints. You may then lead them in a three to five minute stretching exercise. The activity could be done as a freestyle activity that allows older adults to play tennis at their own pace, with peers for casual play or with the help of a tennis instructor.

Due to medications, or falling potential, older adults should be supervised very carefully. Those with restrictions may be able to use special equipment available for the physically challenged. It might be helpful to ask the facility what they have available to support those with limited ability to join in on the tennis activities.

Because tennis can be a highly vigorous form of exercise, all older adults involved in Tennis should be carefully monitored by a physician. No older adult should be allowed to participate in this sport without prior clearance by a physician. If Tennis is offered by a facility/in a rehabilitation setting, a signed release stating physician approval must be documented and on file.

The CDC recommends that older adults participate in moderate-intensity aerobic activity 3-5 days a week for at least 30 minutes. This will help older adults to increase endurance, strength, and balance. It is also recommended that older adults engage in activities that include stretching everyday and strength training activities 2-3 days per week. (CDC, NCCDPHP. Special focus: healthy aging. Chronic Disease Notes and Reports 1999; 12(3):10-11. Insert CDC recommendations obtained from aoa.hhs.gov 2005

* All older adults engaging in activities should have physician approval to engage in physical activities.

Tennis
Cognitive Goals, Objectives, and Methods

Skill	Goal	Objectives Sample	Method Sample
Orientation	Show increased awareness of, time/"timeframe," people, circumstances, and past experiences vs. present experiences, to engage in present-time activities, or for a reminiscing intended question	-will respond with correct answer to two choice questions (Ex: "Are you at the mall or at the sports center?") Or yes/ no answer, will state where they are, time of day, present company of people on own and with the correct answer	Staff will ask residents a series of questions to stimulate focus to the present setting, Or past if reminiscing exercise (Ex: "When have you played tennis before? Where are we?")
Attention	Show increased attention span, task for function, and to engage in meaningful, recreational/fulfilling activities	-will make eye-contact with instructor for _____ sec(s), will verbalize with staff, will read/listen to rules, will say yes/no to show understand	Staff will address or stand in front of resident, make eye-contact, ask questions, or use others methods to get resident's attention/gauge attention
Memory	Show increased memory skills of recall, recognition, retention of information, working memory	-will repeat/recall and retain rules, will repeat /recall how to throw and hit the ball, will remember lesson at next class	Staff will show steps on how to play the game and ask residents to repeat the actions
Language	Show increased ability to communicate use of words, phrases, sentence structure, mprehension, interpretation	-will be asked a question and answer yes/no to a two choice question; will interact with peers and staff, will interpret instructor's request and follow directions	Staff will ask questions to stimu-late a communication (Ex: "Do you want to Tennis?") Or for Interpretation/ Lang. skills (Ex: "Hand me the racket please.")
Cognitive Stimulation (awareness, seeks information in)	Increased stimulus/exposure for visual/ motor memory, cognitive experiences/ awareness and brain stimulation to enhance (function, pragmatics, neuro-plasticity)	-will listen/seek cognitive stimulation, will accept challenge of input information and engage/ interact in game	Staff will set up a game and introduce residents to stimulation experiences
Perceptual Awareness	Show increased abilities of depth perception, visual-spatial awareness, and acuity (for discrimination, comparison, and categorizing), safety	-will gauge distance to hit the ball over the net). will stay within own space on court, next to others, will maneuver around peers, net	-Staff will instruct the residents on where they need to stay in their area -Staff will use the game to help residents understand/practice/ increase depth perception skills
Problem-solving (goes beyond thinking/stimulus and initiates thinking process)	Increase problem-solving ability, processing of information, thinking, reasoning, and use of good judgment and decision-making	-will use good judgment of speed and motor coordination, movement or strength and distance to hit ball; will consider dimensions, force of arm strength to aim/swing; will consider strategies to hit the ball	-Staff will direct the residents on using a series of techniques for tennis -Staff will answer questions regarding understanding of steps and offer the residents challenging strategies for processing info, step judgments -Staff will have residents attempt to swing racket, hit the ball, considering dimensions, strategies
Complete a Task	Increase ability to complete a task		

TABLE 7.1

Recreational Objectives Observation Form
Tennis -Cognitive skills

PATIENT		Dependent (Totally dependent)	High Assistance (25+ ability)	Moderate Assist. (50+ ability)	Mild Assistance (75+ability)	Independent (Totally independent)
SEE CODES BELOW USE OPTIONAL CODES IF APPROPRIATE		1	2	3	4	5
		3 cue/ 2-3 physical	2-3 cues/ 2 physical	2-3 cues/ 1 physical	1-2 cues	Encouragement
97530-Therapeutic activities or	**SKILL**	**GOAL**	**OBJECTIVES** ____times per ____		**METHOD**	**OUTCOME DATE**
97532 Cognitive skills	ORIENTATION					
97532 Cognitive skills	ATTENTION					
97532 Cognitive skills	MEMORY					
97532 Cognitive skills	PROBLEM-SOLVING					
97532 Cognitive skills	COMPLETE A TASK					
97139 Speech Therapy 97532 Cognitive skills	LANGUAGE					
97533	SENSORY STIMULATION/ COGNITIVE STIMULATION					
97532	PERCEPTUAL AWARENESS					

97532-Development of cognitive skills to improve attention, memory, problem-solving, includes compensatory training and/or sensory integrative activities, direct (one-on-one) patient contact by the provider, each 15 minutes; **97530-Therapeutic activities**, direct (one-on-one) patient contact by the provider (use of dynamic activities to improve functional performance), each 15 minutes; **97533-Sensory integration techniques** to enhance sensory processing and promote adaptive responses to environmental demands, direct (one-on-one) patient contact by the provider, each 15 minutes; **97150-Therapeutic procedure(s)**, group (2 or more individuals); **97139-Unlisted therapeutic procedure** (specify) minutes; **97003- occupational therapy evaluation**; **97004- re-evaluation**	Staff Initial Add total score here -Maximum Score 40 pt. each form per activity See scale below or use own/facilities optional score system

(Score 1-8)=1 (9-16) =2 (17-24) =3 (25-32) =4 (33-40) =5 If w/device add d if wish, ex: 1d, 2d, or If using 1-7 scale: (41-48) =6 (49-56)

Tennis
Physical Goals, Objectives, and Methods

Skill	Goal	Objectives Sample	Method Sample
Fine motor skills	Increase fine motor skills, including: using fingers, toes, hand-eye coordination, and dexterity	-will use racket to hit the ball, will pick up ball	Staff will give instructions, and residents will be involved in a game that requires small motor skills
Gross motor skills	Increase large motor skills	-will bend, stretch, jump, hit the ball (may also do from chair)	Staff will give instructions, and residents will be involved in a volleyball game that requires large motor skills
Perceptual speed and motor function	Increase speed and motor ability for function, safety, meaningful/fulfilling activities	-will increase acuity and hit the ball faster (with Dr. approval)	-Staff will give residents instructions on how to play the game -Staff will use varied types of game equipment (balloon or ball) to support resident's ability to hit the ball.
Following step patterns/backwards forward movement	Increase strength, balance, endurance, meaningful/fulfilling activities	-will stand/sit and swing racket to make contact with the ball	Staff will ask residents to walk forwards/backwards and turn during the game while hitting the ball (support device if needed), or can be done sitting in a chair
For clinician/Dr. approved use only	For clinician/Dr. approved use only	-will lift arms, legs, bend, reach (to capacity - set by Dr./clinician), will extend and flex (to capacity - set by clinician)	Staff/clinician will instruct residents to do exercises that include flexing, extending muscles
Balance and Posture (approved by Dr. and capacity tests)	Increase balance and improve body alignment and flexibility	-will maintain posture, will stand and maintain posture	Staff will remind residents of proper posture and ask residents to hold body in straight alignment/ posture
Gait/Following Step patterns/ Backwards/Forward movement	Increase strength, balance, endurance, meaningful/fulfilling activities	-will stand up without losing balance, use correct alignment to stand and swing racket, walk backwards and forward and walk a safe pace (approved by Dr. and capacity tests), If approved clinical specialist: ____ ft. ______________________________	Staff will call residents to the activity and have them walk to activity (w/device if needed) to work on leg strength (if approved by clinician etc.)
Cardio-vascular Workout*	Increase circulation, blood flow, stamina	-will play the game at a safe pace (approved by Dr. and capacity tests), If approved clinical specialist: ______________________________	Staff/clinician will have residents play game (according to doctor approved ability and approved amount of exercise)

TABLE 7.2

Recreational Objectives Observation Form
Tennis-Physical Skills

PATIENT	Dependent (Totally dependent)	High Assistance (25+ ability)	Moderate Assist. (50+ ability)	Mild Assistance (75+ability)	Independent (Totally independent.)
SEE CODES BELOW USE OPTIONAL CODES IF APPROPRIATE	1	2	3	4	5
	3 cue/ 2-3 physical	2-3 cues/ 2 physical	2-3 cues/ 1 physical	1-2 cues	Encouragement

97530- Therapeutic activities or	**SKILL**	**GOAL**	**OBJECTIVES** ____times per ____	**METHOD**	**OUTCOME DATE**			
97530 Therapeutic Activity	FINE MOTOR SKILLS							
97110/ 97530	GROSS MOTOR SKILLS							
97110/ 97530/ cognitive code 97532	PERCEPTUAL SPEED/ MOTOR FUNCTION							
97530 or Gait training 97116-	STEP PATTERNS							
		Licensed/ Clinician	Dr. approved use only	Licensed/ Clinician				
97110	RANGE OF MOTION							
97112	POSTURE AND BALANCE							
97110 Or Gait training 97116-	GAIT (INCLUDES STAIR CLIMBING)							
97110	CARDIO-VASCULAR WORKOUT*							

97110-Therapeutic procedure, one or more areas, each 15 minutes; therapeutic exercises to develop strength and endurance, range of motion, and flexibility; 97112-Neuromuscular reeducation of movement, balance, coordination, kinesthetic sense, posture, and proprioception; **97113-Aquatic therapy** with therapeutic exercises; **97116-Gait training** (includes stair climbing); **97139-Unlisted therapeutic procedure** (specify); **97150 Therapeutic procedure(s)**, group (2 or more individuals); **97750-Physical performance test or measurement** (e.g., musculoskeletal, functional capacity), with written report, each 15 minutes; **97535-Self care/home management training** (e.g., activities of daily living and compensatory training, meal preparation, safety procedures, and instructions in use of adaptive equipment), direct (one-on-one) contact by provider, each 15 minutes; **Physical therapy 97001 evaluation, 97002 Re-evaluation. occupational therapy evaluation 97003, re-evaluation. 97004; Athlete training 97005; re-evaluation 97006**	Staff Initial				
	Add total score here Maximum Score 40 pt. each form per activity				
	See scale below or use own/facilities optional score system				

Score 1-8) =1 (9-16) =2 (17-24) =3 (25-32) =4 (33-40) =5 If w/device add d if wish, ex: 1d, 2d, or If using 1-7 scale: (41-48) =6 (49-56)

Tennis
Socio-emotional Goals, Objectives and Methods

Skill	Goal	Objectives Sample	Method Sample
Socialization/Community Integration	Increase social interactions, meaningful/fulfilling activities	-will interact with peers, will engage in community integration experiences (for social skills), will use manners, social practices	Staff will engage residents in a sport and support/encourage residents to socialize through community integration and being paired w/group for games
Team Playing/Sharing	Increase teamwork/sharing, meaningful/fulfilling activities	-will join in on the game with others and share, wait turn, support peers	Staff will encourage residents to play, form teams, strategize together, include all members in play
Initiative and Motivation	Increase initiative and motivation/wellness, and quality of life	-will choose if they wish to play or not, will try a new technique, will initiate playing on own (or with assistance), will increase amount of practice after stating own goal	-Staff will support and encourage the residents to prepare/join activities for their own personal gains -Staff will offer new techniques to motivate resident's interests and desires
Emotional Gratification	Increase emotional gratification/wellness, and quality of life	-will state that the game was a gratifying experience or will show pleasure by smiling, laughing, deep focus, and involvement during the game	Staff will ask residents if they enjoyed tennis and what they liked through the use of verbal discussion, group discussions or as observed
Sense of Accomplishment	Increase feelings of self-worth, pride, productivity, dignity/wellness, and quality of life	-will use gestures to express pride in self , will talk about their accomplishments while playing he game	Staff will place a chart on the unit wall or hand a paper to the residents that reflect the team scores, the charts/paper etc. will be available for residents to see their personal best
Self-esteem/self-identity	Increase self-esteem, feelings of belonging, dignity, self-worth, integrity, self-identity/wellness, and quality of life	-will state/communicate positive feelings about self and ability to play, will join game to take an active role in health though exercising, will join the game based on own choices	Staff will educate residents on the value of exercise and will encourage residents to join sports games
Fostering Appropriate Behaviors	Increase social interaction, social opportunities and adjustment, safety, using appropriate behaviors during an activity for a calm environment/wellness, and quality of life	-will adjust to the noises, other's movements, surroundings, etc.	-Staff will engage residents in sports to expose residents to sensory stimulating experiences -Staff will support residents as they adjust to the stimulus one step at a time
Sensory Integration/Tolerating Stimulation	Increase sensory processing and enhance awareness of sensations and toleration/adaptation of sensory stimulations and demands	-will join in on tennis lesson, listen and follow instructions, use appropriate behavior for the setting; will wait turn, stand in line quietly; will quiet down when asked	Before class begins, staff will discuss the rules, appropriate behaviors, respect of property, safety, and respect of fellow team players

TABLE 7.3

Recreational Objectives Observation Form
Tennis- Socio-emotional Skills

PATIENT		Dependent (Totally dependent)	High Assistance (25+ ability)	Moderate Assist. (50+ ability)	Mild Assistance (75+ability)	Independent (Totally independent.)
SEE CODES BELOW USE OPTIONAL CODES IF APPROPRIATE		1	2	3	4	5
		3 cue/ 2-3 physical	2-3 cues/ 2 physical	2-3 cues/ 1 physical	1-2 cues	Encouragement
97530- Therapeutic activities or	**SKILL**	**GOAL**	**OBJECTIVES** ____times per ____		**METHOD**	**OUTCOME DATE**
97537 Or 97535	SOCIALIZATION/ COMMUNITY INTEGRATION					
97537 Or 97535	TEAM PLAYING /SHARING					
97537 Or 97535	INITIATIVE AND MOTIVATION					
97537 Or 97535	EMOTIONAL GRATIFICATION					
97537 Or 97535	SENSE OF ACCOMPLISHM ENT					
97537 Or 97535	SELF-ESTEEM/ SELF-IDENTITY					
97537 Or 97535	FOSTERING APPROPRIATE BEHAVIORS					
97533	SENSORY INTEGRATION/ TOLERATING					

97537-Community/work reintegration training (e.g., shopping, transportation, money management, avocational activities and/or work environment/modification analysis, work task analysis), direct (one-on-one) contact by provider, each 15 minutes; **97535-Self care/home management training** (e.g., activities of daily living and compensatory training, meal preparation, safety procedures, and instructions in use of adaptive equipment), direct (one-on-one) contact by provider, each 15 minutes; **97530-Therapeutic activities, direct (one-on-one)** patient contact by the provider (use of dynamic activities to improve functional performance), each 15 minutes; **97150-Therapeutic procedure(s), group (2 or more individuals); 97533-Sensory integration techniques** to enhance sensory processing and promote adaptive responses to environmental demands, direct (one-on-one) patient contact by the provider, each 15 minutes; **occupational therapy evaluation 97003, re-evaluation . 97004**	Staff Initial Add total score here-Maximum Score 40 pt. each form per activity See scale below or use own/facilities optional score system

(Score 1-8)=1 (9-16) =2 (17-24) =3 (25-32) =4 (33-40) =5 If w/device add d if wish, ex: 1d, 2d, or If using 1-7 scale: (41-48) =6 (49-56)

Volleyball/Balloon Volleyball

Objectives and benefits

Cognitive Challenges: attention, memory, language, orientation, following patterns, keeping rhythm, perceptual awareness, and cognitive stimulation

Physical Needs: fine motor skills, gross motor skills, coordination, range of motion, flexibility, posture, balance, backward and forward movement, gait, following step patterns, circulation, cardio-vascular workout

Socio-emotional Needs: socialization, community integration, initiative and motivation, emotional gratification, sense of accomplishment, self-esteem, tolerating stimulation, fostering appropriate behaviors, relaxation, solace and healing

Supplies: Beach ball, tape

Time: 30 minutes

Staff/older adult ratio: 1:6

Instructions: Have older adults warm up for volleyball by leading them in a sub maximal active warm-up first. This will gradually increase their body temperature, blood flow to the muscles, and synovial fluid to the joints. Then you may lead them in a three to five minute stretching exercise.

Have residents sit in chairs that are set up on two sides of the room. Put a piece of tape in the center of the floor. This will be a way to distinguish two separate sides of the volleyball court. One team will start the game by hitting the ball to the players on the opposite side of the "court." Just as is played in real volleyball, the team who does not drop the ball gains points when the opposite team allows the ball to drop to the floor. Let each resident have a turn serving the ball. For patients who have very slow reflexes it is favorable to use balloons, because a balloon moves much slower and can compensate for their slow reaction time. The balloon is also lighter which may help patients suffering from range of motion difficulties.

The CDC recommends that older adults participate in moderate-intensity aerobic activity 3-5 days a week for at least 30 minutes. This will help older adults to increase endurance, strength, and balance. It is also recommended that older adults engage in activities that include stretching everyday and strength training activities 2-3 days per week. (CDC, NCCDPHP. Special focus: healthy aging. Chronic Disease Notes and Reports 1999; 12(3):10-11. Insert CDC recommendations obtained from aoa.hhs.gov 2005

* All older adults engaging in activities should have physician approval to engage in physical activities.

Volleyball/Balloon Volleyball
COGNITIVE GOALS, OBJECTIVES, AND METHODS

Skill	Goal	Objectives Sample	Method Sample
Orientation	Show increased awareness of, time/"timeframe," people, circumstances, and past experiences vs. present experiences, to engage in present-time activities, or for a reminiscing intended question	-will respond with correct answer to two choice questions (Ex: "Are you at the mall or at the sports center?") Or yes/no answer, will state where they are, time of day, present company of people on own and with the correct answer	Staff will ask residents a series of questions to stimulate focus to the present setting, Or past if reminiscing exercise (Ex: "When have you played volleyball before? Where are we?")
Attention	Show increased attention span, task for function, and to engage in meaningful, recreational/fulfilling activities	-will make eye-contact with instructor for _____ sec(s), will verbalize with staff, will read/listen to rules, will say yes/no to show understand	Staff will address or stand in front of resident, make eye-contact, ask questions, or use others methods to get resident's attention/gauge attention
Memory	Show increased memory skills of recall, recognition, retention of information, working memory	-will repeat/recall and retain rules, will repeat /recall how to throw and hit the ball, will remember lesson at next class	Staff will show steps on how to play the game and ask residents to repeat the actions
Language	Show increased ability to communicate use of words, phrases, sentence structure, comprehension, interpretation	-will be asked a question and answer yes/no to a two choice question; will interact with peers and staff, will interpret instructor's request and follow directions	Staff will ask questions to stimulate a communication (Ex: "Do you want to play volleyball?") Or for Interpretation/Lang. skills (Ex: "Hand me the volleyball.")
Cognitive Stimulation (awareness, seeks information in)	Increased stimulus/exposure for visual/ motor memory, cognitive experiences/awareness and brain stimulation to enhance (function, pragmatics, neuro-plasticity)	-will listen/seek cognitive stimulation, will accept challenge of input information and engage/interact in game	Staff will set up a game and introduce residents to stimulation experiences
Perceptual Awareness	Show increased abilities of depth perception, visual-spatial awareness, and acuity (for discrimination, comparison, and categorizing), safety	-will stay in own line (net side). will stay within own space next to others, will maneuver around peers, net	-Staff will instruct the residents on where they need to stay in their area -Staff will use the game to help residents understand/practice/ increase depth perception skills
Problem-solving (goes beyond thinking/stimulus and initiates thinking process)	Increase problem-solving ability, processing of information, thinking, reasoning, and use of good judgment and decision-making	-will use good judgment of speed and motor coordination, movement of the ball off of floor; will consider dimensions, force of arm strength to aim/toss; will consider strategies to hit the ball	-Staff will direct the residents on using a series of techniques for volleyball -Staff will answer questions regarding understanding of steps and offer the residents challenging strategies for processing info, step judgments -Staff will have residents attempt to hit the ball over the net, considering dimensions, strategies
Complete a Task	Increase ability to complete a task		

TABLE 8.1

Recreational Objectives Observation Form
Volleyball/Balloon Volleyball- Cognitive skills

PATIENT		Dependent (Totally dependent)	High Assistance (25+ ability)	Moderate Assist. (50+ ability)	Mild Assistance (75+ability)	Independent (Totally independent)			
SEE CODES BELOW USE OPTIONAL CODES IF APPROPRIATE		1	2	3	4	5			
		3 cue/ 2-3 physical	2-3 cues/ 2 physical	2-3 cues/ 1 physical	1-2 cues	Encouragement			
97530- Therapeutic activities or	**SKILL**	**GOAL**	**OBJECTIVES** ____times per ____		**METHOD**	**OUTCOME DATE**			
97532 Cognitive skills	ORIENTATION								
97532 Cognitive skills	ATTENTION								
97532 Cognitive skills	MEMORY								
97532 Cognitive skills	PROBLEM-SOLVING								
97532 Cognitive skills	COMPLETE A TASK								
97139 Speech Therapy 97532 Cognitive skills	LANGUAGE								
97533	SENSORY STIMULATION/ COGNITIVE STIMULATION								
97532	PERCEPTUAL AWARENESS								

97532-Development of cognitive skills to improve attention, memory, problem-solving, includes compensatory training and/or sensory integrative activities, direct (one-on-one) patient contact by the provider, each 15 minutes; **97530-Therapeutic activities**, direct (one-on-one) patient contact by the provider (use of dynamic activities to improve functional performance), each 15 minutes**; 97533-Sensory integration techniques** to enhance sensory processing and promote adaptive responses to environmental demands, direct (one-on-one) patient contact by the provider, each 15 minutes; **97150-Therapeutic procedure(s)**, group (2 or more individuals); **97139-Unlisted therapeutic procedure** (specify) minutes; **97003- occupational therapy evaluation**; **97004- re-evaluation**	Staff Initial				
	Add total score here -Maximum Score 40 pt. each form per activity				
	See scale below or use own/facilities optional score system				

(Score 1-8)=1 (9-16) =2 (17-24) =3 (25-32) =4 (33-40) =5 If w/device add d if wish, ex: 1d, 2d, or If using 1-7 scale: (41-48) =6 (49-56)

Volleyball/Balloon Volleyball
Physical Goals, Objectives, and Methods

Skill	Goal	Objectives Sample	Method Sample
Fine motor skills	Increase fine motor skills, including: using fingers, toes, hand-eye coordination, and dexterity	-will use hands to hit the ball/balloon, will pick up ball/balloon	Staff will give instructions, and residents will be involved in a game that requires small motor skills
Gross motor skills	Increase large motor skills	-will bend, stretch, jump, hit the ball (may also do from chair)	Staff will give instructions, and residents will be involved in a volleyball game that requires large motor skills
Perceptual speed and motor function	Increase speed and motor ability for function, safety, meaningful/fulfilling activities	-will increase acuity and hit the ball faster (with Dr. approval)	-Staff will give residents instructions on how to play the game -Staff will use varied types of game equipment (balloon or ball) to support resident's ability to hit the ball.
Following step patterns/backwards forward movement	Increase strength, balance, endurance, meaningful/fulfilling activities	-will stand/sit and hold ball, will hit the ball/balloon in the air, will hit the ball as it enters their space	Staff will ask residents to walk forwards/backwards and turn during the game while hitting the ball (support device if needed), or can be done sitting in a chair
Range of motion	Increase range of motion	-will lift arms, legs, bend, reach (to capacity - set by Dr./clinician), will extend and flex (to capacity - set by clinician)	Staff/clinician will instruct residents to do exercises that include flexing, extending muscles
Balance and Posture (approved by Dr. and capacity tests)	Increase balance and improve body alignment and flexibility	-will sit in chair and maintain posture, will stand and maintain posture	Staff will remind residents of proper posture and ask residents to hold body in straight alignment/ posture
Gait/Following Step patterns/ Backwards/Forward movement	Increase strength, balance, endurance, meaningful/fulfilling activities	-will stand up without losing balance and walk a safe pace (approved by Dr. and capacity tests), If approved clinical specialist: ____ ft. ________________________	Staff will call residents to the activity and have them walk to activity (w/device if needed) to work on leg strength (if approved by clinician etc.)
Cardio-vascular Workout*	Increase circulation, blood flow, stamina	-will play the game at a safe pace (approved by Dr. and capacity tests), If approved clinical specialist: ________________________	Staff/clinician will have residents play game (according to doctor approved ability and approved amount of exercise)

TABLE 8.2

Recreational Objectives Observation Form
Volleyball/Balloon Volleyball- Physical Skills

PATIENT		Dependent (Totally dependent)	High Assistance (25+ ability)	Moderate Assist. (50+ ability)	Mild Assistance (75+ability)	Independent (Totally independent.)			
SEE CODES BELOW		1	2	3	4	5			
USE OPTIONAL CODES IF APPROPRIATE		3 cue/ 2-3 physical	2-3 cues/ 2 physical	2-3 cues/ 1 physical	1-2 cues	Encouragement			
97530- Therapeutic activities or	**SKILL**	**GOAL**	**OBJECTIVES** ____times per ____		**METHOD**	**OUTCOME DATE**			
97530 Therapeutic Activity	FINE MOTOR SKILLS								
97110/ 97530	GROSS MOTOR SKILLS								
97110/ 97530/ If under cognitive code 97532	PERCEPTUAL SPEED/ MOTOR FUNCTION								
97530 or Gait training 97116-	STEP PATTERNS								
		Licensed/ Clinician	Dr. approved use only		Licensed/ Clinician				
97110	RANGE OF MOTION								
97112	POSTURE AND BALANCE								
97110 Or Gait training 97116-	GAIT (INCLUDES STAIR CLIMBING)								
97110	CARDIO-VASCULAR WORKOUT*								

97110-Therapeutic procedure, one or more areas, each 15 minutes; therapeutic exercises to develop strength and endurance, range of motion, and flexibility; 97112-Neuromuscular reeducation of movement, balance, coordination, kinesthetic sense, posture, and proprioception; **97113-Aquatic therapy** with therapeutic exercises; **97116-Gait training** (includes stair climbing); **97139-Unlisted therapeutic procedure** (specify); **97150 Therapeutic procedure(s)**, group (2 or more individuals); **97750-Physical performance test or measurement** (e.g., musculoskeletal, functional capacity), with written report, each 15 minutes; **97535-Self care/home management training** (e.g., activities of daily living and compensatory training, meal preparation, safety procedures, and instructions in use of adaptive equipment), direct (one-on-one) contact by provider, each 15 minutes; **Physical therapy 97001 evaluation, 97002 Re-evaluation. occupational therapy evaluation 97003, re-evaluation. 97004; Athlete training 97005; re-evaluation 97006**	Staff Initial				
	Add total score here Maximum Score 40 pt. each form per activity				
	See scale below or use own/facilities optional score system				

Score 1-8) =1 (9-16) =2 (17-24) =3 (25-32) =4 (33-40) =5 If w/device add d if wish, ex: 1d, 2d, or If using 1-7 scale: (41-48) =6 (49-56)

Volleyball/Balloon Volleyball
Socio-emotional Goals, Objectives and Methods

SKILL	GOAL	OBJECTIVES SAMPLE	METHOD SAMPLE
Socialization/Community Integration	Increase social interactions, meaningful/fulfilling activities	-will interact with peers, will engage in community integration experiences (for social skills), will use manners, social practices	Staff will engage residents in a sport and support/encourage residents to socialize through community integration and being paired w/group for games
Team Playing/Sharing	Increase teamwork/sharing, meaningful/fulfilling activities	-will join in on the game with others and share, wait turn, support peers	Staff will encourage residents to play, form teams, strategize together, include all members in play
Initiative and Motivation	Increase initiative and motivation/wellness, and quality of life	-will choose if they wish to play or not, will try a new technique, will initiate playing on own (or with assistance), will increase amount of practice after stating own goal	-Staff will support and encourage the residents to prepare/join activities for their own personal gains -Staff will offer new techniques to motivate resident's interests and desires
Emotional Gratification	Increase emotional gratification/wellness, and quality of life	-will state that the game was a gratifying experience or will show pleasure by smiling, laughing, deep focus, and involvement during the game	Staff will ask residents if they enjoyed the volleyball game and what they liked through the use of verbal discussion, group discussions or as observed
Sense of Accomplishment	Increase feelings of self-worth, pride, productivity, dignity/wellness, and quality of life	-will use gestures to express pride in self , will talk about their accomplishments while playing he game	Staff will place a chart on the unit wall or hand a paper to the residents that reflect the team scores, the charts/paper etc. will be available for residents to see their personal best
Self-esteem/self-identity	Increase self-esteem, feelings of belonging, dignity, self-worth, integrity, self-identity/wellness, and quality of life	-will state/communicate positive feelings about self and ability to play, will join game to take an active role in health though exercising, will join the game based on own choices	Staff will educate residents on the value of exercise and will encourage residents to join sports games
Fostering Appropriate Behaviors	Increase social interaction, social opportunities and adjustment, safety, using appropriate behaviors during an activity for a calm environment/wellness, and quality of life	-will adjust to the noises, other's movements, touch of volleyball/balloon, etc.	-Staff will engage residents in sports to expose residents to sensory stimulating experiences -Staff will support residents as they adjust to the stimulus one step at a time
Sensory Integration/Tolerating Stimulation	Increase sensory processing and enhance awareness of sensations and toleration/adaptation of sensory stimulations and demands	-will join in on volleyball class, listen and follow instructions, use appropriate behavior for the setting; will wait turn, stand in line quietly; will quiet down when asked	Before class begins, staff will discuss the rules, appropriate behaviors, respect of property, safety, and respect of fellow team players

TABLE 8.3

Recreational Objectives Observation Form
Volleyball/balloon Volleyball- Socio-emotional skills

PATIENT	Dependent (Totally dependent)	High Assistance (25+ ability)	Moderate Assist. (50+ ability)	Mild Assistance (75+ability)	Independent (Totally independent.)
SEE CODES BELOW USE OPTIONAL CODES IF APPROPRIATE	1	2	3	4	5
	3 cue/ 2-3 physical	2-3 cues/ 2 physical	2-3 cues/ 1 physical	1-2 cues	Encouragement

97530- Therapeutic activities or	SKILL	GOAL	OBJECTIVES ____times per ____	METHOD	OUTCOME DATE			
97537 Or 97535	SOCIALIZATION/ COMMUNITY INTEGRATION							
97537 Or 97535	TEAM PLAYING /SHARING							
97537 Or 97535	INITIATIVE AND MOTIVATION							
97537 Or 97535	EMOTIONAL GRATIFICATION							
97537 Or 97535	SENSE OF ACCOMPLISHM ENT							
97537 Or 97535	SELF-ESTEEM/ SELF-IDENTITY							
97537 Or 97535	FOSTERING APPROPRIATE BEHAVIORS							
97533	SENSORY INTEGRATION/ TOLERATING							

97537-Community/work reintegration training (e.g., shopping, transportation, money management, avocational activities and/or work environment/modification analysis, work task analysis), direct (one-on-one) contact by provider, each 15 minutes; **97535-Self care/home management training** (e.g., activities of daily living and compensatory training, meal preparation, safety procedures, and instructions in use of adaptive equipment), direct (one-on-one) contact by provider, each 15 minutes; **97530-Therapeutic activities, direct (one-on-one)** patient contact by the provider (use of dynamic activities to improve functional performance), each 15 minutes; **97150-Therapeutic procedure(s), group (2 or more individuals); 97533-Sensory integration techniques** to enhance sensory processing and promote adaptive responses to environmental demands, direct (one-on-one) patient contact by the provider, each 15 minutes; **occupational therapy evaluation 97003, re-evaluation . 97004**	Staff Initial				
	Add total score here-Maximum Score 40 pt. each form per activity				
	See scale below or use own/facilities optional score system				

(Score 1-8)=1 (9-16) =2 (17-24) =3 (25-32) =4 (33-40) =5 If w/device add d if wish, ex: 1d, 2d, or If using 1-7 scale: (41-48) =6 (49-56)

Walking

Objectives and benefits

***Cognitive Challenges**:* attention, memory, language, orientation, following patterns, keeping rhythm, perceptual awareness, and cognitive stimulation

***Physical Needs**:* fine motor skills, gross motor skills, coordination, range of motion, flexibility, posture, balance, backward and forward movement, gait, following step patterns, circulation, cardio-vascular workout

Socio-emotional Needs: socialization, community integration, initiative and motivation, emotional gratification, sense of accomplishment, self-esteem, tolerating stimulation, fostering appropriate behaviors, relaxation, solace and healing

Supplies: Good sneakers, weather-suitable outfit

Time: 20–30 minutes

Staff/older adult ratio: 1:2 It is very important to pay close attention to the whereabouts and safety of the residents while taking a walk. They could fall or wander off. This might be an issue if you have residents with dementia problems. Also, be careful of weather changes while on the walk. Keep in mind the different strengths of the residents. It is best to use caution and have plenty of staff.

Instructions: Have older adults warm up for dancing by leading them in a sub maximal active warm-up first. This will gradually increase their body temperature, blood flow to the muscles, and synovial fluid to the joints. Then you may lead them in a three to five minute stretching exercise. Then just walk and enjoy!

The CDC recommends that older adults participate in moderate-intensity aerobic activity 3-5 days a week for at least 30 minutes. This will help older adults to increase endurance, strength, and balance. It is also recommended that older adults engage in activities that include stretching everyday and strength training activities 2-3 days per week. (CDC, NCCDPHP. Special focus: healthy aging. Chronic Disease Notes and Reports 1999; 12(3): 10-11. Insert CDC recommendations obtained from aoa.hhs.gov 2005

*Walking 30 minutes per day has been shown to be beneficial for those suffering from arthritic conditions. Walking has also been shown to enhance cognitive function.

* All older adults should have physician approval before engage in formalized physical activities

Walking
Cognitive Goals, Objectives, and Methods

SKILL	GOAL	OBJECTIVES SAMPLE	METHOD SAMPLE
Orientation	Show increased awareness of, time/"timeframe," people, circumstances, and past experiences vs. present experiences, to engage in present-time activities, or for a reminiscing intended question	-will respond with correct answer to two choice questions Or yes/no answer, will state where they are, time of day, present company of people on own and with the correct answer	Staff will ask the residents a series of questions to stimulate focus to the present setting, Or past if reminiscing exercise (Ex: "Did you walk or do yard work at home?")
Attention	Show increased attention span, task for function, and to engage in meaningful, recreational/fulfilling activities	-will make eye-contact with staff for _____ sec. will verbalize with staff and instructor	Staff will address or stand in front of resident, make eye-contact, ask questions, or use others methods to get resident's attention/gauge attention (Ex: "Where did I say we where walking to?")
Memory	Show increased memory skills of recall, recognition, retention of information, working memory	-will repeat/recall identification of items on the walk, will recall events when back at the center	-Staff will take residents on a walk and, after, return to the unit -Staff will ask residents to share what they saw -Staff will show residents a special sight when on a trip, and ask them to remember the sight and describe it later at the unit
Language	Show increased ability to communicate use of words, phrases, sentence structure, comprehension, interpretation	-will answer questions and reply with a yes/no when asked questions about what they saw on the trip, will interact with peers and staff	Staff will ask questions to stimulate a communication (Ex: "Tell me, did you see a dog or a cat while walking? Who was walking in front of you? Sara or Jan?")
Cognitive Stimulation (awareness, seeks information in)	Increased stimulus/exposure for visual/ motor memory, cognitive experiences/awareness and brain stimulation to enhance (function, pragmatics, neuroplasticity)	-will look around the streets as they walk, will listen/seek cognitive stimulation, will accept challenge of input information and engage/interact in game	While on a walk, staff talk about an environmental issue or show residents special sights
Perceptual Awareness	Show increased abilities of depth perception, visio-spatical awareness, and acuity (for discrimination, comparison, and categorizing), safety	-will stay within own space next to others, will maneuver around sidewalk etc.	Staff will instruct the residents on where they need to stay within the sidewalk area, and walk with enough distance between each other and objects on the path
Problem-solving (goes beyond thinking/stimulus and initiates thinking process)	Increase problem-solving ability, processing of information, thinking, reasoning, and use of good judgment and decision-making	-will use good judgment on rules, safety of walking, will walk at a pace and rhythm set for all walkers on trip	Staff will talk about the environment and offer the residents educational experiences, stimulating questions to spark thinking, etc., and offer hands on experiences if possible
Complete a task	Increase ability to complete a task	-will recall/retain and sort/gather information, problem-solve, and complete activity	-Staff will explain the procedure/agenda regarding events, understanding to support resident's ability to follow procedures -Staff will instruct, encourage, make use of adaptive devices, if needed, and supply necessary materials and support

TABLE 9.1

Recreational Objectives Observation Form
Walking- Cognitive skills

PATIENT	Dependent (Totally dependent)	High Assistance (25+ ability)	Moderate Assist. (50+ ability)	Mild Assistance (75+ability)	Independent (Totally independent)
SEE CODES BELOW USE OPTIONAL CODES IF APPROPRIATE	1	2	3	4	5
	3 cue/ 2-3 physical	2-3 cues/ 2 physical	2-3 cues/ 1 physical	1-2 cues	Encourageme nt

97530-Therapeutic activities or	SKILL	GOAL	OBJECTIVES ____times per ____	METHOD	OUTCOME DATE			
97532 Cognitive skills or if using Therapeutic Activity code-9753o	ORIENTATION							
97532 Cognitive skills	ATTENTION							
97532 Cognitive skills	MEMORY							
97532 Cognitive skills	PROBLEM-SOLVING							
97532 Cognitive skills	COMPLETE A TASK							
97139 Speech Therapy 97532 Cognitive skills	LANGUAGE							
97533	SENSORY STIMULATION/ COGNITIVE STIMULATION							
97532	PERCEPTUAL AWARENESS							

97532-Development of cognitive skills to improve attention, memory, problem-solving, includes compensatory training and/or sensory integrative activities, direct (one-on-one) patient contact by the provider, each 15 minutes; **97530-Therapeutic activities**, direct (one-on-one) patient contact by the provider (use of dynamic activities to improve functional performance), each 15 minutes; **97533-Sensory integration techniques** to enhance sensory processing and promote adaptive responses to environmental demands, direct (one-on-one) patient contact by the provider, each 15 minutes; **97150-Therapeutic procedure(s)**, group (2 or more individuals); **97139-Unlisted therapeutic procedure** (specify) minutes; **97003- occupational therapy evaluation**; **97004- re-evaluation**	Staff Initial				
	Add total score here -Maximum Score 40 pt. each form per activity				
	See scale below or use own/facilities optional score system				

(Score 1-8)=1 (9-16) =2 (17-24) =3 (25-32) =4 (33-40) =5 If w/device add d if wish, ex: 1d, 2d, or If using 1-7 scale: (41-48) =6 (49-56)

Walking
Physical Goals, Objectives and Methods

SKILL	GOAL	OBJECTIVES SAMPLE	METHOD SAMPLE
Fine motor skills	Increase fine motor skills, including: using fingers, toes, hand-eye coordination, and dexterity	-will flex and stretch fingers during sub maximal warm up for walk	While on a unit walk, staff will stop with the residents and admire and prune the flowers in the garden, do sub maximal warm up before walking
Gross motor skills	Increase large motor skills	-will bend, stretch, walk	Staff will take residents on a walk, and residents will use large motor skills/muscles
Perceptual speed and motor function	Increase speed and motor ability for function, safety, meaningful/fulfilling activities	-will walk at a beginning pace and continue to increase speed (with Dr. approval)	While walking, the staff member will carry watch and observe if the residents have begun to walk at an increased rate and ability
Following step patterns/backwards forward movement	Increase strength, balance, endurance, meaningful/fulfilling activities	-will walk forward	During sub maximal warm-up, staff will ask residents to take a step backwards/forwards (support device if needed), as part of front and back leg strength exercises
Range of Motion	Increase range of motion	-will lift arms, legs (to capacity - set by Dr./clinician), will extend and flex (to capacity -set by Dr./clinician)	Staff will instruct residents to do exercises that include flexing and extending muscles
Balance and Posture (approved by Dr. and capacity tests)	Increase balance and improve body alignment and flexibility	-will maintain adequate posture while walking	While walking, staff will show residents proper posture while walking, and residents will be asked to hold body in straight alignment/posture (Dr. approved)
Gait/Following Step patterns/ Backwards/Forward movement	Increase strength, balance, endurance, meaningful/fulfilling activities	-will stand up without losing balance, and walks a safe pace (approved by Dr. and capacity tests) If approved, clinical specialist: _____ft. ________________________________	Staff will ask residents to walk as a measure to strengthen leg muscles to benefit balance and gait
Cardio-vascular Workout*	Increase circulation, blood flow, stamina	-will walk at a safe pace (approved by Dr. and capacity tests) If approved, clinical specialist: ________________________________	Staff will offer walking opportunities to enhance walking/cardio-vascular workout (according to ability and approved by Dr.)

TABLE 9.2

Recreational Objectives Observation Form
Walking - Physical Skills

PATIENT		Dependent (Totally dependent)	High Assistance (25+ ability)	Moderate Assist. (50+ ability)	Mild Assistance (75+ability)	Independent (Totally independent.)
SEE CODES BELOW USE OPTIONAL CODES IF APPROPRIATE		1	2	3	4	5
		3 cue/ 2-3 physical	2-3 cues/ 2 physical	2-3 cues/ 1 physical	1-2 cues	Encouragement
97530- Therapeutic activities or	SKILL	GOAL	OBJECTIVES ____times per ____		METHOD	OUTCOME DATE
97530 Therapeutic Activity	FINE MOTOR SKILLS					
97110/ 97530	GROSS MOTOR SKILLS					
97110/ 97530/ If under cognitive code 97532	PERCEPTUAL SPEED/ MOTOR FUNCTION					
97530 or Gait training 97116-	STEP PATTERNS					
		Licensed/ Clinician	Dr. approved use only		Licensed/ Clinician	
97110	RANGE OF MOTION					
97112	POSTURE AND BALANCE					
97110 Or Gait training 97116-	GAIT (INCLUDES STAIR CLIMBING)					
97110	CARDIO-VASCULAR WORKOUT*					

97110-Therapeutic procedure, one or more areas, each 15 minutes; therapeutic exercises to develop strength and endurance, range of motion, and flexibility; 97112-Neuromuscular reeducation of movement, balance, coordination, kinesthetic sense, posture, and proprioception; **97113-Aquatic therapy** with therapeutic exercises; **97116-Gait training** (includes stair climbing); **97139-Unlisted therapeutic procedure** (specify); **97150 Therapeutic procedure(s)**, group (2 or more individuals); **97750-Physical performance test or measurement** (e.g., musculoskeletal, functional capacity), with written report, each 15 minutes; **97535-Self care/home management training** (e.g., activities of daily living and compensatory training, meal preparation, safety procedures, and instructions in use of adaptive equipment), direct (one-on-one) contact by provider, each 15 minutes; **Physical therapy 97001 evaluation, 97002 Re-evaluation. occupational therapy evaluation 97003, re-evaluation. 97004; Athlete training 97005; re-evaluation 97006**

Staff Initial

Add total score here Maximum Score 40 pt. each form per activity

See scale below or use own/facilities optional score system

Score 1-8) =1 (9-16) =2 (17-24) =3 (25-32) =4 (33-40) =5 If w/device add d if wish, ex: 1d, 2d, or If using 1-7 scale: (41-48) =6 (49-56)

Walking
Socio-emotional Goals, Objectives, and Methods

SKILL	GOAL	OBJECTIVES SAMPLE	METHOD SAMPLE
Socialization/Community Integration	Increase social interactions, meaningful/fulfilling activities	-will interact with peers, will engage in community integration experiences (for social skills), will use manners, social practices	Staff will take residents on a walk and support/encourage them to socialize through community integration and being paired w/other walkers
Team Playing/Sharing	Increase teamwork/sharing, meaningful/fulfilling activities	-will join in on the game with others and share, wait turn, support peers, and show compassion, will listen to each other's laughs and sorrows	Staff will encourage residents to talk, share a story or joke with others, and show compassion by listening to each other and including each other in activity
Initiative and Motivation	Increase initiative and motivation/wellness, and quality of life	-will choose if they wish to walk, will try a new walking terrain, will initiate walking on own (or with assistance), will increase amount of walking after stating own goal	-Staff will support/encourage the resident to prepare for walk by having proper shoes, a drink, etc., and be ready for the walk in a timely fashion for their own personal gains of joining walkers -Staff will offer new routes to motivate continued walking
Emotional Gratification	Increase emotional gratification/wellness, and quality of life	-will state that the game was a gratifying experience, or will show pleasure by smiling, laughing, focus and involvement during the walk	Staff will ask residents if they enjoyed walking and what they liked through verbal discussion, writing, group discussions
Sense of Accomplishment	Increase feelings of self-worth, pride, productivity, dignity/wellness, and quality of life	-will use gestures to express pride in self, will talk about their accomplishments of walking length, speed	Staff will place a chart on the unit wall or hand a paper to the resident that reflects the residents' walk time, etc. -This info will be made available for residents to see their personal best/increased walking ability, length of walks, etc.
Self-esteem/self-identity	Increase self-esteem, feelings of belonging, dignity, self-worth, integrity, self-identity/wellness, and quality of life	-will state positive feelings about self and ability to walk, will join walk to take an active role in health though exercising, will join the game based on own choices	Staff will educate residents on the value of walking and exercise, and residents will be encouraged to continue walking activities
Sensory Integration/Tolerating Stimulation	Increase sensory processing and enhance awareness of sensations and toleration/adaptation of sensory stimulations and demands	-will adjust to the environmental sounds, sights, smells, tactile experiences (and, if a snack from store, taste)	-Staff will take residents on a walk, and residents will be exposed to sensory stimulating experiences -Staff will support residents as they adjust to the stimulus
Sensory Integration/Tolerating Stimulation	Increase social interaction, social opportunities and adjustment, safety, using appropriate behaviors during an activity for a calm environment/wellness, and quality of life	-will join in on exercise class, listen and follow instructions, use appropriate behavior for the setting; will wait turn, stand in line quietly; will quiet down when asked	Before walk begins, staff will discuss the rules, appropriate behaviors, respect of property, safety, and respect of fellow walkers while on the walk

TABLE 9.3

Recreational Objectives Observation Form

Walking - Socio-emotional Skills

PATIENT	Dependent (Totally dependent)	High Assistance (25+ ability)	Moderate Assist. (50+ ability)	Mild Assistance (75+ability)	Independent (Totally independent.)
SEE CODES BELOW USE OPTIONAL CODES IF APPROPRIATE	1	2	3	4	5
	3 cue/ 2-3 physical	2-3 cues/ 2 physical	2-3 cues/ 1 physical	1-2 cues	Encouragement

97530- Therapeutic activities or	**SKILL**	**GOAL**	**OBJECTIVES** ____times per ____	**METHOD**	**OUTCOME DATE**			
97537 Or 97535	SOCIALIZATION/ COMMUNITY INTEGRATION							
97537 Or 97535	TEAM PLAYING /SHARING							
97537 Or 97535	INITIATIVE AND MOTIVATION							
97537 Or 97535	EMOTIONAL GRATIFICATION							
97537 Or 97535	SENSE OF ACCOMPLISHM ENT							
97537 Or 97535	SELF-ESTEEM/ SELF-IDENTITY							
97537 Or 97535	FOSTERING APPROPRIATE BEHAVIORS							
97533	SENSORY INTEGRATION/ TOLERATING							

97537-Community/work reintegration training (e.g., shopping, transportation, money management, avocational activities and/or work environment/modification analysis, work task analysis), direct (one-on-one) contact by provider, each 15 minutes; **97535-Self care/home management training** (e.g., activities of daily living and compensatory training, meal preparation, safety procedures, and instructions in use of adaptive equipment), direct (one-on-one) contact by provider, each 15 minutes; **97530-Therapeutic activities, direct (one-on-one)** patient contact by the provider (use of dynamic activities to improve functional performance), each 15 minutes; **97150-Therapeutic procedure(s), group (2 or more individuals); 97533-Sensory integration techniques** to enhance sensory processing and promote adaptive responses to environmental demands, direct (one-on-one) patient contact by the provider, each 15 minutes; **occupational therapy evaluation 97003, re-evaluation . 97004**	Staff Initial				
	Add total score here-Maximum Score 40 pt. each form per activity				
	See scale below or use own/facilities optional score system				

(Score 1-8)=1 (9-16) =2 (17-24) =3 (25-32) =4 (33-40) =5 If w/device add d if wish, ex: 1d, 2d, or If using 1-7 scale: (41-48) =6 (49-56)

Yoga

Objectives and benefits

***Cognitive Challenges**:* attention, memory, language, orientation, following patterns, keeping rhythm, perceptual awareness, and cognitive stimulation

***Physical Needs**:* fine motor skills, gross motor skills, coordination, range of motion, flexibility, posture, balance, backward and forward movement, gait, following step patterns, circulation, cardio-vascular workout

Socio-emotional Needs: socialization, community integration, initiative and motivation, emotional gratification, sense of accomplishment, self-esteem, tolerating stimulation, fostering appropriate behaviors, relaxation, solace and healing

Supplies: Meditation tapes and/or aromatherapy supplies

Time: 20–30 minutes

Staff/older adult ratio: 1:6 or as assessed per needs of individuals or group

Instructions: Have the residents join together in a circle. Have them warm up for Yoga by leading them in a sub maximal active warm-up first. This will gradually increase their body temperature, blood flow to the muscles, and synovial fluid to the joints. Then you may lead them in a three to five minute stretching exercise.

Explain the benefits of yoga and what they will do during a yoga exercise. You can use meditation tapes or soothing sounds to encourage relaxation. Demonstrate breathing and body positioning of the yoga experience. The staff member doing yoga can model and encourage slow, gentle, and relaxed movements. Have residents do the exercise with your assistance.

The CDC recommends that older adults participate in moderate-intensity aerobic activity 3-5 days a week for at least 30 minutes. This will help older adults to increase endurance, strength, and balance. It is also recommended that older adults engage in activities that include stretching everyday and strength training activities 2-3 days per week. (CDC, NCCDPHP. Special focus: healthy aging. Chronic Disease Notes and Reports 1999; 12(3): 10-11. Insert CDC recommendations obtained from aoa.hhs.gov 2005

*Walking 30 minutes per day has been shown to be beneficial for those suffering from arthritic conditions. Walking has also been shown to enhance cognitive function.

* All older adults should have physician approval before engage in formalized physical activities

Yoga
Cognitive Goals, Objectives and Methods

SKILL	GOAL	OBJECTIVES SAMPLE	METHOD SAMPLE
Orientation	Show increased awareness of, time/"timeframe," people, circumstances, and past experiences vs. present experiences, to engage in present-time activities, or for a reminiscing intended question	-will respond with correct answer to two choice questions, will state where they are, time of day, present company of people on own and with correct answer	-Staff will ask residents a series of questions to stimulate focus to the present setting, and then challenge with imagery picturing to help residents relax (Ex: "Imagine you are by a tree sitting in the grass.") -Staff will also ask questions to gauge/stabilize orientation to moment (Ex: "Are you at the mall or at the activity center?")
Attention	Show increased attention span, task for function, and to engage in meaningful, recreational/fulfilling activities	-will make eye-contact with yoga instructor for _____ sec., will verbalize with staff and instructor, will read/listen to rules, will say yes/no to show understand	Staff will address or stand in front of resident, make eye-contact, ask questions, or use others forms to get resident's attention/gauge attention (Ex: observe if residents are trying to do positioning asked to do)
Memory	Show increased memory skills of recall, recognition, retention of information, working memory	-will repeat/recall movements learned, will repeat/recall how to do steps, will remember lesson at next class	Staff will show steps on yoga positions and ask residents to repeat the actions, then ask resident to repeat the action 5-to-10 minutes later, the follow day, etc.
Language	Show increased ability to communicate use of words, phrases, sentence structure, comprehension, interpretation	-will be asked two choice question or yes/no, will interpret instructor's request and follow	Staff will ask questions to stimulate communication or have residents hum as they relax their bodies and release all excess tension
Cognitive Stimulation (awareness, seeks information in)	Increased stimulus/exposure for visual/ motor memory, cognitive experiences/awareness and brain stimulation to enhance (function, pragmatics, neuro-plasticity)	-will look around the room, will interact with peers, will listen/seek cognitive stimulation, will accept challenge of input information and engage/interact in game	Staff will ask residents to do own imagery exercise while doing yoga positioning, breathing, etc.
Perceptual Awareness	Show increased abilities of depth perception, visual-spatial awareness, and acuity (for discrimination, comparison, and categorizing), safety	-will stay within own space next to others, will be aware of own body in relation to self, others, objects	Staff will instruct the residents on where they need to stay in their own space (portions to other areas)
Problem-solving (goes beyond thinking/stimulus and initiates thinking process)	Increase problem-solving ability, processing of information, thinking, reasoning, and use of good judgment and decision-making	-will use good judgment of speed and motor coordination, movement rhythm of yoga, breathing; will stretch, flex, and move arms and legs in order of instruction	Staff will direct the residents on using a series of techniques for Yoga. Staff will answer questions regarding understanding of steps and offer the residents challenging strategies for processing info. Staff will guide residents on how to breath correctly and position according to rhythm of yoga movements
Complete a Task	Increase ability to complete a task	-will recall/retain and sort/gather information, problem-solve, and complete activity	-Staff will explain the procedure/agenda regarding yoga and guide residents in ability to follow/complete yoga. -Staff will instruct, encourage, make use of adaptive devices, if needed, and supply necessary materials and support

TABLE 10.1

Recreational Objectives Observation Form
Yoga - Cognitive skills

PATIENT		Dependent (Totally dependent)	High Assistance (25+ ability)	Moderate Assist. (50+ ability)	Mild Assistance (75+ability)	Independent (Totally independent)
SEE CODES BELOW USE OPTIONAL CODES IF APPROPRIATE		1	2	3	4	5
		3 cue/ 2-3 physical	2-3 cues/ 2 physical	2-3 cues/ 1 physical	1-2 cues	Encouragement
97530- Therapeutic activities or	**SKILL**	**GOAL**	**OBJECTIVES** ____times per ____		**METHOD**	**OUTCOME DATE**
97532 Cognitive skills	ORIENTATION					
97532 Cognitive skills	ATTENTION					
97532 Cognitive skills	MEMORY					
97532 Cognitive skills	PROBLEM-SOLVING					
97532 Cognitive skills	COMPLETE A TASK					
97139 Speech Therapy 97532 Cognitive skills	LANGUAGE					
97533	SENSORY STIMULATION/ COGNITIVE STIMULATION					
97532	PERCEPTUAL AWARENESS					

97532-Development of cognitive skills to improve attention, memory, problem-solving, includes compensatory training and/or sensory integrative activities, direct (one-on-one) patient contact by the provider, each 15 minutes; **97530-Therapeutic activities**, direct (one-on-one) patient contact by the provider (use of dynamic activities to improve functional performance), each 15 minutes; **97533-Sensory integration techniques** to enhance sensory processing and promote adaptive responses to environmental demands, direct (one-on-one) patient contact by the provider, each 15 minutes; **97150-Therapeutic procedure(s)**, group (2 or more individuals); **97139-Unlisted therapeutic procedure** (specify) minutes; **97003- occupational therapy evaluation**; **97004- re-evaluation**	Staff Initial Add total score here -Maximum Score 40 pt. each form per activity See scale below or use own/facilities optional score system

(Score 1-8)=1 (9-16) =2 (17-24) =3 (25-32) =4 (33-40) =5 If w/device add d if wish, ex: 1d, 2d, or If using 1-7 scale: (41-48) =6 (49-56)

Yoga
Physical Goals, Objectives, and Methods

Skill	Goal	Objectives Sample	Method Sample
Fine motor skills	Increase fine motor skills, including: using fingers, toes, hand-eye coordination, and dexterity	-will move fingers in motion to the yoga exercise	Staff will give instructions on the steps to a particular yoga routine and include small motor abilities
Gross motor skills	Increase large motor skills	-will bend, stretch, turn and do Yoga movements	Staff will give instructions on the steps to a particular yoga routine and include large motor abilities
Perceptual speed and motor function	Increase speed and motor ability for function, safety, meaningful/fulfilling activities	-will do a slow style dance, will do a moderate style yoga routine (with Dr. approval)	Staff will introduce new movements to increase perceptual speed and motor skills
Following step patterns/backwards forward movement	Increase strength, balance, endurance, meaningful/fulfilling activities	-will walk forward during yoga, will turn, change direction of path; will walk backwards, will walk backwards and forwards, will walk backwards, forwards, turn, move all directions	Staff will ask residents to move forwards/backwards and turn (with support device if needed) during yoga routine
Range of motion	Increase range of motion	-will lift arms, legs, trunk (to capacity - set by Dr./clinician), will extend and flex (to capacity - set by clinician)	Staff will instruct residents to do exercises that include flexing, extending muscles
Balance and Posture (approved by Dr. and capacity tests)	Increase balance and improve body alignment and flexibility	-will hold on to a railing and show proper posture for 3 min., will stand to do yoga routine using proper alignment/posture	While doing yoga staff will show residents proper posture and ask residents to hold body in straight alignment/posture for at 3 minutes (then increase)
Gait/Following Step patterns/ Backwards/Forward movement	Increase strength, balance, endurance, meaningful/fulfilling activities	-will stand up, without losing balance, and walk at a safe pace (approved by Dr. and capacity tests), If approved, clinical specialist: _____ ft. ______________________________	Staff will show residents the proper posture / balance and gait for yoga steps, and have them hold body in straight alignment/posture (may hold on to railing for safety or use device if needed) (with Dr. approval)
Cardio-vascular Workout*	Increase circulation, blood flow, stamina	-will dance at a safe pace (approved by Dr. and capacity tests), If approved, clinical specialist: ______________________________	Staff will have residents do routine (according to ability

TABLE 10.2

Recreational Objectives Observation Form
Yoga- Physical Skills

PATIENT		Dependent (Totally dependent)	High Assistance (25+ ability)	Moderate Assist. (50+ ability)	Mild Assistance (75+ability)	Independent (Totally independent.)
SEE CODES BELOW USE OPTIONAL CODES IF APPROPRIATE		1	2	3	4	5
		3 cue/ 2-3 physical	2-3 cues/ 2 physical	2-3 cues/ 1 physical	1-2 cues	Encouragement
97530- Therapeutic activities or	**SKILL**	**GOAL**	**OBJECTIVES** ____times per ____		**METHOD**	**OUTCOME DATE**
97530 Therapeutic Activity	FINE MOTOR SKILLS					
97110/ 97530	GROSS MOTOR SKILLS					
97110/ 97530/ If under cognitive code 97532	PERCEPTUAL SPEED/ MOTOR FUNCTION					
97530 or Gait training 97116-	STEP PATTERNS					
		Licensed/ Clinician	Dr. approved use only		Licensed/ Clinician	
97110	RANGE OF MOTION					
97112	POSTURE AND BALANCE					
97110 Or Gait training 97116-	GAIT (INCLUDES STAIR CLIMBING)					
97110	CARDIO-VASCULAR WORKOUT*					

97110-Therapeutic procedure, one or more areas, each 15 minutes; therapeutic exercises to develop strength and endurance, range of motion, and flexibility; 97112-Neuromuscular reeducation of movement, balance, coordination, kinesthetic sense, posture, and proprioception; **97116-Gait training** (includes stair climbing); **97139-Unlisted therapeutic procedure** (specify); **97150 Therapeutic procedure(s)**, group (2 or more individuals); **97750-Physical performance test or measurement** (e.g., musculoskeletal, functional capacity), with written report, each 15 minutes; **97535-Self care/home management training** (e.g., activities of daily living and compensatory training, meal preparation, safety procedures, and instructions in use of adaptive equipment), direct (one-on-one) contact by provider, each 15 minutes; **Physical therapy 97001 evaluation, 97002 Re-evaluation. occupational therapy evaluation 97003, re-evaluation. 97004; Athlete training 97005; re-evaluation 97006**	Staff Initial	
	Add total score here Maximum Score 40 pt. each form per activity	
	See scale below or use own/facilities optional score system	

Score 1-8) =1 (9-16) =2 (17-24) =3 (25-32) =4 (33-40) =5 If w/device add d if wish, ex: 1d, 2d, or If using 1-7 scale: (41-48) =6 (49-56)

Yoga

SOCIO-EMOTIONAL GOALS, OBJECTIVES AND METHODS

SKILL	GOAL	OBJECTIVES SAMPLE	METHOD SAMPLE
Socialization/Community Integration	Increase social interactions, meaningful/fulfilling activities	-will interact with peers, will engage in community integration experiences (for social skills), will use manners, social practices	Staff will take residents to a yoga class and support/encourage them to socialize through community integration and being paired w/other residents interested in yoga
Team Playing/Sharing	Increase teamwork/sharing, meaningful/fulfilling activities	-will join in on yoga activity with others and share, wait turn, support peers _____ time(s) this week	Staff will encourage residents to sit quietly together and experience yoga class/relaxation activity
Initiative and Motivation	Increase initiative and motivation/wellness, and quality of life	-will choose if they wish to yoga or not, will choose if wishes to join in with group, will try a new technique, will do yoga moves on own or with assistance	Staff will support/encourage the resident to prepare for yoga (loose relaxed clothing) for their own personal gains in the healing soothing activity of yoga; will offer new yoga techniques/music, etc. to motivate
Emotional Gratification	Increase emotional gratification/wellness, and quality of life	-will state that the class is a gratifying experience, or will show pleasure by smiling, laughing, deep focus on activity	Staff will ask residents if they enjoyed the yoga class and what they liked through verbal discussion, writing, group discussions
Sense of Accomplishment	Increase feelings of self-worth, pride, productivity, dignity/wellness, and quality of life	-will use gestures to express pride in self, will talk about leaning yoga	Staff will ask resident to share what they gained while partaking in the yoga exercise
Self-esteem/self-identity	Increase self-esteem, feelings of belonging, dignity, self-worth, integrity, self-identity/wellness, and quality of life	-will state/communicate positive feelings about self, will join yoga class to take an active role in maintaining health though exercising, will join class based on own choices	Staff will educate residents on the value of exercise/relaxation methods and continued use of the activities
Sensory Integration/Tolerating Stimulation	Increase sensory processing and enhance awareness of sensations and toleration/adaptation of sensory stimulations and demands	-will join in on yoga class, will listen and follow instructions, use appropriate behavior for the setting; will wait turn, stand in line quietly, will quiet down when asked -will relax _____ time(s) this week	-Staff will take residents to a yoga class and residents will be exposed to sensory stimulating experiences -Staff will support residents as they adjust to the stimulus one step at a time
Fostering Appropriate Behaviors	Increase social interaction, social opportunities and adjustment, safety, using appropriate behaviors during an activity for a calm environment/wellness, and quality of life	asked -will relax _____ time(s) this week	Before yoga class begins, staff will discuss the rules, appropriate behaviors, respect of property, safety, and respect of fellow peers/instructor

Table 10.3

Recreational Objectives Observation Form
Yoga- Socio-emotional Skills

Patient	Dependent (Totally dependent)	High Assistance (25+ ability)	Moderate Assist. (50+ ability)	Mild Assistance (75+ability)	Independent (Totally independent.)
SEE CODES BELOW USE OPTIONAL CODES IF APPROPRIATE	1	2	3	4	5
	3 cue/ 2-3 physical	2-3 cues/ 2 physical	2-3 cues/ 1 physical	1-2 cues	Encouragement

97530- Therapeutic activities or	**Skill**	**Goal**	**Objectives** ____times per ____	**Method**	**Outcome Date**			
97537 Or 97535	Socialization/ Community Integration							
97537 Or 97535	Team Playing /Sharing							
97537 Or 97535	Initiative and Motivation							
97537 Or 97535	Emotional Gratification							
97537 Or 97535	Sense of Accomplishment							
97537 Or 97535	Self-esteem/ Self-identity							
97537 Or 97535	Fostering Appropriate Behaviors							
97533	Sensory Integration/ Tolerating							

97537-Community/work reintegration training (e.g., shopping, transportation, money management, avocational activities and/or work environment/modification analysis, work task analysis), direct (one-on-one) contact by provider, each 15 minutes; **97535-Self care/home management training** (e.g., activities of daily living and compensatory training, meal preparation, safety procedures, and instructions in use of adaptive equipment), direct (one-on-one) contact by provider, each 15 minutes; **97530-Therapeutic activities, direct (one-on-one)** patient contact by the provider (use of dynamic activities to improve functional performance), each 15 minutes; **97150-Therapeutic procedure(s), group (2 or more individuals); 97533-Sensory integration techniques** to enhance sensory processing and promote adaptive responses to environmental demands, direct (one-on-one) patient contact by the provider, each 15 minutes; **occupational therapy evaluation 97003, re-evaluation . 97004**	Staff Initial				
	Add total score here-Maximum Score 40 pt. each form per activity				
	See scale below or use own/facilities optional score system				

(Score 1-8)=1 (9-16) =2 (17-24) =3 (25-32) =4 (33-40) =5 If w/device add d if wish, ex: 1d, 2d, or If using 1-7 scale: (41-48) =6 (49-56)

Games/Educational Activities

(Primary cognitive stimulation)

Research has shown activities that help cognition of sensory/motor and speed processing will be geared towards help in visual and motor memory, discrimination, comparison, and categorizing areas. Reminiscing activities may help improve memory skills. Long-term studies (Arbuckle and others, 1998) have consistently showed that stimulating the brain with activities helps cognitive function in a similar way exercise helps muscle function.

Bingo

Objectives and benefits:

Cognitive Challenges**:** attention, memory, language, orientation, following patterns, obeying rules, letter and number recognition and recall.

Physical Needs**:** fine motor skills, possible gross motor skills, hand-eye coordination, perceptual speed and motor function, grasping small objects.

Socio-emotional Needs**:** socialization, community integration, awareness of others, team playing, emotional gratification, tolerating stimulation, fostering appropriate behaviors.

Supplies: Large print Bingo boards, large chips for easier grasp to pick up and place on the bingo boards.

Time: 30 minutes

Staff/older adult ratio: 1:10 or as assessed per needs of individuals or group

Instructions: Have one board and plenty of chips for each resident. You can have a staff member call out number/letter from a bowl or let one resident do this if they would like. When they have covered the appropriate number of spaces, they need to call out bingo. If unable to verify through speech, a bell may be placed by them to ring or jingle. If you have residents with restricted arm use or sight, it is okay to have a staff member play for them, they will still be able to win because they possessed the winning board and this will bring a sense of joy to anyone. You can have a winner's token if you like.

Research has shown activities that help cognition of sensory/motor and speed processing will be geared towards help in visual and motor memory, discrimination, comparison, and categorizing areas and may help improve memory skills. Long-term studies (Arbuckle and others, 1998) have consistently showed that stimulating the brain with activities helps cognitive function in a similar way exercise helps muscle function.

BINGO
COGNITIVE GOALS, OBJECTIVE AND METHODS

SKILL	GOAL	OBJECTIVES SAMPLE	METHOD SAMPLE
Orientation	Show increased awareness of, time/"timeframe," people, circumstances, and past experiences vs. present experiences, to engage in present-time activities, or for a reminiscing intended question	-will respond with correct answer to two choice questions Or yes/no answer, will state where they are, time of day, present company of people on own and with correct answer _____ times a week	Staff will ask residents a series of questions to stimulate focus to the present setting (Ex: "Today is bingo day. Do you know what day of the week it is?"), Or past, if reminiscing exercise (Ex: "Who have you played bingo with when you lived at home: your friend Helen or Bonnie?")
Attention	Show increased attention span, task for function, and to engage in meaningful, recreational/fulfilling activities	-will make eye-contact with staff for _____ sec., will verbalize with staff and instructor, will read/listen to game rules, will say yes/no or initiate action to do the action required/to show listening	Staff will address or stand in front of resident, make eye-contact, ask questions, or use others forms to get resident's attention
Memory	Show increased memory skills of recall, recognition, retention of information, working memory	-will repeat/recall letters/numbers and will repeat when asked (Ex: "What numbers/letters do you have?"), will repeat/recall how to place cards on board, will remember how to play at next class	Staff will show steps on how to play bingo and teach the steps of game
Language	Show increased ability to communicate use of words, phrases, sentence structure, comprehension, interpretation	-will interact with Peers and staff, will call out bingo/game words, etc. when asked, will recognize and interpret the numbers, letters, and colors and state them/point	Staff will ask questions to stimulate a communication (Ex: "Do you want to use the chips or an ink marker to fill in the called out bingo numbers/letters?") Or make a command to - Interpretation/Lang. skills
Cognitive Stimulation (awareness, seeks information in)	Increased stimulus/exposure for visual/ motor memory, cognitive experiences/awareness and brain stimulation to enhance (function, pragmatics, neuroplasticity)	-will look around the room, will be engaged in game w/peers and interact, will listen/seek cognitive stimulation, will accept challenge of input information and engage/interact in bingo game	Staff will set up a bingo game and have residents exposed to letter/number recognition, critical thinking, recognizing patterns, categories, discriminating, and comparing
Perceptual Awareness	Show increased abilities of depth perception, visio-spatial awareness, and acuity (for discrimination, comparison, and categorizing), safety	-will place chips/game piece on correct space on board, will stay within own space, will maneuver/pick up items, will put items away in proper containers associated with areas	Staff will instruct the residents on where they need to stay in their space, or bingo card space
Problem-solving (goes beyond thinking/stimulus and initiates thinking process)	Increase problem-solving ability, processing of information, thinking, reasoning, and use of good judgment and decision-making	-will problem-solve and process information regarding rules of game, strategies/patterns to win, will place chips on board when number/letter is called, and be ready when next set called, will call out " I win" or some form of communication if numbers/letters match, will watch their board to see if game pieces fall in a pattern, will discriminate, and compare for winning game, will follow patterns/rhythm of game	-Staff will direct the residents on techniques of the game/materials -Staff will answer questions regarding understanding of steps, and offer the residents challenging strategies for processing info, step judgments -Staff will name off bingo numbers/letters, and residents will follow cue/rhythm by filling in spaces
Complete a Task	Increase ability to complete a task	will recall/retain and sort/gather information, problem-solve, and complete activity	Staff will support resident's ability to follow procedure through instruction, encouragement, and supplying adaptive devices, if needed, and necessary materials and support

TABLE 11.1

Recreational Objectives Observational Form
Bingo- Cognitive skills

PATIENT		Dependent (Totally dependent)	High Assistance (25+ ability)	Moderate Assist. (50+ ability)	Mild Assistance (75+ability)	Independent (Totally independent)
SEE CODES BELOW USE OPTIONAL CODES IF APPROPRIATE		1	2	3	4	5
		3 cue/ 2-3 physical	2-3 cues/ 2 physical	2-3 cues/ 1 physical	1-2 cues	Encouragement
97530- Therapeutic activities or	**SKILL**	**GOAL**	**OBJECTIVES** ____times per ____		**METHOD**	**OUTCOME DATE**
97532 Cognitive skills	Orientation					
97532 Cognitive skills	Attention					
97532 Cognitive skills	Memory					
97532 Cognitive skills	Problem-Solving					
97532 Cognitive skills	Complete a Task					
97139 Speech Therapy 97532 Cognitive skills	Language					
97533	Sensory Stimulation/ Cognitive Stimulation					
97532	Perceptual Awareness					

97532-Development of cognitive skills to improve attention, memory, problem-solving, includes compensatory training and/or sensory integrative activities, direct (one-on-one) patient contact by the provider, each 15 minutes; **97530-Therapeutic activities**, direct (one-on-one) patient contact by the provider (use of dynamic activities to improve functional performance), each 15 minutes; **97533-Sensory integration techniques** to enhance sensory processing and promote adaptive responses to environmental demands, direct (one-on-one) patient contact by the provider, each 15 minutes; **97150-Therapeutic procedure(s)**, group (2 or more individuals); **97139-Unlisted therapeutic procedure** (specify) minutes; **97003- occupational therapy evaluation**; **97004- re-evaluation**	Staff Initial
	Add total score here -Maximum Score 40 pt. each form per activity
	See scale below or use own/facilities optional score system

(Score 1-8)=1 (9-16) =2 (17-24) =3 (25-32) =4 (33-40) =5 If w/device add d if wish, ex: 1d, 2d, or If using 1-7 scale: (41-48) =6 (49-56)

Bingo
Physical Goals, Objectives, and Methods

SKILL	GOAL	OBJECTIVES SAMPLE	METHOD SAMPLE
Fine Motor Skills	Increase fine motor skills, meaningful/fulfilling activities	-will pick up bingo chips, use bingo magnetic brush	-Staff will give residents boards, chips, or markers -When the letters and number are called out, they will pick up chips, etc.
Hand-Eye Coordination	Increase hand-eye coordination	-will place the chips on the proper square, write their name on the top of page; will place game pieces on the board	Staff will instruct residents to put their name on paper form of bingo pages and use ink markers or chips to dot in the bingo number/letter called
Gross Motor Skills	Increase large motor skills, meaningful/fulfilling activities	-will walk to table or walk to table with device (independent if does on own w/device)	Staff will ask/support residents to come to bingo, do a mild stretch before beginning the game
Perceptual Speed and Motor Function	Increase speed and motor ability for function, safety, meaningful /fulfilling activities	-will react and place pieces on the board and increase speed of reaction	Staff will decrease the amount of time waited between calling out bingo numbers/letters

TABLE 11.2

Recreational Objectives Observational Form

BINGO - PHYSICAL SKILLS

PATIENT		Dependent (Totally dependent)	High Assistance (25+ ability)	Moderate Assist. (50+ ability)	Mild Assistance (75+ability)	Independent (Totally independent)
SEE CODES BELOW USE OPTIONAL CODES IF APPROPRIATE		1	2	3	4	5
		3 cue/ 2-3 physical	2-3 cues/ 2 physical	2-3 cues/ 1 physical	1-2 cues	Encouragement
97530-Therapeutic activities or	**SKILL**	**GOAL**	**OBJECTIVES** ____times per ____		**METHOD**	**OUTCOME DATE**
Therapeutic Activity 97530	FINE MOTOR SKILLS					
97530	EYE-HAND COORDINATION					
97110/ 97530	GROSS MOTOR SKILLS					
97530 If under cognitive code 97532	PERCEPTUAL SPEED/MOTOR FUNCTION					

97530 Therapeutic activities, direct (one on one) patient contact by the provider (use of dynamic activities to improve functional performance),each 15 minutes; **97110 Therapeutic procedure**, **one or more areas**, each 15 minutes; therapeutic exercises to develop strength and endurance, range of motion and flexibility; ; **97150 Therapeutic procedure(s), group (2 or more individuals**; **97535-Self care/home management training** (e.g., activities of daily living and compensatory training, meal preparation, safety procedures, and instructions in use of adaptive equipment), direct (one-on-one) contact by provider, each 15 minutes; **Physical therapy 97001 evaluation, 97002 Re-evaluation. occupational therapy evaluation 97003, re-evaluation. 97004**	Staff Initials
	Add total score here Maximum Score 20 pt. each form per activity
	See scale below or use own/facilities optional score system

(Score 1-4)=1 (5-8) =2 (9-12) =3 (13-16) =4 (17-20) =5 If w/device add d if wish, ex: 1d, 2d, or If using 1-7 scale: (21-24) =6 (25-28) =7

Bingo
Socio-emotional Goals, Objectives, and Methods

SKILL	GOAL	OBJECTIVES SAMPLE	METHOD SAMPLE
Socialization/Community Integration	Increase social interactions, meaningful/fulfilling activities	-will interact with peers, will engage in community integration experiences (for social skills), will use manners and social practices (for community adaptation), will buy own bingo cards, will sit at table along with people in public place	Staff will offer residents a game of bingo and support/encourage them to socialize through community integration and being paired w/other residents playing game
Team Playing/Sharing	Increase teamwork/sharing, meaningful/fulfilling activities	-will join in game with others and share, wait turn, support peers	Staff will encourage residents to share items, take turns, strategize as a team, include all team members
Initiative and Motivation	Increase initiative and motivation/wellness, and quality of life	-will choose ,if they wish, to play the game, will do all moves on own or with assistance (as a sign of motivation to play)	Staff will support/encourage the resident to pursue games of choice
Emotional Gratification	Increase emotional gratification/wellness, and quality of life	-will state that the game is a gratifying experience, or will show pleasure by smiling, laughing, deep focus on game	Staff will ask residents if they enjoyed the game and what they liked through the use of verbal discussion, writing, group discussions
Sense of Accomplishment	Increase feelings of self-worth, pride, productivity, dignity/wellness, and quality of life	-will use gestures to express pride in self , will talk about their accomplishments of winning, show winning board	Staff will ask resident to share what they gained by partaking in the game (Ex: "I felt a feeling of…")
Self-esteem/self-identity	Increase self-esteem, feelings of belonging, dignity, self-worth, integrity, self-identity/wellness, and quality of life	-will state/communicate positive feelings about self and ability to play, will take an active role in health though games/simulating activity, will join the game based on own choices	Staff will educate residents on the value of mind exercises/games and continued use of the activities
Sensory Integration/Tolerating Stimulation	Increase sensory processing and enhance awareness of sensations and toleration/adaptation of sensory stimulations and demands	-will adjust to the smell, noise, lights, peers in the room during game and stay (does not ask to leave, does not become agitated)	-Staff will offer residents sensory stimulating experiences -Staff will support residents as they adjust to the stimulus one step at a time
Fostering Appropriate Behaviors	Increase social interaction, social opportunities and adjustment, safety, using appropriate behaviors during an activity for a calm environment/wellness, and quality of life	-will join in on game, listen and follow instructions, use appropriate behavior for the setting; will wait turn, stand in line quietly; will quiet down when asked	Before game begins, staff will discuss the rules, appropriate behaviors, respect of property, safety, and respect of fellow peers/instructor

TABLE 11.3

Recreational Objectives Observational Form
Bingo- Socio-emotional Skills

PATIENT	Dependent (Totally dependent)	High Assistance (25+ ability)	Moderate Assist. (50+ ability)	Mild Assistance (75+ability)	Independent (Totally independent.)
SEE CODES BELOW USE OPTIONAL CODES IF APPROPRIATE	1	2	3	4	5
	3 cue/ 2-3 physical	2-3 cues/ 2 physical	2-3 cues/ 1 physical	1-2 cues	Encouragement

97530-Therapeutic activities or	SKILL	GOAL	OBJECTIVES ____times per ____	METHOD	OUTCOME DATE			
97537 Or 97535	SOCIALIZATION/ COMMUNITY INTEGRATION							
97537 Or 97535	TEAM PLAYING /SHARING							
97537 Or 97535	INITIATIVE AND MOTIVATION							
97537 Or 97535	EMOTIONAL GRATIFICATION							
97537 Or 97535	SENSE OF ACCOMPLISHM ENT							
97537 Or 97535	SELF-ESTEEM/ SELF-IDENTITY							
97537 Or 97535	FOSTERING APPROPRIATE BEHAVIORS							
97533	SENSORY INTEGRATION/ TOLERATING							

97537-Community/work reintegration training (e.g., shopping, transportation, money management, avocational activities and/or work environment/modification analysis, work task analysis), direct (one-on-one) contact by provider, each 15 minutes; **97535-Self care/home management training** (e.g., activities of daily living and compensatory training, meal preparation, safety procedures, and instructions in use of adaptive equipment), direct (one-on-one) contact by provider, each 15 minutes; **97530-Therapeutic activities, direct (one-on-one)** patient contact by the provider (use of dynamic activities to improve functional performance), each 15 minutes; **97150-Therapeutic procedure(s), group (2 or more individuals)**; **97533-Sensory integration techniques** to enhance sensory processing and promote adaptive responses to environmental demands, direct (one-on-one) patient contact by the provider, each 15 minutes; **occupational therapy evaluation 97003, re-evaluation . 97004**	Staff Initial				
	Add total score here-Maximum Score 40 pt. each form per activity				
	See scale below or use own/facilities optional score system				

(Score 1-8)=1 (9-16) =2 (17-24) =3 (25-32) =4 (33-40) =5 If w/device add d if wish, ex: 1d, 2d, or If using 1-7 scale: (41-48) =6 (49-56)

Board Games

Objectives and benefits:

***Cognitive Challenges*:** attention, memory, language, orientation, following patterns, obeying rules, letter and number recognition and recall.

***Physical Needs*:** fine motor skills, possible gross motor skills, hand-eye coordination, perceptual speed and motor function, grasping small objects.

***Socio-emotional Needs*:** socialization, community integration, awareness of others, team playing, emotional gratification, tolerating stimulation, fostering appropriate behaviors.

Supplies: Board games, playing cards. You may need two of some games for larger groups.

Time: 30–45 minutes. This is an activity that can be scheduled once a week.

Staff/older adult ratio: 1:8

Instructions: Let the older adults choose a game. Follow the game rules. You could even improvise games such as Family Feud, Yahtzee, and Boggle. You can also do simple card games; these could be a great opportunity for residents to teach each other their favorite games such as Bridge or Panicle.

Research has shown activities that help cognition of sensory/motor and speed processing will be geared towards help in visual and motor memory, discrimination, comparison, and categorizing areas and may help improve memory skills. Long-term studies (Arbuckle and others, 1998) have consistently showed that stimulating the brain with activities helps cognitive function in a similar way exercise helps muscle function.

Board Games

COGNITIVE GOALS, OBJECTIVES, AND METHODS

SKILL	GOAL	OBJECTIVES SAMPLE	METHOD SAMPLE
Orientation	Show increased awareness of, time/"timeframe," people, circumstances, and past experiences vs. present experiences, to engage in present-time activities, or for a reminiscing intended question	-will respond with correct answer to two choice questions Or yes/no answer, will state where they are, time of day, present company of people on own and with the correct answer _____ times a week	Staff will ask residents a series of questions to stimulate focus to the present setting and circumstances (Ex: "Who are you playing Boggle with? Are you playing with new or old friends?"), Or past if reminiscing exercise (Ex: "Have you played boggle before?")
Attention	Show increased attention span, task for function, and to engage in meaningful, recreational/fulfilling activities	-will make eye-contact with staff for _____ sec(s), will verbalize with staff and instructor, will read/listen to game rules, will say yes/no or initiate action to do the action required/to show listening	Staff will address, direct, or stand in front of resident, and make eye contact, ask questions, or use other methods to get resident's attention and gauge listening ability
Memory	Show increased memory skills of recall, recognition, retention of information, working memory	-will repeat/recall letters and numbers and will repeat when asked "What numbers/letters do you have?; will repeat/recall how to place cards on board, will remember how to play at next class	Staff will show steps on how to play
Language	Show increased ability to communicate use of words, phrases, sentence structure, comprehension, interpretation	-will interact with peers and staff, will call out game words, etc. when letters/numbers match, will call out " I win" or use some form of communication	Staff will ask questions to stimulate a communication (Ex: "Do you want to play Boggle or Scrabble?") Or make a command to gauge Interpretation/Lang. skills
Cognitive Stimulation (awareness, seeks information in)	Increased stimulus/exposure for visual/ motor memory, cognitive experiences/awareness and brain stimulation to enhance (function, pragmatics, neuro-plasticity)	-will look around the room, will engage in game w/peers and interact, will listen/seek cognitive stimulation, will accept challenge of input information and engage/interact in board game	Staff will set up a game and have residents exposed to letter/number recognition, word play, critical thinking, recognizing patterns, categories, discriminating, and comparing
Perceptual Awareness	Show increased abilities of depth perception, visual-spatial awareness, and acuity (for discrimination, comparison, and categorizing), safety	-will place chips/game piece on correct space on board, will stay within own space ,will maneuver and pick up items, will put items away in proper containers associated with areas	Staff will instruct the residents on where they need to stay in their space or game space
Problem-solving (goes beyond thinking/stimulus and initiates thinking process)	Increase problem-solving ability, processing of information, thinking, reasoning, and use of good judgment and decision-making	-will problem-solve and process information regarding rules of game, strategies, and patterns to win; will place chips on board when number/letter is called and be ready when next set is called; will follow patterns/rhythm of game	-Staff will direct the residents on techniques of the game/materials. ---- Staff will answer questions regarding understanding of steps and offer the residents challenging strategies for processing info and step judgments -Staff will use games that require a pattern/rhythms, and residents will follow cue/rhythm
Complete a Task	Increase ability to complete a task	will recall/retain and sort/gather information, problem-solve, and complete activity	Staff will support resident's ability to follow procedure through instruction, encouragement, and supplying adaptive devices, if needed, and necessary materials and support

TABLE 12.1

Recreational Objectives Observational Form
Board Games- Cognitive Skills

PATIENT		Dependent (Totally dependent)	High Assistance (25+ ability)	Moderate Assist. (50+ ability)	Mild Assistance (75+ability)	Independent (Totally independent)
SEE CODES BELOW USE OPTIONAL CODES IF APPROPRIATE		1	2	3	4	5
		3 cue/ 2-3 physical	2-3 cues/ 2 physical	2-3 cues/ 1 physical	1-2 cues	Encouragement
97530- Therapeutic activities or	**SKILL**	**GOAL**	**OBJECTIVES** ____times per ____		**METHOD**	**OUTCOME DATE**
97532 Cognitive skills	ORIENTATION					
97532 Cognitive skills	ATTENTION					
97532 Cognitive skills	MEMORY					
97532 Cognitive skills	PROBLEM-SOLVING					
97532 Cognitive skills	COMPLETE A TASK					
97139 Speech Therapy 97532 Cognitive skills	LANGUAGE					
97533	SENSORY STIMULATION/ COGNITIVE STIMULATION					
97532	PERCEPTUAL AWARENESS					

97532-Development of cognitive skills to improve attention, memory, problem-solving, includes compensatory training and/or sensory integrative activities, direct (one-on-one) patient contact by the provider, each 15 minutes; **97530-Therapeutic activities**, direct (one-on-one) patient contact by the provider (use of dynamic activities to improve functional performance), each 15 minutes; **97533-Sensory integration techniques** to enhance sensory processing and promote adaptive responses to environmental demands, direct (one-on-one) patient contact by the provider, each 15 minutes; **97150-Therapeutic procedure(s)**, group (2 or more individuals); **97139-Unlisted therapeutic procedure** (specify) minutes; **97003- occupational therapy evaluation**; **97004- re-evaluation**	Staff Initial	
	Add total score here -Maximum Score 40 pt. each form per activity	
	See scale below or use own/facilities optional score system	

(Score 1-8)=1 (9-16) =2 (17-24) =3 (25-32) =4 (33-40) =5 If w/device add d if wish, ex: 1d, 2d, or If using 1-7 scale: (41-48) =6 (49-56)

Board Games
Physical Goals, Objectives, and Methods

SKILL	GOAL	OBJECTIVES SAMPLE	METHOD SAMPLE
Fine Motor Skills	Increase fine motor skills, meaningful/fulfilling activities	-will pick up dice, word dice	-Staff will give residents boards, dice, or other game pieces -When the letters and number are called out, they will pick up chips, etc.
Hand-Eye Coordination	Increase hand-eye coordination	-will place the dice and pieces on the proper square, write their name on the top of page; will place game pieces on board	Staff will instruct residents to put their name on paper form of bingo pages and use ink markers to dot in the bingo number/letter called or if chips /place on
Gross Motor Skills	Increase large motor skills, meaningful/fulfilling activities	-will walk to table or walk to table with device (independent if they do it on own w/device)	Staff will engage residents in a mild sub maximal warm up before sitting for the game
Perceptual Speed and Motor Function	Increase speed and motor ability for function, safety, meaningful /fulfilling activities	-will react and place pieces on the board and increase speed of reaction and placing chips on board.	Staff will decrease the amount of time waited between calling out words, numbers, and letters

TABLE 12.2

Recreational Objectives Observational Form
Board Games- Physical Skills

PATIENT		Dependent (Totally dependent)	High Assistance (25+ ability)	Moderate Assist. (50+ ability)	Mild Assistance (75+ability)	Independent (Totally independent)
SEE CODES BELOW USE OPTIONAL CODES IF APPROPRIATE		1	2	3	4	5
		3 cue/ 2-3 physical	2-3 cues/ 2 physical	2-3 cues/ 1 physical	1-2 cues	Encouragement
97530-Therapeutic activities or	**SKILL**	**GOAL**	**OBJECTIVES** ____times per ____		**METHOD**	**OUTCOME DATE**
Therapeutic Activity 97530	FINE MOTOR SKILLS					
97530	EYE-HAND COORDINATION					
97110/ 97530	GROSS MOTOR SKILLS					
97530 If under cognitive code 97532	PERCEPTUAL SPEED/MOTOR FUNCTION					

97530 Therapeutic activities, direct (one on one) patient contact by the provider (use of dynamic activities to improve functional performance),each 15 minutes; **97110 Therapeutic procedure, one or more areas**, each 15 minutes; therapeutic exercises to develop strength and endurance, range of motion and flexibility; ; **97150 Therapeutic procedure(s), group (2 or more individuals**; **97535-Self care/home management training** (e.g., activities of daily living and compensatory training, meal preparation, safety procedures, and instructions in use of adaptive equipment), direct (one-on-one) contact by provider, each 15 minutes; **Physical therapy 97001 evaluation, 97002 Re-evaluation. occupational therapy evaluation 97003, re-evaluation. 97004**	Staff Initials
	Add total score here Maximum Score 20 pt. each form per activity
	See scale below or use own/facilities optional score system

(Score 1-4)=1 (5-8) =2 (9-12) =3 (13-16) =4 (17-20) =5 If w/device add d if wish, ex: 1d, 2d, or If using 1-7 scale: (21-24) =6 (25-28) =7

Board Games

Socio-emotional Goals, Objectives, and Methods

Skill	Goal	Objectives Sample	Method Sample
Socialization/Community Integration	Increase social interactions, meaningful/fulfilling activities	-will interact with peers, will engage in community integration experiences (for community adaptation and social skills), will use manners, social practices (for community adaptation)	Staff will offer residents a game and support/encourage residents to socialize through community integration and being paired w/other residents playing game
Team Playing/Sharing	Increase teamwork/sharing, meaningful/fulfilling activities	-will join in game with others and share, wait turn, support peers _____ time(s) this week.	Staff will encourage residents to share items, take turns, strategize as a team, include all team members
Initiative and Motivation	Increase initiative and motivation/wellness, and quality of life	-will choose ,if they wish, to play the game, will do all moves on own or with assistance (as a sign of motivation to play)	Staff will support/encourage the resident to pursue games of choice
Emotional Gratification	Increase emotional gratification/wellness, and quality of life	-will state that the game is a gratifying experience, or will show pleasure by smiling, laughing, deep focus on activity.	Staff will ask residents if they enjoyed the game and what they liked through verbal discussion, writing, group discussions
Sense of Accomplishment	Increase feelings of self-worth, pride, productivity, dignity/wellness, and quality of life	-will use gestures to express pride in self, will talk about their accomplishments of winning, show winning sets	Staff will ask residents to share what they gained by partaking in the game (Ex: "I felt a sense/feeling of…")
Self-esteem/self-identity	Increase self-esteem, feelings of belonging, dignity, self-worth, integrity, self-identity/wellness, and quality of life	-will state/communicate positive feelings about self and ability to play, will take an active role in health though games/simulating activity, will join the game based on own choices	Staff will educate residents on the value of mind exercise methods and continued use of the activities
Sensory Integration/Tolerating Stimulation	Increase sensory processing and enhance awareness of sensations and toleration/adaptation of sensory stimulations and demands	-will adjust to the smell, noise, lights, peers in the room during game and stay (does not ask to leave, does not become agitated)	-Staff will offer residents sensory stimulating experiences -Staff will support residents as they adjust to the stimulus
Fostering Appropriate Behaviors	Increase social interaction, social opportunities and adjustment, safety, using appropriate behaviors during an activity for a calm environment/wellness, and quality of life	-will join in on game, listen and follow instructions, use appropriate behavior for the setting; will wait turn, stand in line quietly; will quiet down when asked	Before game begins, staff will discuss the rules, appropriate behaviors, respect of property, safety, and respect of fellow peers/instructor

TABLE 12.3

Recreational Objectives Observational Form
Board Games- Socio-emotional Skills

PATIENT	Dependent (Totally dependent)	High Assistance (25+ ability)	Moderate Assist. (50+ ability)	Mild Assistance (75+ability)	Independent (Totally independent.)
SEE CODES BELOW USE OPTIONAL CODES IF APPROPRIATE	1	2	3	4	5
	3 cue/ 2-3 physical	2-3 cues/ 2 physical	2-3 cues/ 1 physical	1-2 cues	Encouragement

97530-Therapeutic activities or	SKILL	GOAL	OBJECTIVES ____times per ____	METHOD	OUTCOME DATE			
97537 Or 97535	SOCIALIZATION/ COMMUNITY INTEGRATION							
97537 Or 97535	TEAM PLAYING /SHARING							
97537 Or 97535	INITIATIVE AND MOTIVATION							
97537 Or 97535	EMOTIONAL GRATIFICATION							
97537 Or 97535	SENSE OF ACCOMPLISHM ENT							
97537 Or 97535	SELF-ESTEEM/ SELF-IDENTITY							
97537 Or 97535	FOSTERING APPROPRIATE BEHAVIORS							
97533	SENSORY INTEGRATION/ TOLERATING							

97537-Community/work reintegration training (e.g., shopping, transportation, money management, avocational activities and/or work environment/modification analysis, work task analysis), direct (one-on-one) contact by provider, each 15 minutes; **97535-Self care/home management training** (e.g., activities of daily living and compensatory training, meal preparation, safety procedures, and instructions in use of adaptive equipment), direct (one-on-one) contact by provider, each 15 minutes; **97530-Therapeutic activities, direct (one-on-one)** patient contact by the provider (use of dynamic activities to improve functional performance), each 15 minutes; **97150-Therapeutic procedure(s), group (2 or more individuals); 97533-Sensory integration techniques** to enhance sensory processing and promote adaptive responses to environmental demands, direct (one-on-one) patient contact by the provider, each 15 minutes; **occupational therapy evaluation 97003, re-evaluation . 97004**	Staff Initial				
	Add total score here-Maximum Score 40 pt. each form per activity				
	See scale below or use own/facilities optional score system				

(Score 1-8)=1 (9-16) =2 (17-24) =3 (25-32) =4 (33-40) =5 If w/device add d if wish, ex: 1d, 2d, or If using 1-7 scale: (41-48) =6 (49-56)

Computers/Interactive Games

Objectives and benefits:

Cognitive Challenges**:** attention, memory, language, orientation, following patterns, obeying rules, letter and number recognition and recall.

Physical Needs**:** fine motor skills, possible gross motor skills, hand-eye coordination, perceptual speed and motor function, grasping small objects.

Socio-emotional Needs**:** socialization, community integration, awareness of others, team playing, emotional gratification, tolerating stimulation, fostering appropriate behaviors.

Supplies: Computer games or other interactive games

Time: As long as desired. If possible, it could be set up and available throughout the day. There may also be times when the computer can be used in conjunction with an activity, perhaps as a way to talk about current events.

Staff/older adult ratio: As assessed per needs of individuals or group. Generally this is an individual activity.

Instructions: Set up a computer or interactive game. This would work well in a community room or home. Show the adults how to start the games. Offer help as needed. Learning how to run a computer may be very overwhelming to older adults, but the computer can be an incredibly valuable resource to them as well.

Research has shown activities that help cognition of sensory/motor and speed processing will be geared towards help in visual and motor memory, discrimination, comparison, and categorizing areas and may help improve memory skills. Long-term studies (Arbuckle and others, 1998) have consistently showed that stimulating the brain with activities helps cognitive function in a similar way exercise helps muscle function.

Computer/ Interactive Games
Cognitive Goals, Objectives, and Methods

Skill	Goal	Objectives Sample	Method Sample
Orientation	Show increased awareness of, time/"timeframe," people, circumstances, and past experiences vs. present experiences, to engage in present-time activities, or for a reminiscing intended question	-will respond with correct answer to two choice questions Or yes/no answer, will state where they are, time of day, present company of people on own and with the correct answer _____ times a week	Staff will ask residents a series of questions to stimulate focus to the present setting (Ex: "Today we will play computer games. Do you know what day it is?") Or past if reminiscing exercise (Ex: "Have you played Computer games before? When?")
Attention	Show increased attention span, task for function, and to engage in meaningful, recreational/fulfilling activities	-will make eye-contact with staff for _____ sec., will verbalize with staff and instructor, will read/listen to game rules, will say yes/no or initiate action to do the action required/to show listening	Staff will address or stand in front of resident, make eye-contact, ask questions, or use other methods to get resident's attention
Memory	Show increased memory skills of recall, recognition, retention of information, working memory	-will repeat/recall the rules of the computer game, will repeat/recall how to use the joystick/keyboard, will remember how to play at next class	Staff will show steps on how to play the computer game and teach the steps of game
Language	Show increased ability to communicate use of words, phrases, sentence structure, comprehension, interpretation	-will interact with peers and staff, will verbally explain how the game is played, etc., will recognize/interpret, will discriminate the numbers, objects, letters, reading materials and state them/point	Staff will ask questions to stimulate a communication (Ex: "Do you want to use the joystick or mouse pad? Which game /program would you like to use? Or make a command to (Interpretation/Lang. skills)
Cognitive Stimulation (awareness, seeks information in)	Increased stimulus/exposure for visual/ motor memory, cognitive experiences/awareness and brain stimulation to enhance (function, pragmatics, neuro-plasticity)	-will look around the room, be engaged in game w/ peers/interact listens/seeks cognitive stimulation, will accept challenge of input information and engage/interact in computer game or educational programs	Staff will set up a game/educational program and have residents exposed to letter/number recognition, critical thinking, recognizing patterns, categories, discriminating, and comparing, educational materials
Perceptual Awareness	Show increased abilities of depth perception, visual-spatial awareness, and acuity (for discrimination, comparison, and categorizing), safety	-will place mouse at select area to imitate movement on screen, will stay within own space, will maneuver/pick up items, will put items away in proper containers associated with computer materials	Staff will instruct the residents on where they need to stay in their space, or table space
Problem-solving (goes beyond thinking/stimulus and initiates thinking process)	Increase problem-solving ability, processing of information, thinking, reasoning, and use of good judgment and decision-making	-will problem-solve and process information regarding rules of game, strategies, and patterns to win; will call out "I win" if win game. or -will use the computer for educational purposes requiring problem solving abilities	-Staff will direct the residents on techniques of the game/materials -Staff will answer questions regarding understanding of steps and offer the residents challenging strategies for processing info -Staff will use games that require letter/number recognition, critical thinking, recognizing patterns, categories, discriminating, and comparing; and residents will follow cue/rhythm
Complete a Task	Increase ability to complete a task	will recall/retain and sort/gather information, problem-solve, and complete activity	Staff will support resident's ability to follow procedure through instruction, encouragement; and supplying adaptive devices, if needed, and necessary materials and support

TABLE 13.1

Recreational Objectives Observational Form

Computer/Interactive Games- Cognitive skills

PATIENT	Dependent (Totally dependent)	High Assistance (25+ ability)	Moderate Assist. (50+ ability)	Mild Assistance (75+ability)	Independent (Totally independent)
SEE CODES BELOW USE OPTIONAL CODES IF APPROPRIATE	1	2	3	4	5
	3 cue/ 2-3 physical	2-3 cues/ 2 physical	2-3 cues/ 1 physical	1-2 cues	Encouragement

97530-Therapeutic activities or	**SKILL**	**GOAL**	**OBJECTIVES** ____times per ____	**METHOD**	**OUTCOME DATE**			
97532 Cognitive skills	ORIENTATION							
97532 Cognitive skills	ATTENTION							
97532 Cognitive skills	MEMORY							
97532 Cognitive skills	PROBLEM-SOLVING							
97532 Cognitive skills	COMPLETE A TASK							
97139 Speech Therapy 97532 Cognitive skills	LANGUAGE							
97533	SENSORY STIMULATION/ COGNITIVE STIMULATION							
97532	PERCEPTUAL AWARENESS							

97532-Development of cognitive skills to improve attention, memory, problem-solving, includes compensatory training and/or sensory integrative activities, direct (one-on-one) patient contact by the provider, each 15 minutes; **97530-Therapeutic activities**, direct (one-on-one) patient contact by the provider (use of dynamic activities to improve functional performance), each 15 minutes; **97533-Sensory integration techniques** to enhance sensory processing and promote adaptive responses to environmental demands, direct (one-on-one) patient contact by the provider, each 15 minutes; **97150-Therapeutic procedure(s)**, group (2 or more individuals); **97139-Unlisted therapeutic procedure** (specify) minutes; **97003- occupational therapy evaluation**; **97004- re-evaluation**	Staff Initial				
	Add total score here -Maximum Score 40 pt. each form per activity				
	See scale below or use own/facilities optional score system				

(Score 1-8)=1 (9-16) =2 (17-24) =3 (25-32) =4 (33-40) =5 If w/device add d if wish, ex: 1d, 2d, or If using 1-7 scale: (41-48) =6 (49-56)

Computer/Interactive Games
Physical Goals, Objectives, and Methods

SKILL	GOAL	OBJECTIVES SAMPLE	METHOD SAMPLE
Fine Motor Skills	Increase fine motor skills, meaningful/fulfilling activities	-will use fingers on keyboard	-Staff will give residents computer games that require use of fine motor skills such as a keyboard
Hand-Eye Coordination	Increase hand-eye coordination	-will use mouse pad, joystick	-Staff will give residents computer games that require use of fine motor skills such as a keyboard
Gross Motor Skills	Increase large motor skills, meaningful/fulfilling activities	-will walk to table or to table with device (independent if they do it on own w/device)	Staff will have residents walk to game do a mild stretch before beginning the game
Perceptual Speed and Motor Function	Increase speed and motor ability for function, safety, meaningful /fulfilling activities	-will react to required commands on the computer screen and increase speed of reaction time.	Staff will offer computer games requiring quicker reaction times to increase resident's reaction time.

TABLE 13.2

Recreational Objectives Observational Form

Computer/Interactive Games- Physical Skills

PATIENT	Dependent (Totally dependent)	High Assistance (25+ ability)	Moderate Assist. (50+ ability)	Mild Assistance (75+ability)	Independent (Totally independent)
	1	2	3	4	5
SEE CODES BELOW USE OPTIONAL CODES IF APPROPRIATE	3 cue/ 2-3 physical	2-3 cues/ 2 physical	2-3 cues/ 1 physical	1-2 cues	Encouragement

97530- Therapeutic activities or	SKILL	GOAL	OBJECTIVES ____times per ____	METHOD	OUTCOME DATE			
Therapeutic Activity 97530	FINE MOTOR SKILLS							
97530	EYE-HAND COORDINATION							
97110/ 97530	GROSS MOTOR SKILLS							
97530 If under cognitive code 97532	PERCEPTUAL SPEED/MOTOR FUNCTION							

97530 Therapeutic activities, direct (one on one) patient contact by the provider (use of dynamic activities to improve functional performance),each 15 minutes; **97110 Therapeutic procedure, one or more areas**, each 15 minutes; therapeutic exercises to develop strength and endurance, range of motion and flexibility; ; **97150 Therapeutic procedure(s), group (2 or more individuals**; **97535-Self care/home management training** (e.g., activities of daily living and compensatory training, meal preparation, safety procedures, and instructions in use of adaptive equipment), direct (one-on-one) contact by provider, each 15 minutes; **Physical therapy 97001 evaluation, 97002 Re-evaluation. occupational therapy evaluation 97003, re-evaluation. 97004**	Staff Initials				
	Add total score here Maximum Score 20 pt. each form per activity				
	See scale below or use own/facilities optional score system				

(Score 1-4)=1 (5-8) =2 (9-12) =3 (13-16) =4 (17-20) =5 If w/device add d if wish, ex: 1d, 2d, or If using 1-7 scale: (21-24) =6 (25-28) =7

Computer/Interactive Games

SOCIO-EMOTIONAL GOALS, OBJECTIVES, AND METHODS

SKILL	GOAL	OBJECTIVES SAMPLE	METHOD SAMPLE
Socialization/Community Integration	Increase social interactions, meaningful/fulfilling activities	-will interact with peers, will engage in community integration experiences (for community adaptation and social skills), will use manners, social practices (for community adaptation)	Staff will offer residents a computer game and support/encourage residents to socialize through community integration and or being paired w/other residents playing game
Team Playing/Sharing	Increase teamwork/sharing, meaningful/fulfilling activities	-will join in game/use of computer programs with others and share, wait turn, support peers _____ time(s) this week	Staff will encourage residents to share items, take turns, strategize as a team, include all team members
Initiative and Motivation	Increase initiative and motivation/wellness, and quality of life	-will choose if they wish to play game, will do all moves on own or with assistance (as a sign of motivation to play)	Staff will support and encourage the resident to pursue games/ educational programs of choice
Emotional Gratification	Increase emotional gratification/wellness, and quality of life	-will state that the computer program/game is a gratifying experience, or will show pleasure by smiling, laughing, deep focus on activity.	Staff will ask residents if they enjoyed the game and what they liked through verbal discussion, writing, group discussions
Sense of Accomplishment	Increase feelings of self-worth, pride, productivity, dignity/wellness, and quality of life	-will use gestures to express pride in self, will talk about their accomplishments of completing an educational class, computer game	Staff will ask residents to share what they gained by partaking in the game (Ex: "I felt a feeling pride in my ability to use a computer.")
Self-esteem/self-identity	Increase self-esteem, feelings of belonging, dignity, self-worth, integrity, self-identity/wellness, and quality of life	-will state/communicate positive feelings about self and ability to play, will take an active role in health though games/simulating activity, will join the game based on own choices	-Staff will educate residents on the value of mind exercises and continued use of the activities
Fostering Appropriate Behaviors	Increase social interaction, social opportunities and adjustment, safety, using appropriate behaviors during an activity for a calm environment/wellness, and quality of life	-will adjust to the smell, noise, lights, peers in the room during game, and stay (does not ask to leave, does not become distracting)	-Staff will offer residents sensory stimulating experiences -Staff will support residents as they adjust to the stimulus
Sensory Integration/Tolerating Stimulation	Increase sensory processing and enhance awareness of sensations and toleration/adaptation of sensory stimulations and demands	-will join in on game, listen and follow instructions, use appropriate behavior for the setting; will wait turn, stand in line quietly; will quiet down when asked	Before game begins, staff will discuss the rules, appropriate behaviors, respect of property, safety, and respect of fellow peers/instructor

TABLE 13.3

Recreational Objectives Observational Form

COMPUTER/ INTERACTIVE GAMES- SOCIO-EMOTIONAL SKILLS

PATIENT	Dependent (Totally dependent)	High Assistance (25+ ability)	Moderate Assist. (50+ ability)	Mild Assistance (75+ability)	Independent (Totally independent.)
SEE CODES BELOW USE OPTIONAL CODES IF APPROPRIATE	1	2	3	4	5
	3 cue/ 2-3 physical	2-3 cues/ 2 physical	2-3 cues/ 1 physical	1-2 cues	Encouragement

97530-Therapeutic activities or	SKILL	GOAL	OBJECTIVES ____times per ____	METHOD	OUTCOME DATE			
97537 Or 97535	SOCIALIZATION/ COMMUNITY INTEGRATION							
97537 Or 97535	TEAM PLAYING /SHARING							
97537 Or 97535	INITIATIVE AND MOTIVATION							
97537 Or 97535	EMOTIONAL GRATIFICATION							
97537 Or 97535	SENSE OF ACCOMPLISHMENT							
97537 Or 97535	SELF-ESTEEM/ SELF-IDENTITY							
97537 Or 97535	FOSTERING APPROPRIATE BEHAVIORS							
97533	SENSORY INTEGRATION/ TOLERATING							

97537-Community/work reintegration training (e.g., shopping, transportation, money management, avocational activities and/or work environment/modification analysis, work task analysis), direct (one-on-one) contact by provider, each 15 minutes; **97535-Self care/home management training** (e.g., activities of daily living and compensatory training, meal preparation, safety procedures, and instructions in use of adaptive equipment), direct (one-on-one) contact by provider, each 15 minutes; **97530-Therapeutic activities, direct (one-on-one)** patient contact by the provider (use of dynamic activities to improve functional performance), each 15 minutes; **97150-Therapeutic procedure(s), group (2 or more individuals); 97533-Sensory integration techniques** to enhance sensory processing and promote adaptive responses to environmental demands, direct (one-on-one) patient contact by the provider, each 15 minutes; **occupational therapy evaluation 97003, re-evaluation . 97004**	Staff Initial				
	Add total score here-Maximum Score 40 pt. each form per activity				
	See scale below or use own/facilities optional score system				

(Score 1-8)=1 (9-16) =2 (17-24) =3 (25-32) =4 (33-40) =5 If w/device add d if wish, ex: 1d, 2d, or If using 1-7 scale: (41-48) =6 (49-56)

Concentration

Objectives and benefits:

Cognitive Challenges: attention, memory, language, orientation, following patterns, obeying rules, letter and number recognition and recall.

Physical Needs: fine motor skills, possible gross motor skills, hand-eye coordination, perceptual speed and motor function, grasping small objects.

Socio-emotional Needs: socialization, community integration, awareness of others, team playing, emotional gratification, tolerating stimulation, fostering appropriate behaviors.

.

Supplies: One deck of cards with letters, numbers, or pictures on them

Time: 20–30 minutes

Staff/older adult ratio: 1:8 or as assessed per needs of individuals or group

Instructions: Place the cards down on a large table, allow the residents to take turns. Let the first older adult pick one card and try to match it with another card. Continue giving everyone a chance to try until all the cards are matched. Add the scores.

> Research has shown activities that help cognition of sensory/motor and speed processing will be geared towards help in visual and motor memory, discrimination, comparison, and categorizing areas and may help improve memory skills. Long-term studies (Arbuckle and others, 1998) have consistently showed that stimulating the brain with activities helps cognitive function in a similar way exercise helps muscle function.

Concentration
Cognitive Goals, Objectives, and Methods

Skill	Goal	Objectives Sample	Method Sample
Orientation	Show increased awareness of, time/"timeframe," people, circumstances, and past experiences vs. present experiences, to engage in present-time activities, or for a reminiscing intended question	-will respond with correct answer to two choice questions Or yes/no answer, will state where they are, time of day, present company of people on own and with the correct answer _____ times a week	Staff will ask residents a series of questions to stimulate focus to the present setting (Ex: "Today we will play a game of concentration. Do you know what day it is?") Or past if reminiscing exercise (Ex: "Have you played Concentration before? When?")
Attention	Show increased attention span, task for function, and to engage in meaningful, recreational/fulfilling activities	-will make eye-contact with staff for _____ sec., will verbalize with staff and instructor, will read/listen to game rules, will say yes/no or initiate action to do the action required/to show listening	Staff will address or stand in front of resident, make eye-contact, ask questions, or use other methods to get resident's attention
Memory	Show increased memory skills of recall, recognition, retention of information, working memory	-will repeat/recall letters and numbers and will repeat when asked "What numbers or letters do you have?", will repeat/recall how to place cards on board, will remember how to play at next class	Staff will show steps on how to play Concentration and teach the steps of game
Language	Show increased ability to communicate use of words, phrases, sentence structure, comprehension, interpretation	-will interact with peers and staff, will call out game words, etc., will recognize/interpret, will discriminate the numbers, letters, and colors, and state them/point	Staff will ask questions to stimulate a communication (Ex: "Do you want to use matching flowers or matching animals? Or make a command to (Interpretation/Lang. skills)
Cognitive Stimulation (awareness, seeks information in)	Increased stimulus/exposure for visual/ motor memory, cognitive experiences/awareness and brain stimulation to enhance (function, pragmatics, neuroplasticity)	-will look around the room, be engaged in game w/ peers/interact listens/seeks cognitive stimulation, will accept challenge of input information and engage/interact in board game	Staff will set up a game and have residents exposed to letter/number recognition, critical thinking, recognizing patterns, categories, discriminating, and comparing
Perceptual Awareness	Show increased abilities of depth perception, visio-spatical awareness, and acuity (for discrimination, comparison, and categorizing), safety	-will place cards on top of other matching cards, will stay within own space, will maneuver/pick up items, will put items away in proper containers associated with areas	Staff will instruct the residents on where they need to stay in their space, or table space
Problem-solving (goes beyond thinking/stimulus and initiates thinking process)	Increase problem-solving ability, processing of information, thinking, reasoning, and use of good judgment and decision-making	-will problem-solve and process information regarding rules of game, strategies, and patterns to win; will call out " I win" if letters and numbers match	-Staff will direct the residents on techniques of the game/materials -Staff will answer questions regarding understanding of steps and offer the residents challenging strategies for processing info -Staff will use games that require letter/number recognition, critical thinking, recognizing patterns, categories, discriminating, and comparing; and residents will follow cue/rhythm
Complete a Task	Increase ability to complete a task	will recall/retain and sort/gather information, problem-solve, and complete activity	Staff will support resident's ability to follow procedure through instruction, encouragement; and supplying adaptive devices, if needed, and necessary materials and support

TABLE 14.1

Recreational Objectives Observational Form
Concentration- Cognitive skills

PATIENT		Dependent (Totally dependent)	High Assistance (25+ ability)	Moderate Assist. (50+ ability)	Mild Assistance (75+ability)	Independent (Totally independent)			
SEE CODES BELOW USE OPTIONAL CODES IF APPROPRIATE		1	2	3	4	5			
		3 cue/ 2-3 physical	2-3 cues/ 2 physical	2-3 cues/ 1 physical	1-2 cues	Encouragement			
97530- Therapeutic activities or	**SKILL**	**GOAL**	**OBJECTIVES** ____times per ____		**METHOD**	**OUTCOME DATE**			
97532 Cognitive skills	ORIENTATION								
97532 Cognitive skills	ATTENTION								
97532 Cognitive skills	MEMORY								
97532 Cognitive skills	PROBLEM-SOLVING								
97532 Cognitive skills	COMPLETE A TASK								
97139 Speech Therapy 97532 Cognitive skills	LANGUAGE								
97533	SENSORY STIMULATION/ COGNITIVE STIMULATION								
97532	PERCEPTUAL AWARENESS								

97532-Development of cognitive skills to improve attention, memory, problem-solving, includes compensatory training and/or sensory integrative activities, direct (one-on-one) patient contact by the provider, each 15 minutes; **97530-Therapeutic activities**, direct (one-on-one) patient contact by the provider (use of dynamic activities to improve functional performance), each 15 minutes; **97533-Sensory integration techniques** to enhance sensory processing and promote adaptive responses to environmental demands, direct (one-on-one) patient contact by the provider, each 15 minutes; **97150-Therapeutic procedure(s)**, group (2 or more individuals); **97139-Unlisted therapeutic procedure** (specify) minutes; **97003- occupational therapy evaluation**; **97004- re-evaluation**	Staff Initial				
	Add total score here -Maximum Score 40 pt. each form per activity				
	See scale below or use own/facilities optional score system				

(Score 1-8)=1 (9-16) =2 (17-24) =3 (25-32) =4 (33-40) =5 If w/device add d if wish, ex: 1d, 2d, or If using 1-7 scale: (41-48) =6 (49-56)

Concentration
Physical Goals, Objectives, and Methods

Skill	Goal	Objectives Sample	Method Sample
Fine Motor Skills	Increase fine motor skills, meaningful/fulfilling activities	-will pick up and shuffle cards	-Staff will give residents cards -Staff will say" go" and resident will turn over cards and search until they find the matching card
Hand-Eye Coordination	Increase hand-eye coordination	-will place the cards on top of matching card	Staff will instruct residents to put the matching card on top of the other card
Gross Motor Skills	Increase large motor skills, meaningful/fulfilling activities	-will walk to table or to table with device (independent if they do it on own w/device)	Staff will have residents walk to game do a mild stretch before beginning the game
Perceptual Speed and Motor Function	Increase speed and motor ability for function, safety, meaningful /fulfilling activities	-will react and place matching cards, and increase speed of reaction time.	Staff will decrease the amount of time waited between calling out "go" and residents' time to match the cards

Table 14.2

Recreational Objectives Observational Form
Concentration- Physical Skills

<table>
<tr><td colspan="2">Patient</td><td>Dependent (Totally dependent)</td><td>High Assistance (25+ ability)</td><td>Moderate Assist. (50+ ability)</td><td>Mild Assistance (75+ability)</td><td colspan="4">Independent (Totally independent)</td></tr>
<tr><td colspan="2">SEE CODES BELOW
USE OPTIONAL CODES IF APPROPRIATE</td><td>1</td><td>2</td><td>3</td><td>4</td><td colspan="4">5</td></tr>
<tr><td colspan="2"></td><td>3 cue/
2-3 physical</td><td>2-3 cues/
2 physical</td><td>2-3 cues/
1 physical</td><td>1-2 cues</td><td colspan="4">Encouragement</td></tr>
<tr><td>97530-Therapeutic activities or</td><td>Skill</td><td>Goal</td><td colspan="2">Objectives
____times per ____</td><td>Method</td><td colspan="4">Outcome Date</td></tr>
<tr><td>Therapeutic Activity 97530</td><td>Fine motor skills</td><td></td><td colspan="2"></td><td></td><td></td><td></td><td></td><td></td></tr>
<tr><td>97530</td><td>Eye-Hand Coordination</td><td></td><td colspan="2"></td><td></td><td></td><td></td><td></td><td></td></tr>
<tr><td>97110/
97530</td><td>Gross motor skills</td><td></td><td colspan="2"></td><td></td><td></td><td></td><td></td><td></td></tr>
<tr><td>97530
If under cognitive code 97532</td><td>Perceptual speed/motor function</td><td></td><td colspan="2"></td><td></td><td></td><td></td><td></td><td></td></tr>
<tr><td colspan="5" rowspan="3">97530 Therapeutic activities, direct (one on one) patient contact by the provider (use of dynamic activities to improve functional performance),each 15 minutes; 97110 Therapeutic procedure, one or more areas, each 15 minutes; therapeutic exercises to develop strength and endurance, range of motion and flexibility; ; 97150 Therapeutic procedure(s), group (2 or more individuals; 97535-Self care/home management training (e.g., activities of daily living and compensatory training, meal preparation, safety procedures, and instructions in use of adaptive equipment), direct (one-on-one) contact by provider, each 15 minutes; Physical therapy 97001 evaluation, 97002 Re-evaluation. occupational therapy evaluation 97003, re-evaluation. 97004</td><td colspan="5">Staff Initials</td></tr>
<tr><td>Add total score here
Maximum Score 20 pt. each form per activity</td><td></td><td></td><td></td><td></td></tr>
<tr><td>See scale below
or use own/facilities optional score system</td><td></td><td></td><td></td><td></td></tr>
</table>

(Score 1-4)=1 (5-8) =2 (9-12) =3 (13-16) =4 (17-20) =5 If w/device add d if wish, ex: 1d, 2d, or If using 1-7 scale: (21-24) =6 (25-28) =7

Concentration
Socio-emotional Goals, Objectives, and Methods

Skill	Goal	Objectives Sample	Method Sample
Socialization/Community Integration	Increase social interactions, meaningful/fulfilling activities	-will interact with peers, will engage in community integration experiences (for community adaptation and social skills), will use manners, social practices (for community adaptation)	Staff will offer residents a game and support/encourage residents to socialize through community integration and being paired w/other residents playing game
Team Playing/Sharing	Increase teamwork/sharing, meaningful/fulfilling activities	-will join in game with others and share, wait turn, support peers _____ time(s) this week	Staff will encourage residents to share items, take turns, strategize as a team, include all team members
Initiative and Motivation	Increase initiative and motivation/wellness, and quality of life	-will choose if they wish to play game, will do all moves on own or with assistance (as a sign of motivation to play)	Staff will support and encourage the resident to pursue games of choice
Emotional Gratification	Increase emotional gratification/wellness, and quality of life	-will state that the game is a gratifying experience, or will show pleasure by smiling, laughing, deep focus on activity.	Staff will ask residents if they enjoyed the game and what they liked through verbal discussion, writing, group discussions
Sense of Accomplishment	Increase feelings of self-worth, pride, productivity, dignity/wellness, and quality of life	-will use gestures to express pride in self, will talk about their accomplishments of winning and show winning sets	Staff will ask residents to share what they gained by partaking in the game (Ex: "I felt a feeling pride in my ability to find the card.")
Self-esteem/self-identity	Increase self-esteem, feelings of belonging, dignity, self-worth, integrity, self-identity/wellness, and quality of life	-will state/communicate positive feelings about self and ability to play, will take an active role in health though games/simulating activity, will join the game based on own choices	-Staff will educate residents on the value of mind exercises/relaxation methods and continued use of the activities
Sensory Integration/Tolerating Stimulation	Increase sensory processing and enhance awareness of sensations and toleration/adaptation of sensory stimulations and demands	-will adjust to the smell, noise, lights, peers in the room during game, and stay (does not ask to leave, does not become agitated or distractive to others)	-Staff will offer residents sensory stimulating experiences -Staff will support residents as they adjust to the stimulus
Fostering Appropriate Behaviors	Increase social interaction, social opportunities and adjustment, safety, using appropriate behaviors during an activity for a calm environment/wellness, and quality of life	-will join in on game, listen and follow instructions, use appropriate behavior for the setting; will wait turn, stand in line quietly; will quiet down when asked	Before game begins, staff will discuss the rules, appropriate behaviors, respect of property, safety, and respect of fellow peers/instructor

TABLE 14.3

Recreational Objectives Observational Form
Concentration- Socio-emotional Skills

PATIENT		Dependent (Totally dependent)	High Assistance (25+ ability)	Moderate Assist. (50+ ability)	Mild Assistance (75+ability)	Independent (Totally independent.)
SEE CODES BELOW USE OPTIONAL CODES IF APPROPRIATE		1	2	3	4	5
		3 cue/ 2-3 physical	2-3 cues/ 2 physical	2-3 cues/ 1 physical	1-2 cues	Encouragement
97530- Therapeutic activities or	SKILL	GOAL	OBJECTIVES ____times per ____		METHOD	OUTCOME DATE
97537 Or 97535	SOCIALIZATION/ COMMUNITY INTEGRATION					
97537 Or 97535	TEAM PLAYING /SHARING					
97537 Or 97535	INITIATIVE AND MOTIVATION					
97537 Or 97535	EMOTIONAL GRATIFICATION					
97537 Or 97535	SENSE OF ACCOMPLISHM ENT					
97537 Or 97535	SELF-ESTEEM/ SELF-IDENTITY					
97537 Or 97535	FOSTERING APPROPRIATE BEHAVIORS					
97533	SENSORY INTEGRATION/ TOLERATING					

97537-Community/work reintegration training (e.g., shopping, transportation, money management, avocational activities and/or work environment/modification analysis, work task analysis), direct (one-on-one) contact by provider, each 15 minutes; **97535-Self care/home management training** (e.g., activities of daily living and compensatory training, meal preparation, safety procedures, and instructions in use of adaptive equipment), direct (one-on-one) contact by provider, each 15 minutes; **97530-Therapeutic activities, direct (one-on-one)** patient contact by the provider (use of dynamic activities to improve functional performance), each 15 minutes; **97150-Therapeutic procedure(s), group (2 or more individuals); 97533-Sensory integration techniques** to enhance sensory processing and promote adaptive responses to environmental demands, direct (one-on-one) patient contact by the provider, each 15 minutes; **occupational therapy evaluation 97003, re-evaluation . 97004**	Staff Initial Add total score here-Maximum Score 40 pt. each form per activity See scale below or use own/facilities optional score system

(Score 1-8)=1 (9-16) =2 (17-24) =3 (25-32) =4 (33-40) =5 If w/device add d if wish, ex: 1d, 2d, or If using 1-7 scale: (41-48) =6 (49-56)

Good Sense

Objectives and benefits:

Cognitive Challenges: attention, memory, language, orientation, following patterns, obeying rules, letter and number recognition and recall.

Physical Needs: fine motor skills, possible gross motor skills, hand-eye coordination, perceptual speed and motor function, grasping small objects.

Socio-emotional Needs: socialization, community integration, awareness of others, team playing, emotional gratification, tolerating stimulation, fostering appropriate behaviors.

.

Supplies: A variety of tactile objects, sound objects, smelling objects, tasting objects, sequence or associated objects for the sight sense part of game. A note pad if you plan to add up points to have real winners of the game.

Time: 30 minutes

Staff/older adult ratio: 1:8 or as assessed per needs of individuals or group. All levels of function may join in.

Instructions: Sit residents in a circle. After they are all in a circle, place a variety of items in a bag. You may place a light cover over eyes in the form of a blind fold out of construction paper that looks like glasses.

Give each older adult a turn putting their hand in the bag and guessing the items inside. Generally three items would be good. They may guess the items and gain points for each item guessed correctly. In the end add up the points and award a small token or privilege to the „sharpest winner of the day."

If you are doing this activity without blindfolds, you may want to use associated objects which work together to make something. For example, for a bag that contains a small ball, a picture of a baseball bat, and a baseball game ticket the answer would be „baseball" or „items that represent baseball."

You can also use this game as a way to look back at history. For example, a theme based on the 40s or music from the 40s. The residents will love reminiscing and it works very well for recalling and retaining memories.

When doing a game that involves items that are messy, such as food, it is better to do this activity at a table setting.

> Research has shown activities that help cognition of sensory/motor and speed processing will be geared towards help in visual and motor memory, discrimination, comparison, and categorizing areas and may help improve memory skills. Long-term studies (Arbuckle and others, 1998) have consistently showed that stimulating the brain with activities helps cognitive function in a similar way exercise helps muscle function.

Good Sense
Cognitive Goals, Objectives, and Methods

Skill	Goal	Objectives Sample	Method Sample
Orientation	Show increased awareness of, time/"timeframe," people, circumstances, and past experiences vs. present experiences, to engage in present-time activities, or for a reminiscing intended question	-will respond with correct answer to two choice questions Or yes/no answer, will state where they are, time of day, present company of people on own and with the correct answer _____ times a week	Staff will ask residents a series of questions to stimulate focus to the present setting (Ex: "Do you know what time it is? Is it 12 o'clock or 5 o'clock in the afternoon?") Or past if reminiscing exercise (Ex: "Where do you live? Where did you live?")
Attention	Show increased attention span, task for function, and to engage in meaningful, recreational/fulfilling activities	-will make eye-contact with staff for _____ sec., will verbalize with staff and instructor, will read/listen to game rules, will say yes/no or initiate action to do the action required/to show listening	Staff will address or stand in front of resident, make eye-contact, ask questions, or use other methods to get resident's attention
Memory	Show increased memory skills of recall, recognition, retention of information, working memory	-will retain/repeat/recall associated items, will remember how to play at next class	Staff will show steps on how to play a game and teach the steps of game.
Language	Show increased ability to communicate use of words, phrases, sentence structure, comprehension, interpretation	-will interact with peers and staff; will call out associated items/words, etc. when asked, will recognize/interpret item's use and state them/point out associated categories	Staff will ask questions to stimulate a communication (Ex: "Tell us how the items you took out of the bag are associated.") Or make a command to - Interpretation/Lang. skills
Cognitive Stimulation (awareness, seeks information in)	Increased stimulus/exposure for visual/ motor memory, cognitive experiences/awareness and brain stimulation to enhance (function, pragmatics, neuroplasticity)	-will look around the room, be engaged in game w/peers and interact, will listen/seek cognitive stimulation, will accept challenge of input information and engage/interact in board game	-Staff will put 12 items in a bag. Residents will feel items in the bag. If resident guesses item, they can keep it and try to match to other items in the bag, or guess associated items right away. -Staff will encourage residents to think of associated items.
Perceptual Awareness	Show increased abilities of depth perception, visio-spatical awareness, and acuity (for discrimination, comparison, and categorizing), safety	-will place items in space on table, will stay within own space at, will maneuver/pick up item, will put items away in proper containers associated with area	Staff will have items in a bag, and residents will reach into the bag, feel items, and take items out
Problem-solving (goes beyond thinking/stimulus and initiates thinking process)	Increase problem-solving ability, processing of information, thinking, reasoning, and use of good judgment and decision-making	-will feel items in the bag, will guess items, will pull items from bag to see if correct, will place items on table after hearing a 1-2-3 rhythm each time, will follow patterns/rhythm of game	-Staff will direct the residents on techniques of the game/materials -Staff will answer questions regarding understanding of steps -Staff will call out ready, set, go, and resident will place hand in bag, feel items for 1 minute and then try to guess item.
Complete a Task	Increase ability to complete a task	will recall/retain and sort/gather information, problem-solve, and complete activity	Staff will support resident's ability to follow procedure through instruction, encouragement; and supplying adaptive devices if needed, and necessary materials and support

TABLE 15.1

Recreational Objectives Observational Form
Good Sense- Cognitive skills

PATIENT		Dependent (Totally dependent)	High Assistance (25+ ability)	Moderate Assist. (50+ ability)	Mild Assistance (75+ability)	Independent (Totally independent)
SEE CODES BELOW USE OPTIONAL CODES IF APPROPRIATE		1	2	3	4	5
		3 cue/ 2-3 physical	2-3 cues/ 2 physical	2-3 cues/ 1 physical	1-2 cues	Encouragement
97530- Therapeutic activities or	SKILL	GOAL	OBJECTIVES ____times per ____		METHOD	OUTCOME DATE
97532 Cognitive skills	ORIENTATION					
97532 Cognitive skills	ATTENTION					
97532 Cognitive skills	MEMORY					
97532 Cognitive skills	PROBLEM-SOLVING					
97532 Cognitive skills	COMPLETE A TASK					
97139 Speech Therapy 97532 Cognitive skills	LANGUAGE					
97533	SENSORY STIMULATION/ COGNITIVE STIMULATION					
97532	PERCEPTUAL AWARENESS					

97532-Development of cognitive skills to improve attention, memory, problem-solving, includes compensatory training and/or sensory integrative activities, direct (one-on-one) patient contact by the provider, each 15 minutes; **97530-Therapeutic activities**, direct (one-on-one) patient contact by the provider (use of dynamic activities to improve functional performance), each 15 minutes; **97533-Sensory integration techniques** to enhance sensory processing and promote adaptive responses to environmental demands, direct (one-on-one) patient contact by the provider, each 15 minutes; **97150-Therapeutic procedure(s)**, group (2 or more individuals); **97139-Unlisted therapeutic procedure** (specify) minutes; **97003- occupational therapy evaluation**; **97004- re-evaluation**	Staff Initial
	Add total score here -Maximum Score 40 pt. each form per activity
	See scale below or use own/facilities optional score system

(Score 1-8)=1 (9-16) =2 (17-24) =3 (25-32) =4 (33-40) =5 If w/device add d if wish, ex: 1d, 2d, or If using 1-7 scale: (41-48) =6 (49-56)

Good Sense
Physical Goals, Objectives, and Methods

Skill	Goal	Objectives Sample	Method Sample
Fine Motor Skills	Increase fine motor skills, meaningful/fulfilling activities	-will pick up bingo chips, use bingo magnetic brush	Staff will give residents associated items in a bag, residents will take items from the bag, manipulate items, guess item
Hand-Eye Coordination	Increase hand-eye coordination	-will place the chips on the proper square, write their name on the top of page, will place game pieces on board	Staff will give residents items that require manipulation of the item to guess what it is, and then place the item on the board
Gross Motor Skills	Increase large motor skills, meaningful/fulfilling activities	-will walk to table or walk to table with device (independent if they do on own w/device)	Staff will call residents to an activity and do a mild stretch before beginning the game
Perceptual Speed and Motor Function	Increase speed and motor ability for function, safety, meaningful /fulfilling activities	-will react and place pieces on the board, and increase speed of reaction and placing chips/item on board.	Staff will decrease the amount of time waited between manipulation of the items to guess association/item and time allowed

TABLE 15.2

Recreational Objectives Observational Form
Good Sense- Physical Skills

PATIENT		Dependent (Totally dependent)	High Assistance (25+ ability)	Moderate Assist. (50+ ability)	Mild Assistance (75+ability)	Independent (Totally independent)
SEE CODES BELOW USE OPTIONAL CODES IF APPROPRIATE		1	2	3	4	5
		3 cue/ 2-3 physical	2-3 cues/ 2 physical	2-3 cues/ 1 physical	1-2 cues	Encouragement
97530- Therapeutic activities or	**SKILL**	**GOAL**	**OBJECTIVES** ____times per ____		**METHOD**	**OUTCOME DATE**
Therapeutic Activity 97530	FINE MOTOR SKILLS					
97530	EYE-HAND COORDINATION					
97110/ 97530	GROSS MOTOR SKILLS					
97530 If under cognitive code 97532	PERCEPTUAL SPEED/MOTOR FUNCTION					

97530 Therapeutic activities, direct (one on one) patient contact by the provider (use of dynamic activities to improve functional performance),each 15 minutes; **97110 Therapeutic procedure**, **one or more areas**, each 15 minutes; therapeutic exercises to develop strength and endurance, range of motion and flexibility; ; **97150 Therapeutic procedure(s), group (2 or more individuals**; **97535-Self care/home management training** (e.g., activities of daily living and compensatory training, meal preparation, safety procedures, and instructions in use of adaptive equipment), direct (one-on-one) contact by provider, each 15 minutes; **Physical therapy 97001 evaluation, 97002 Re-evaluation. occupational therapy evaluation 97003, re-evaluation. 97004**	Staff Initials
	Add total score here Maximum Score 20 pt. each form per activity
	See scale below or use own/facilities optional score system

(Score 1-4)=1 (5-8) =2 (9-12) =3 (13-16) =4 (17-20) =5 If w/device add d if wish, ex: 1d, 2d, or If using 1-7 scale: (21-24) =6 (25-28) =7

Good Sense
Socio-emotional Goals, Objectives, and Methods

Skill	Goal	Objectives Sample	Method Sample
Socialization/Community Integration	Increase social interactions, meaningful/fulfilling activities	-will interact with one or more residents/staff/peers, will engage in community integration experiences (for community adaptation and social skills), will use manners, social practices (for community adaptation)	Staff will offer residents an activity and encourage residents to socialize through community integration and being paired during group games
Team Playing/Sharing	Increase teamwork/sharing, meaningful/fulfilling activities	-will join in game with others and share, wait turn, support peers _____ time(s) this week	Staff will encourage residents to play, share, form teams, strategize together
Initiative and Motivation	Increase initiative and motivation/wellness, and quality of life	-will choose if they wish to play the game, will do all moves on own or with assistance (as a sign of motivation to play)	-Staff will encourage the resident to prepare to come to the game in a timely fashion for their own personal gains of playing the game -Staff will offer new techniques to motivate
Emotional Gratification	Increase emotional gratification/wellness, and quality of life	-will state that the game is a gratifying experience, or will show pleasure by smiling, laughing, deep focus on game	Staff will ask residents if they enjoyed the activity and what they liked through verbal discussion, group discussions
Sense of Accomplishment	Increase feelings of self-worth, pride, productivity, dignity/wellness, and quality of life	-will use gestures to express pride in self, will talk about their accomplishments of winning	Staff will place a chart on the unit wall listing the "sharpest winner of the day," the chart will be available for residents to see their personal best and wins
Self-esteem/self-identity	Increase self-esteem, feelings of belonging, dignity, self-worth, integrity, self-identity/wellness, and quality of life	-will state/communicate positive feelings about self and ability to play, will take an active role in health though games/simulating activity, will join the game based on own choices	Staff will educate residents on the value of challenging brain games/exercise and encourage residents to participate in games
Sensory Integration/Tolerating Stimulation	Increase sensory processing and enhance awareness of sensations and toleration/adaptation of sensory stimulations and demands	-will adjust to the smell, noise, lights, peers in the room during game and stay (does not ask to leave, does not become agitated)	-During activity time, staff will expose residents to sensory stimulating experiences of varied texture items -Staff will support residents as they adjust to the stimulus
Fostering Appropriate Behaviors	Increase social interaction, social opportunities and adjustment, safety, using appropriate behaviors during an activity for a calm environment/wellness, and quality of life	-will join in on game, listen and follow instructions, use appropriate behavior for the setting; will wait turn, stand in line quietly; will quiet down when asked	Before activity begins, staff will discuss the rules, appropriate behaviors, respect of property, safety, and respect of fellow peers

TABLE 15.3

Recreational Objectives Observational Form
Good Sense- Socio-emotional Skills

PATIENT		Dependent (Totally dependent)	High Assistance (25+ ability)	Moderate Assist. (50+ ability)	Mild Assistance (75+ability)	Independent (Totally independent.)
SEE CODES BELOW USE OPTIONAL CODES IF APPROPRIATE		1	2	3	4	5
		3 cue/ 2-3 physical	2-3 cues/ 2 physical	2-3 cues/ 1 physical	1-2 cues	Encouragement

97530- Therapeutic activities or	SKILL	GOAL	OBJECTIVES ____times per ____	METHOD	OUTCOME DATE			
97537 Or 97535	SOCIALIZATION/ COMMUNITY INTEGRATION							
97537 Or 97535	TEAM PLAYING /SHARING							
97537 Or 97535	INITIATIVE AND MOTIVATION							
97537 Or 97535	EMOTIONAL GRATIFICATION							
97537 Or 97535	SENSE OF ACCOMPLISHM ENT							
97537 Or 97535	SELF-ESTEEM/ SELF-IDENTITY							
97537 Or 97535	FOSTERING APPROPRIATE BEHAVIORS							
97533	SENSORY INTEGRATION/ TOLERATING							

97537-Community/work reintegration training (e.g., shopping, transportation, money management, avocational activities and/or work environment/modification analysis, work task analysis), direct (one-on-one) contact by provider, each 15 minutes; **97535-Self care/home management training** (e.g., activities of daily living and compensatory training, meal preparation, safety procedures, and instructions in use of adaptive equipment), direct (one-on-one) contact by provider, each 15 minutes; **97530-Therapeutic activities, direct (one-on-one)** patient contact by the provider (use of dynamic activities to improve functional performance), each 15 minutes; **97150-Therapeutic procedure(s), group (2 or more individuals); 97533-Sensory integration techniques** to enhance sensory processing and promote adaptive responses to environmental demands, direct (one-on-one) patient contact by the provider, each 15 minutes; **occupational therapy evaluation 97003, re-evaluation . 97004**	Staff Initial				
	Add total score here-Maximum Score 40 pt. each form per activity				
	See scale below or use own/facilities optional score system				

(Score 1-8)=1 (9-16) =2 (17-24) =3 (25-32) =4 (33-40) =5 If w/device add d if wish, ex: 1d, 2d, or If using 1-7 scale: (41-48) =6 (49-56)

Memory

Objectives and benefits:

***Cognitive Challenges*:** attention, memory, language, orientation, following patterns, obeying rules, letter and number recognition and recall.

***Physical Needs*:** fine motor skills, possible gross motor skills, hand-eye coordination, perceptual speed and motor function, grasping small objects.

***Socio-emotional Needs*:** socialization, community integration, awareness of others, team playing, emotional gratification, tolerating stimulation, fostering appropriate behaviors.

.

Supplies: A variety of items

Time: 30 minutes

Staff/older adult ratio: 1:8 or as assessed per needs of individuals or group

Instructions: Have the older adults sit in a circle. Divide them into two groups. Start by showing them four items, and then hide the items from view. Allow one team to go first and attempt to identify what the items were. If they miss items, allow the other team to guess. Give one point for each right answer. Increase the number of items as many as you can. Have them take turns and keep score.

Research has shown activities that help cognition of sensory/motor and speed processing will be geared towards help in visual and motor memory, discrimination, comparison, and categorizing areas and may help improve memory skills. Long-term studies (Arbuckle and others, 1998) have consistently showed that stimulating the brain with activities helps cognitive function in a similar way exercise helps muscle function.

Memory
Cognitive Goals, Objectives, and Methods

Skill	Goal	Objectives Sample	Method Sample
Orientation	Show increased awareness of, time/"timeframe," people, circumstances, and past experiences vs. present experiences, to engage in present-time activities, or for a reminiscing intended question	-will respond with correct answer to two choice questions Or yes/no answer, will state where they are, time of day, present company of people on own and with the correct answer _____ times a week	Staff will ask residents a series of questions to stimulate focus to the present setting (Ex: "Today is Monday. Do you know what day of the week it is? Do we swim on Mondays or play memory challenge games?"), Or past if reminiscing exercise (Ex: "Did you ever watch Jeopardy? When?")
Attention	Show increased attention span, task for function, and to engage in meaningful, recreational/fulfilling activities	-will make eye-contact with staff for _____ sec., will verbalize with staff and instructor, will read/listen to game rules, will say yes/no or initiate action to do the action required and to they are listening	Staff will address or stand in front of resident, make eye-contact, ask questions, or use others methods to get resident's attention (Ex: "How do we play this game?")
Memory	Show increased memory skills of recall, recognition, retention of information, working memory	-will repeat/recall items, will remember how to play at next class	Staff will show steps on how to play game and teach the steps of game
Language	Show increased ability to communicate use of words, phrases, sentence structure, comprehension, interpretation	-will interact with peers and staff, will call out items shown, etc.	Staff will ask questions to stimulate a communication (Ex: "Do you want to use items for the memory challenge or remember a set of words?") Or make a command (Ex: "Put the items back on the table.") Interpretation/Lang. skills
Cognitive Stimulation (awareness, seeks information in)	Increased stimulus/exposure for visual/ motor memory, cognitive experiences/awareness and brain stimulation to enhance (function, pragmatics, neuroplasticity)	-will look around the room, be engaged in game w/peers and interact, will listen/seek cognitive stimulation, will accept challenge of input information and engage/interact in game	Staff will set up a game and have residents exposed to letter/number recognition, critical thinking, recognizing patterns, categories, discriminating and comparing to remember associations
Perceptual Awareness	Show increased abilities of depth perception, visio-spatical awareness, and acuity (for discrimination, comparison, and categorizing), safety	-will stay within own space at table, will put items away in proper containers associated with areas	Staff will instruct the residents on where they need to stay in their space (proportion to area)
Problem-solving (goes beyond thinking/stimulus and initiates thinking process)	Increase problem-solving ability, processing of information, thinking, reasoning, and use of good judgment and decision-making	-will look at items, will state items after taken out of view, will remember items using some memory strategy (Ex: associated items, colors)	Staff will name off memory items using a clock rhythm of time, and residents will follow cue/rhythm to answer seen (Ex: 1,2,3 and name items)
Complete a Task	Increase ability to complete a task	will recall/retain and sort/gather information, problem-solve, and complete activity	Staff will support resident's ability to follow procedure through instruction, encouragement, adaptive devices if needed, and supply necessary materials and support

TABLE 16.1

Recreational Objectives Observational Form
Memory- Cognitive skills

PATIENT	Dependent (Totally dependent)	High Assistance (25+ ability)	Moderate Assist. (50+ ability)	Mild Assistance (75+ability)	Independent (Totally independent)
SEE CODES BELOW USE OPTIONAL CODES IF APPROPRIATE	1	2	3	4	5
	3 cue/ 2-3 physical	2-3 cues/ 2 physical	2-3 cues/ 1 physical	1-2 cues	Encouragement

97530-Therapeutic activities or	SKILL	GOAL	OBJECTIVES ____times per ____	METHOD	OUTCOME DATE			
97532 Cognitive skills	ORIENTATION							
97532 Cognitive skills	ATTENTION							
97532 Cognitive skills	MEMORY							
97532 Cognitive skills	PROBLEM-SOLVING							
97532 Cognitive skills	COMPLETE A TASK							
97139 Speech Therapy 97532 Cognitive skills	LANGUAGE							
97533	SENSORY STIMULATION/ COGNITIVE STIMULATION							
97532	PERCEPTUAL AWARENESS							

97532-Development of cognitive skills to improve attention, memory, problem-solving, includes compensatory training and/or sensory integrative activities, direct (one-on-one) patient contact by the provider, each 15 minutes; **97530-Therapeutic activities**, direct (one-on-one) patient contact by the provider (use of dynamic activities to improve functional performance), each 15 minutes; **97533-Sensory integration techniques** to enhance sensory processing and promote adaptive responses to environmental demands, direct (one-on-one) patient contact by the provider, each 15 minutes; **97150-Therapeutic procedure(s)**, group (2 or more individuals); **97139-Unlisted therapeutic procedure** (specify) minutes; **97003- occupational therapy evaluation**; **97004- re-evaluation**	Staff Initial				
	Add total score here -Maximum Score 40 pt. each form per activity				
	See scale below or use own/facilities optional score system				

(Score 1-8)=1 (9-16) =2 (17-24) =3 (25-32) =4 (33-40) =5 If w/device add d if wish, ex: 1d, 2d, or If using 1-7 scale: (41-48) =6 (49-56)

Memory
Physical Goals, Objectives, and Methods

Skill	Goal	Objectives Sample	Method Sample
Fine Motor Skills	Increase fine motor skills, meaningful/fulfilling activities	-will pick up items to examine before items are removed	Staff will allow the residents to feel/manipulate the items which they will remember when the items are removed
Hand-Eye Coordination	Increase hand-eye coordination	-will place items back on table in proper spot	Staff will instruct residents to place items back in a circle on the table where they found the item
Gross Motor Skills	Increase large motor skills, meaningful/fulfilling activities	-will walk to table alone or walk to table with device (independent if does on own w/device)	Staff will offer activity in room that residents can walk to (device/support if needed) and have residents do a mild stretch before beginning the game
Perceptual Speed and Motor Function	Increase speed and motor ability for function, safety, meaningful /fulfilling activities	-will react and answer name of items for motor memory	Staff will decrease the amount of time waited between calling out remembered items

TABLE 16.2

Recreational Objectives Observational Form
Memory- Physical Skills

PATIENT		Dependent (Totally dependent)	High Assistance (25+ ability)	Moderate Assist. (50+ ability)	Mild Assistance (75+ability)	Independent (Totally independent)
		1	2	3	4	5
SEE CODES BELOW USE OPTIONAL CODES IF APPROPRIATE		3 cue/ 2-3 physical	2-3 cues/ 2 physical	2-3 cues/ 1 physical	1-2 cues	Encourageme nt
97530- Therapeutic activities or	**SKILL**	**GOAL**	**OBJECTIVES** ____times per ____		**METHOD**	**OUTCOME DATE**
Therapeutic Activity 97530	FINE MOTOR SKILLS					
97530	EYE-HAND COORDINATION					
97110/ 97530	GROSS MOTOR SKILLS					
97530 If under cognitive code 97532	PERCEPTUAL SPEED/MOTOR FUNCTION					

97530 Therapeutic activities, direct (one on one) patient contact by the provider (use of dynamic activities to improve functional performance),each 15 minutes; **97110 Therapeutic procedure, one or more areas**, each 15 minutes; therapeutic exercises to develop strength and endurance, range of motion and flexibility; ; **97150 Therapeutic procedure(s), group (2 or more individuals; 97535-Self care/home management training** (e.g., activities of daily living and compensatory training, meal preparation, safety procedures, and instructions in use of adaptive equipment), direct (one-on-one) contact by provider, each 15 minutes; **Physical therapy 97001 evaluation, 97002 Re-evaluation. occupational therapy evaluation 97003, re-evaluation. 97004**	Staff Initials
	Add total score here Maximum Score 20 pt. each form per activity
	See scale below or use own/facilities optional score system

(Score 1-4)=1 (5-8) =2 (9-12) =3 (13-16) =4 (17-20) =5 If w/device add d if wish, ex: 1d, 2d, or If using 1-7 scale: (21-24) =6 (25-28) =7

Memory
Socio-emotional Goals, Objectives, and Methods

Skill	Goal	Objectives Sample	Method Sample
Socialization/Community Integration	Increase social interactions, meaningful/fulfilling activities	-will interact with peers, will engage in community integration experiences (for community adaptation), will use manners, social practices	Staff will offer activities that support/encourage residents to socialize through community integration and group games
Team Playing/Sharing	Increase teamwork/sharing, meaningful/fulfilling activities	-will join in game with others and share, wait turn, support peers _____ time(s) this week	Staff will encourage/support residents to share, form teams, strategize together, show patience/compassion, and include all team players
Initiative and Motivation	Increase initiative and motivation/wellness, and quality of life	-will choose if wishes to play the game, will state answers verbally or with assistance (communication board, etc.) as a sign of motivation to play	Staff will support/encourage the resident to prepare for activity in timely fashion for their own personal attendance at activity time -Staff will offer new techniques to motivate, stimulate interest
Emotional Gratification	Increase emotional gratification/wellness, and quality of life	-will state that the game is a gratifying experience or will show pleasure by smiling, laughing, deep focus on activity.	Staff will ask residents if they enjoyed the activity and what they liked through verbal discussion, group discussions
Sense of Accomplishment	Increase feelings of self-worth, pride, productivity, dignity/wellness, and quality of life	-will use gestures to express pride in self, will talk about their accomplishments of having a sharp memory	A chart on the unit wall or a paper handed to the residents' reflecting memory skills/wins will be available for residents to see their personal best/wins
Self-esteem/self-identity	Increase self-esteem, feelings of belonging, dignity, self-worth, integrity, self-identity/wellness, and quality of life	-will state/communicate positive feelings about self and ability to play, will take an active role in health though games/simulating activity, will join the game based on own choices	Staff will educate residents on the value of memory exercise, and will encourage to continue to do activities **-Staff will design a wall chart showing memory game wins/scores
Sensory Integration/Tolerating Stimulation	Increase sensory processing and enhance awareness of sensations and toleration/adaptation of sensory stimulations and demands	-will adjust to the smell, noise, lights, and peers in the room during game and stay (does not ask to leave, does not become agitated (excessive movements, screaming, etc.)	Staff will offer residents challenging memory games and expose them to sensory stimulating experiences
Fostering Appropriate Behaviors	Increase social interaction, social opportunities and adjustment, safety, using appropriate behaviors during an activity for a calm environment/wellness, and quality of life	-will join in on game, listen and follow instructions, use appropriate behavior for the setting; will wait turn, stand in line quietly; will quiet down when asked	Before activity begins, staff will discuss the pool rules, appropriate behaviors, respect of property and safety, and respect of fellow swimmers while activity.

TABLE 16.3

Recreational Objectives Observational Form

Memory- Socio-emotional Skills

PATIENT	Dependent (Totally dependent)	High Assistance (25+ ability)	Moderate Assist. (50+ ability)	Mild Assistance (75+ability)	Independent (Totally independent.)
SEE CODES BELOW USE OPTIONAL CODES IF APPROPRIATE	1	2	3	4	5
	3 cue/ 2-3 physical	2-3 cues/ 2 physical	2-3 cues/ 1 physical	1-2 cues	Encouragement

97530- Therapeutic activities or	**SKILL**	**GOAL**	**OBJECTIVES** ____times per ____	**METHOD**	**OUTCOME DATE**			
97537 Or 97535	SOCIALIZATION/ COMMUNITY INTEGRATION							
97537 Or 97535	TEAM PLAYING /SHARING							
97537 Or 97535	INITIATIVE AND MOTIVATION							
97537 Or 97535	EMOTIONAL GRATIFICATION							
97537 Or 97535	SENSE OF ACCOMPLISHM ENT							
97537 Or 97535	SELF-ESTEEM/ SELF-IDENTITY							
97537 Or 97535	FOSTERING APPROPRIATE BEHAVIORS							
97533	SENSORY INTEGRATION/ TOLERATING							

97537-Community/work reintegration training (e.g., shopping, transportation, money management, avocational activities and/or work environment/modification analysis, work task analysis), direct (one-on-one) contact by provider, each 15 minutes; **97535-Self care/home management training** (e.g., activities of daily living and compensatory training, meal preparation, safety procedures, and instructions in use of adaptive equipment), direct (one-on-one) contact by provider, each 15 minutes; **97530-Therapeutic activities, direct (one-on-one)** patient contact by the provider (use of dynamic activities to improve functional performance), each 15 minutes; **97150-Therapeutic procedure(s), group (2 or more individuals); 97533-Sensory integration techniques** to enhance sensory processing and promote adaptive responses to environmental demands, direct (one-on-one) patient contact by the provider, each 15 minutes; **occupational therapy evaluation 97003, re-evaluation . 97004**	Staff Initial				
	Add total score here-Maximum Score 40 pt. each form per activity				
	See scale below or use own/facilities optional score system				

(Score 1-8)=1 (9-16) =2 (17-24) =3 (25-32) =4 (33-40) =5 If w/device add d if wish, ex: 1d, 2d, or If using 1-7 scale: (41-48) =6 (49-56)

Ongoing Puzzles

Objectives and benefits:

Cognitive Challenges: attention, memory, language, orientation, following patterns, obeying rules, letter and number recognition and recall.

Physical Needs: fine motor skills, possible gross motor skills, hand-eye coordination, perceptual speed and motor function, grasping small objects.

Socio-emotional Needs: socialization, community integration, awareness of others, team playing, emotional gratification, tolerating stimulation, fostering appropriate behaviors.

Supplies: puzzles with various themes and levels

Time: As long as desired

Staff/older adult ratio: Mainly a project that residents can do as they wish, with no assistance needed. However, some residents will need assistance. Many have trouble with hand tremors/vision and may need some guidance. Make sure each resident is given an opportunity to participate.

Instructions: Place three puzzles in a few areas. Let the residents know they are free to work on the puzzles at their leisure. Explain they are all free to work on any puzzle. The idea is for the puzzles to be something one person can do a bit of, and then another person to do a bit more. Puzzles should remain out and available everyday. New puzzles should be put out as older ones are completed.

Research has shown activities that help cognition of sensory/motor and speed processing will be geared towards help in visual and motor memory, discrimination, comparison, and categorizing areas and may help improve memory skills. Long-term studies (Arbuckle and others, 1998) have consistently showed that stimulating the brain with activities helps cognitive function in a similar way exercise helps muscle function.

Ongoing Puzzles
Cognitive Goals, Objectives, and Methods

Skill	Goal	Objectives	Method
Orientation	Show increased awareness of, time/"timeframe," people, circumstances, and past experiences vs. present experiences, to engage in present-time activities, or for a reminiscing intended question	-will respond with correct answer to two choice questions Or yes/no answer, will state where they are, time of day, present company of people on own and with the correct answer _____ times a week	Staff will ask residents a series of questions to stimulate focus to the present setting (Ex: "Is that a new puzzle or an old one?")
Attention	Show increased attention span, task for function, and to engage in meaningful, recreational/fulfilling activities	-will make eye-contact with staff for _____ sec. -will verbalize with staff and instructor, will read/listen to game rules, will say yes/no or initiate action to do the action required	Staff will address or stand in front of resident, make eye-contact, ask questions, or use others forms to get resident's attention
Memory	Show increased memory skills of recall, recognition, retention of information, working memory	-will repeat/recall pictures to form puzzle and will repeat when asked, will repeat/recall how to place puzzle pieces on the board, will remember how to play at next class	Staff will show steps on how to complete a section of the puzzle and ask resident to repeat the process
Language	Show increased ability to communicate use of words, phrases, sentence structure, comprehension, interpretation	-will interact with peers, will answer question (Ex: "Is that a puzzle of a dog or cat?")	Staff will ask questions to stimulate a communication (Ex: "Do you want to do the cat or dog puzzle?")
Cognitive Stimulation (awareness, seeks information in)	Increased stimulus/exposure for visual/ motor memory, cognitive experiences/awareness and brain stimulation to enhance (function, pragmatics, neuroplasticity)	-will look around the room, be engaged in game w/peers, will listen/seek cognitive stimulation, will accept challenge of input information and engage/interact in a challenging puzzle	Staff will set up puzzles and have residents exposed to picture recognition, critical thinking, recognizing patterns, categories, discriminating, and comparing
Perceptual Awareness	Show increased abilities of depth perception, visio-spatial awareness, and acuity (for discrimination, comparison, and categorizing), safety	-will place puzzle pieces in proper space on board, will stay within own space, will maneuver/pick up items, will put items away in proper containers associated with areas	Staff will offer residents puzzles which help the resident to practice use of perceptual abilities
Problem-solving (goes beyond thinking/stimulus and initiates thinking process)	Increase problem-solving ability, processing of information, thinking, reasoning, and use of good judgment and decision-making	-will problem-solve and process information regarding strategies/patterns to complete the puzzle, will consider ways to place puzzle pieces in proper spots, show a pattern/category; will discriminate, compare, will follow patterns	-Staff will direct the residents on techniques of the game/materials. -Staff will answer questions regarding understanding of steps and offer the residents challenging strategies for processing info
Complete a Task	Increase ability to complete a task	will recall/retain and sort/gather information, problem-solve, and complete activity	Staff will support resident's ability to follow procedure through instruction, encourage; and supply adaptive devices, if needed, and necessary materials and support

TABLE 17.1

Recreational Objectives Observational Form
Ongoing Puzzles- Cognitive skills

PATIENT	Dependent (Totally dependent)	High Assistance (25+ ability)	Moderate Assist. (50+ ability)	Mild Assistance (75+ability)	Independent (Totally independent)
SEE CODES BELOW USE OPTIONAL CODES IF APPROPRIATE	1	2	3	4	5
	3 cue/ 2-3 physical	2-3 cues/ 2 physical	2-3 cues/ 1 physical	1-2 cues	Encouragement

97530- Therapeutic activities or	SKILL	GOAL	OBJECTIVES ____times per ____	METHOD	OUTCOME DATE			
97532 Cognitive skills	ORIENTATION							
97532 Cognitive skills	ATTENTION							
97532 Cognitive skills	MEMORY							
97532 Cognitive skills	PROBLEM-SOLVING							
97532 Cognitive skills	COMPLETE A TASK							
97139 Speech Therapy 97532 Cognitive skills	LANGUAGE							
97533	SENSORY STIMULATION/ COGNITIVE STIMULATION							
97532	PERCEPTUAL AWARENESS							

97532-Development of cognitive skills to improve attention, memory, problem-solving, includes compensatory training and/or sensory integrative activities, direct (one-on-one) patient contact by the provider, each 15 minutes; **97530-Therapeutic activities**, direct (one-on-one) patient contact by the provider (use of dynamic activities to improve functional performance), each 15 minutes; **97533-Sensory integration techniques** to enhance sensory processing and promote adaptive responses to environmental demands, direct (one-on-one) patient contact by the provider, each 15 minutes; **97150-Therapeutic procedure(s)**, group (2 or more individuals); **97139-Unlisted therapeutic procedure** (specify) minutes; **97003- occupational therapy evaluation**; **97004- re-evaluation**	Staff Initial				
	Add total score here -Maximum Score 40 pt. each form per activity				
	See scale below or use own/facilities optional score system				

(Score 1-8)=1 (9-16) =2 (17-24) =3 (25-32) =4 (33-40) =5 If w/device add d if wish, ex: 1d, 2d, or If using 1-7 scale: (41-48) =6 (49-56)

Ongoing Puzzles
Physical Goals, Objectives, and Methods

Skill	Goal	Objectives Sample	Method Sample
Fine Motor Skills	Increase fine motor skills, meaningful/fulfilling activities	-will pick up puzzle pieces and insert the pieces on the board	Staff will give small puzzles to use fine motor skills
Hand-Eye Coordination	Increase hand-eye coordination	-will place puzzle pieces in the proper space	Staff will offer small puzzles to the residents to enhance hand-eye coordination
Gross Motor Skills	Increase large motor skills, meaningful/fulfilling activities	-will walk to table or walk to table with device (independent if does on own w/device)	Staff will ask/support residents to come/walk to the table and do a mild stretch before beginning the game
Perceptual Speed and Motor Function	Increase speed and motor ability for function, safety, meaningful /fulfilling activities	-will react and place pieces on the board and increase speed of reaction	Staff will decrease the amount of time waited between allotted time to complete a section of the puzzle

TABLE 17.2

Recreational Objectives Observational Form
Ongoing Puzzles- Physical Skills

PATIENT		Dependent (Totally dependent)	High Assistance (25+ ability)	Moderate Assist. (50+ ability)	Mild Assistance (75+ability)	Independent (Totally independent)
SEE CODES BELOW USE OPTIONAL CODES IF APPROPRIATE		1	2	3	4	5
		3 cue/ 2-3 physical	2-3 cues/ 2 physical	2-3 cues/ 1 physical	1-2 cues	Encouragement
97530- Therapeutic activities or	SKILL	GOAL	OBJECTIVES ____times per ____		METHOD	OUTCOME DATE
Therapeutic Activity 97530	FINE MOTOR SKILLS					
97530	EYE-HAND COORDINATION					
97110/ 97530	GROSS MOTOR SKILLS					
97530 If under cognitive code 97532	PERCEPTUAL SPEED/MOTOR FUNCTION					

97530 Therapeutic activities, direct (one on one) patient contact by the provider (use of dynamic activities to improve functional performance),each 15 minutes; **97110 Therapeutic procedure, one or more areas**, each 15 minutes; therapeutic exercises to develop strength and endurance, range of motion and flexibility; ; **97150 Therapeutic procedure(s), group (2 or more individuals**; **97535-Self care/home management training** (e.g., activities of daily living and compensatory training, meal preparation, safety procedures, and instructions in use of adaptive equipment), direct (one-on-one) contact by provider, each 15 minutes; **Physical therapy 97001 evaluation, 97002 Re-evaluation. occupational therapy evaluation 97003, re-evaluation. 97004**

Staff Initials	
Add total score here Maximum Score 20 pt. each form per activity	
See scale below or use own/facilities optional score system	

(Score 1-4)=1 (5-8) =2 (9-12) =3 (13-16) =4 (17-20) =5 If w/device add d if wish, ex: 1d, 2d, or If using 1-7 scale: (21-24) =6 (25-28) =7

Ongoing Puzzles
Socio-emotional Goals, Objectives, and Methods

Skill	Goal	Objectives Sample	Method Sample
Socialization/Community Integration	Increase social interactions, meaningful/fulfilling activities	-will interact with peers, will engage in community integration experiences (for social skills), will use manners, social practices (for community adaptation), will sit at table along with people in public place	Staff will offer residents puzzles and support/encourage to socialize, through community integration and being paired w/other residents playing game
Team Playing/Sharing	Increase teamwork/sharing, meaningful/fulfilling activities	-will join in game with others and share, wait turn, support peers	Staff will encourage residents to share items, take turns, strategize as a team, include all team members
Initiative and Motivation	Increase initiative and motivation/wellness, and quality of life	-will choose if wishes to take part in the ongoing puzzle, will do all moves on own or with assistance (as a sign of motivation to play)	Staff will support/encourage the resident to pursue games of choice
Emotional Gratification	Increase emotional gratification/wellness, and quality of life	-will state that the puzzle is a gratifying experience, or will show pleasure by smiling, laughing, deep focus on activity	Staff will ask residents if they enjoyed the game and what they liked through the use of verbal discussion, writing, group discussions
Sense of Accomplishment	Increase feelings of self-worth, pride, productivity, dignity/wellness, and quality of life	-will use gestures to express pride in self, will talk about their accomplishments of filling in the puzzle pieces/board	Staff will ask resident to share what they gained by partaking in the game (Ex: "I felt a feeling of…")
Self-esteem/self-identity	Increase self-esteem, feelings of belonging, dignity, self-worth, integrity, self-identity/wellness, and quality of life	-will state/communicate positive feelings about self and ability to play, will take an active role in health though games/simulating activity, will join the game based on own choices	Staff will educate residents on the value of mind exercises/games and continued use of the activities
Sensory Integration/Tolerating Stimulation	Increase sensory processing and enhance awareness of sensations and toleration/adaptation of sensory stimulations and demands	-will adjust to the smell, noise, lights, peers in the room during game, and stays (does not ask to leave, does not become agitated)	-Staff will offer residents sensory stimulating experiences -Staff will support residents as they adjust to the stimulus one step at a time
Fostering Appropriate Behaviors	Increase social interaction, social opportunities and adjustment, safety, using appropriate behaviors during an activity for a calm environment/wellness, and quality of life	-will join in on sharing an ongoing puzzle, listen and follow instructions, use appropriate behavior for the setting; will wait turn, will quiet down when asked	Before putting out the puzzles, staff will discuss the rules, appropriate behaviors, respect of property, safety, and respect of fellow peers/instructor

Table 17.3

Recreational Objectives Observational Form
Ongoing Puzzles- Socio-Emotional Skills

Patient	Dependent (Totally dependent)	High Assistance (25+ ability)	Moderate Assist. (50+ ability)	Mild Assistance (75+ability)	Independent (Totally independent.)
SEE CODES BELOW USE OPTIONAL CODES IF APPROPRIATE	1	2	3	4	5
	3 cue/ 2-3 physical	2-3 cues/ 2 physical	2-3 cues/ 1 physical	1-2 cues	Encouragement

97530- Therapeutic activities or	**Skill**	**Goal**	**Objectives** ____times per ____	**Method**	**Outcome Date**			
97537 Or 97535	Socialization/ Community Integration							
97537 Or 97535	Team Playing /Sharing							
97537 Or 97535	Initiative and Motivation							
97537 Or 97535	Emotional Gratification							
97537 Or 97535	Sense of Accomplishm ent							
97537 Or 97535	Self-esteem/ Self-identity							
97537 Or 97535	Fostering Appropriate Behaviors							
97533	Sensory Integration/ Tolerating							

97537-Community/work reintegration training (e.g., shopping, transportation, money management, avocational activities and/or work environment/modification analysis, work task analysis), direct (one-on-one) contact by provider, each 15 minutes; **97535-Self care/home management training** (e.g., activities of daily living and compensatory training, meal preparation, safety procedures, and instructions in use of adaptive equipment), direct (one-on-one) contact by provider, each 15 minutes; **97530-Therapeutic activities, direct (one-on-one)** patient contact by the provider (use of dynamic activities to improve functional performance), each 15 minutes; **97150-Therapeutic procedure(s), group (2 or more individuals); 97533-Sensory integration techniques** to enhance sensory processing and promote adaptive responses to environmental demands, direct (one-on-one) patient contact by the provider, each 15 minutes; **occupational therapy evaluation 97003, re-evaluation . 97004**	Staff Initial				
	Add total score here-Maximum Score 40 pt. each form per activity				
	See scale below or use own/facilities optional score system				

(Score 1-8)=1 (9-16) =2 (17-24) =3 (25-32) =4 (33-40) =5 If w/device add d if wish, ex: 1d, 2d, or If using 1-7 scale: (41-48) =6 (49-56)

Creative /Expressive Arts

(High cognitive stimulation, socio-emotional/variable physical stimulation/tangible art forms)

Research has shown activities that help cognition of sensory/motor and speed processing will be geared towards help in visual and motor memory, discrimination, comparison, and categorizing areas. Reminiscing activities may help improve memory skills. Long-term studies (Arbuckle and others, 1998) have consistently showed that stimulating the brain with activities helps cognitive function in a similar way exercise helps muscle function. Staying productive and involved in stimulating activities has been shown to enhance socio-emotional wellness

Current Events

Objectives and benefits:

***Cognitive Challenges*:** attention, memory, language, orientation, education

***Physical Needs*:** if done with art component: fine motor skills, gross motor skills, hand-eye coordination, and manipulation of materials

***Socio-emotional Needs*:** socialization, community integration, sharing information, initiative and motivation, emotional gratification, fostering appropriate behaviors

Supplies: Magazines, books, online information, television, radio

Time: 30 minutes

Staff/older adult ratio: As assessed per needs of individuals or group

Instructions: Give each older adult the opportunity to share some news or event that they have read or heard about. Pass articles or newspapers clippings around the room. Encourage them to share an item in the news or a personal event. You can use the articles to discuss their feelings and attitudes on current events.

> Research has shown activities that help cognition of sensory/motor and speed processing will be geared towards help in visual and motor memory, discrimination, comparison, and categorizing areas. Reminiscing activities may help improve memory skills. Long-term studies (Arbuckle and others, 1998) have consistently showed that stimulating the brain with activities helps cognitive function in a similar way exercise helps muscle function. Staying productive and involved in stimulating activities has been shown to enhance socio-emotional wellness

Current Events
Cognitive Goals, Objectives, and Methods

Skill	Goal	Objectives Sample	Method Sample
Orientation	Show increased awareness of, time/"timeframe," people, circumstances, and past experiences vs. present experiences, to engage in present-time activities, or for a reminiscing intended question	-will respond with correct answer to two choice questions (Ex: "Are you at the mall or at the activity center?") Or yes/no answer, will state where they are, time of day, present company of people on own and with the correct answer	Staff will ask residents a series of questions to stimulate focus to the present setting (Ex: "What year is it? Who is the president?") Or past if reminiscing exercise (Ex: "Who was the president during the Korean Conflict?")
Attention	Show increased attention span, task for function, and to engage in meaningful, recreational/fulfilling activities	-will make eye-contact with staff for _____ sec., will verbalize with staff and instructor, will verbally share talents	Staff will address or stand in front of resident, make eye-contact, ask questions, or use others methods to get resident's attention (Ex: "What side of the room did I say we'd start on?")
Memory	Show increased memory skills of recall, recognition, retention of information, working memory	-will recall current events, news, stories, thoughts on life, or new activity	Staff will offer current events activity to support residents in memory exercises, current news for orientation and retention
Language	Show increased ability to communicate use of words, phrases, sentence structure, comprehension, interpretation	-will be asked a question and answer yes or no, will be asked questions about the news (past and present), will interact with peers and staff, will interpret instructor's request to share and follow through with sharing	Staff will ask questions to stimulate a communication (Ex: "What do you think about the Alaskan pipe line and our gas resources?")
Cognitive Stimulation (awareness, seeks information in)	Increased stimulus/exposure for visual/ motor memory, cognitive experiences/awareness and brain stimulation to enhance (function, pragmatics, neuroplasticity)	-will engage in sharing articles and events or learning about news items, will look around the room, be engaged in game w/peers and interact, will listen/seek cognitive stimulation, will accept challenge of input information and engage/interact in current events activity	Staff will offer current event activities to allow residents to share topics, critical thinking, feelings, and strategies on topics, etc.
Perceptual Awareness	Show increased abilities of depth perception, visio-spatical awareness, and acuity (for discrimination, comparison, and categorizing), safety	-will use perceptual awareness while showing, sharing, viewing, and touching items; will discriminate, compare, categorize; will put items away	Staff will ask residents to visually place items on the current event board next to said categories
Problem-solving (goes beyond thinking/stimulus and initiates thinking process)	Increase problem-solving ability, processing of information, thinking, reasoning, and use of good judgment and decision-making	-will read interesting articles and talk about their opinion or information learned, will cut out articles and share, will problem-solve, think, reason and process information regarding use of comparisons, discrimination, categorizing, and questioning new material/current events	Staff will offer current event activities to allow residents to share topics, critical thinking, feelings, and strategies on topics, etc.
Complete a Task	Increase ability to complete a task	will recall/retain and sort/gather information, problem-solve, and complete activity	-Staff will give instruction on sharing current events and direction of the person to share, amount of time given to share, and will offer reflection and feedback time -Staff will support resident's ability to follow procedure through instruction, encourage, and supply adaptive devices/programs, if needed, and necessary materials and support

TABLE 18.1

Recreational Objectives Observational Form

Current Events- Cognitive skills

PATIENT		Dependent (Totally dependent)	High Assistance (25+ ability)	Moderate Assist. (50+ ability)	Mild Assistance (75+ability)	Independent (Totally independent)			
SEE CODES BELOW USE OPTIONAL CODES IF APPROPRIATE		1	2	3	4	5			
		3 cue/ 2-3 physical	2-3 cues/ 2 physical	2-3 cues/ 1 physical	1-2 cues	Encouragement			
97530- Therapeutic activities or	**SKILL**	**GOAL**	**OBJECTIVES** ____times per ____		**METHOD**	**OUTCOME DATE**			
97532 Cognitive skills	ORIENTATION								
97532 Cognitive skills	ATTENTION								
97532 Cognitive skills	MEMORY								
97532 Cognitive skills	PROBLEM-SOLVING								
97532 Cognitive skills	COMPLETE A TASK								
97139 Speech Therapy 97532 Cognitive skills	LANGUAGE								
97533	SENSORY STIMULATION/ COGNITIVE STIMULATION								
97532	PERCEPTUAL AWARENESS								
97532-Development of cognitive skills to improve attention, memory, problem-solving, includes compensatory training and/or sensory integrative activities, direct (one-on-one) patient contact by the provider, each 15 minutes; **97530-Therapeutic activities**, direct (one-on-one) patient contact by the provider (use of dynamic activities to improve functional performance), each 15 minutes**; 97533-Sensory integration techniques** to enhance sensory processing and promote adaptive responses to environmental demands, direct (one-on-one) patient contact by the provider, each 15 minutes; **97150-Therapeutic procedure(s**), group (2 or more individuals); **97139-Unlisted therapeutic procedure** (specify) minutes; **97003- occupational therapy evaluation**; **97004- re-evaluation**					Staff Initial				
					Add total score here -Maximum Score 40 pt. each form per activity				
					See scale below or use own/facilities optional score system				

(Score 1-8)=1 (9-16) =2 (17-24) =3 (25-32) =4 (33-40) =5 If w/device add d if wish, ex: 1d, 2d, or If using 1-7 scale: (41-48) =6 (49-56)

Current Events
Physical Goals, Objectives, and Methods

Skill	Goal	Objectives Sample	Method Sample
Fine Motor Skills	Increase fine motor skills, meaningful/fulfilling activities	-will pick up items, use fingers and dexterity, etc.	-Staff will give papers, scissors, glue, markers, and put news paper articles out
Hand-Eye Coordination	Increase hand-eye coordination	-will paste, cut, glue current event items onto a board	Staff will instruct residents to put their name on the top of the page, and cut out magazine articles
Gross Motor Skills	Increase large motor skills, meaningful/fulfilling activities	-will lift larger item, bend, etc.	Staff will engage residents in a five minute sub maximal warm-up for mild exercise
Perceptual Speed and Motor Function	Increase speed and motor ability for function, safety, meaningful /fulfilling activities	-will increase speed of actions by doing activities	Staff will give residents 5 minutes to add current events on to their construction paper/or to cut articles out, and will decrease amount of time as residents' abilities increase to increase reaction time for cutting, etc.

TABLE 18.2

Recreational Objectives Observational Form
Current Events- Physical Skills

PATIENT		Dependent (Totally dependent)	High Assistance (25+ ability)	Moderate Assist. (50+ ability)	Mild Assistance (75+ability)	Independent (Totally independent)
SEE CODES BELOW USE OPTIONAL CODES IF APPROPRIATE		1	2	3	4	5
		3 cue/ 2-3 physical	2-3 cues/ 2 physical	2-3 cues/ 1 physical	1-2 cues	Encouragement
97530- Therapeutic activities or	**SKILL**	**GOAL**	**OBJECTIVES** ____times per ____		**METHOD**	**OUTCOME DATE**
Therapeutic Activity 97530	FINE MOTOR SKILLS					
97530	EYE-HAND COORDINATION					
97110/ 97530	GROSS MOTOR SKILLS					
97530 If under cognitive code 97532	PERCEPTUAL SPEED/MOTOR FUNCTION					

97530 Therapeutic activities, direct (one on one) patient contact by the provider (use of dynamic activities to improve functional performance),each 15 minutes; **97110 Therapeutic procedure**, **one or more areas**, each 15 minutes; therapeutic exercises to develop strength and endurance, range of motion and flexibility; ; **97150 Therapeutic procedure(s), group (2 or more individuals**; **97535-Self care/home management training** (e.g., activities of daily living and compensatory training, meal preparation, safety procedures, and instructions in use of adaptive equipment), direct (one-on-one) contact by provider, each 15 minutes; **Physical therapy 97001 evaluation, 97002 Re-evaluation. occupational therapy evaluation 97003, re-evaluation. 97004**	Staff Initials
	Add total score here Maximum Score 20 pt. each form per activity
	See scale below or use own/facilities optional score system

(Score 1-4)=1 (5-8) =2 (9-12) =3 (13-16) =4 (17-20) =5 If w/device add d if wish, ex: 1d, 2d, or If using 1-7 scale: (21-24) =6 (25-28) =7

Current Events
Socio-emotionalGoals, Objectives, and Methods

Skill	Goal	Objectives Sample	Method Sample
Socialization/Community Integration	Increase social interactions, meaningful/fulfilling activities	-will interact with peers, will engage in community integration experiences (for community adaptation and social skills), will use manners, share, practice social skills	Staff will offer Current Events activity to support/encourage residence to socialize, through community integration and being paired group
Team Playing/Sharing	Increase teamwork/sharing, meaningful/fulfilling activities	-will join in and share talents, listen as others share, show articles, wait turn, support peers _____ time(s) this week.	Staff will offer magazines, newspapers and articles,; encourage online participation and news sites
Initiative and Motivation	Increase initiative and motivation/wellness, and quality of life	-will choose if wishes to share, will listen and comment about articles shared s as presented	Staff will support/encourage the resident to prepare to share articles, etc. for their own personal gains of sharing interesting information
Emotional Gratification	Increase emotional gratification/wellness, and quality of life	-will state that sharing current events or learning is a gratifying experience, or will show pleasure by smiling, laughing, deep focus on activities/articles	Staff will ask residents if they enjoy current event activities and what they liked through verbal discussion, group discussions
Sense of Accomplishment	Increase feelings of self-worth, pride, productivity, dignity/wellness, and quality of life	-will use gestures to express pride in self, will talk about information they have learned	Articles the residents have shared will be posted on the bulletin board
Self-esteem/self-identity	Increase self-esteem, feelings of belonging, dignity, self-worth, integrity, self-identity/wellness, and quality of life	-will state/communicate positive feelings about self, will join in on sharing important news and take an active role in health though intellectual conversations, will join class based on own choices	-Staff will educate residents on the value of sharing current events, and learning new information -Staff will encourage residents to share -Staff will post articles the residents have shared on the bulletin board
Fostering Appropriate Behaviors	Increase social interaction, social opportunities and adjustment, safety, using appropriate behaviors during an activity for a calm environment/wellness, and quality of life	-will adjust to peers, challenging conversations; will taste new meals, other's cooking, other activities _____ time(s) this week	-Staff will ask residents to share articles/events and expose them to sensory stimulating visual articles or items residents bring to group to share (tactile stimulation, etc.) -Staff will support residents as they adjust to the stimulus
Sensory Integration/Tolerating Stimulation	Increase sensory processing and enhance awareness of sensations and toleration/adaptation of sensory stimulations and demands	-will join in on class, share, listen to others, use appropriate behavior for the setting; will wait turn, sit quietly, and listen will quiet down when asked	Before activity begins, staff will discuss the rules, appropriate behaviors, respect of property, safety, and respect of fellow swimmers while activity.

TABLE 18.3

Recreational Objectives Observational Form
Current Events- Socio-emotional Skills

PATIENT	Dependent (Totally dependent)	High Assistance (25+ ability)	Moderate Assist. (50+ ability)	Mild Assistance (75+ability)	Independent (Totally independent.)
SEE CODES BELOW USE OPTIONAL CODES IF APPROPRIATE	1	2	3	4	5
	3 cue/ 2-3 physical	2-3 cues/ 2 physical	2-3 cues/ 1 physical	1-2 cues	Encouragement

97530-Therapeutic activities or	SKILL	GOAL	OBJECTIVES ____times per ____	METHOD	OUTCOME DATE			
97537 Or 97535	SOCIALIZATION/ COMMUNITY INTEGRATION							
97537 Or 97535	TEAM PLAYING /SHARING							
97537 Or 97535	INITIATIVE AND MOTIVATION							
97537 Or 97535	EMOTIONAL GRATIFICATION							
97537 Or 97535	SENSE OF ACCOMPLISHMENT							
97537 Or 97535	SELF-ESTEEM/ SELF-IDENTITY							
97537 Or 97535	FOSTERING APPROPRIATE BEHAVIORS							
97533	SENSORY INTEGRATION/ TOLERATING							

97537-Community/work reintegration training (e.g., shopping, transportation, money management, avocational activities and/or work environment/modification analysis, work task analysis), direct (one-on-one) contact by provider, each 15 minutes; **97535-Self care/home management training** (e.g., activities of daily living and compensatory training, meal preparation, safety procedures, and instructions in use of adaptive equipment), direct (one-on-one) contact by provider, each 15 minutes; **97530-Therapeutic activities, direct (one-on-one)** patient contact by the provider (use of dynamic activities to improve functional performance), each 15 minutes; **97150-Therapeutic procedure(s), group (2 or more individuals); 97533-Sensory integration techniques** to enhance sensory processing and promote adaptive responses to environmental demands, direct (one-on-one) patient contact by the provider, each 15 minutes; **occupational therapy evaluation 97003, re-evaluation . 97004**	Staff Initial				
	Add total score here-Maximum Score 40 pt. each form per activity				
	See scale below or use own/facilities optional score system				

(Score 1-8)=1 (9-16) =2 (17-24) =3 (25-32) =4 (33-40) =5 If w/device add d if wish, ex: 1d, 2d, or If using 1-7 scale: (41-48) =6 (49-56)

Music Activity

Objectives and benefits:

Cognitive Challenges: attention, memory, language, orientation, following patterns, keeping rhythm, cognitive stimulation

Physical Needs: fine motor skills, gross motor skills, hand-eye coordination, perceptual speed and motor function, breathing, vocal/larynx stimulation, muscle stimulation

Socio-emotional Needs: socialization, community integration, initiative and motivation, self-expression, emotional gratification, sense of accomplishment, tolerating stimulation, fostering appropriate behaviors

Supplies: Keyboard or any instrument the older adults will enjoy listening to, a pre-taped song to sing along to, and possibly a Karaoke machine. A musical movie is also a nice treat.

Time: As long as desired

Staff/older adult ratio: As assessed per needs of individuals or group

Instructions: Have residents come to a circle. If there is a theme, holiday, or special occasion, play chosen songs from staff or residents. Have staff members play instruments and encourage residents to join in. If the staff is singing, the older adults will feel it is okay to sing as well and it will be a real joy for them.

Research has shown activities that help cognition of sensory/motor and speed processing will be geared towards help in visual and motor memory, discrimination, comparison, and categorizing areas. Reminiscing activities may help improve memory skills. Long-term studies (Arbuckle and others, 1998) have consistently showed that stimulating the brain with activities helps cognitive function in a similar way exercise helps muscle function. Staying productive and involved in stimulating activities has been shown to enhance socio-emotional wellness

Music
Cognitive Goals, Objectives, and Methods

Skill	Goal	Objectives Sample	Method Sample
Orientation	Show increased awareness of, time/"timeframe," people, circumstances, and past experiences vs. present experiences, to engage in present-time activities, or for a reminiscing intended question	-will respond with correct answer to two choice question Or yes/no answer; will state where they are, time of day, present company of people on own and with the correct answer	Staff will ask residents a series of questions to stimulate focus to the present setting (Ex: "Do you know what kind of music the kids listen to today"? Are you at the opera or on the unit?") Or past if reminiscing exercise (Ex: "What was your favorite music in the 50's, etc?") (memory and orientation exercise)
Attention	Show increased attention span, task for function, and to engage in meaningful, recreational/fulfilling activities	-will make eye-contact with staff for _____ sec., will verbalize with staff and instructor, will read/listen to rules, will say yes/no to show they understand or do the action	Staff will address or stand in front of resident, make eye-contact, ask questions, or use others forms to get resident's attention (Ex: "What kind of music are we going to listen to?")
Memory	Show increased memory skills of recall, recognition, retention of information, working memory	-will repeat/recall the music, will repeat/recall how to sing a verse, will remember will music later or at next class	Staff will ask residents to name popular music from different time frames or teach a new song and ask residents to repeat it
Language	Show increased ability to communicate use of words, phrases, sentence structure, comprehension, interpretation	-will be asked a question and answer yes/no, will be asked to sing/say the words to the song, will interact/sing with peers and staff, will interpret instructor's request and follow	-Staff will ask questions to stimulate a communication (Ex: "What are the words to that song"? Or for Interpretation/Lang. skills -Staff will show the resident the step-by-step words to the song and ask residents to sing the whole song
Cognitive Stimulation (awareness, seeks information in)	Increased stimulus/exposure for visual/ motor memory, cognitive experiences/awareness and brain stimulation to enhance (function, pragmatics, neuroplasticity)	-will look around the room, will be engaged in game w/peers and interact, will listen/seek cognitive stimulation, will accept challenge of input information and engage/interact in music activity	Staff will set up a music tape and have residents listen to the song or make up their own songs
Perceptual Awareness	Show increased abilities of depth perception, visio-spatial awareness, and acuity (for discrimination, comparison, and categorizing), safety	-will sing when music instructor/staff points to group they are in; as staff raises arms they can raise voice	Staff will instruct the residents on where they need to stay/ sit during a music event
Problem-solving (goes beyond thinking/stimulus and initiates thinking process)	Increase problem-solving ability, processing of information, thinking, reasoning, and use of good judgment and decision-making	-will follow rhythm and tones of music and play instrument in rhythm, will read words and sing songs, will read music if possible, will play instrument (bells, tangerine, etc.), will sing learned verses	Staff will show the resident the step-by-step words to the song and ask residents to sing the whole song
Complete a Task	Increase ability to complete a task	-will recall/retain and sort/gather information, problem-solve, and complete activity	Staff will support resident's ability to follow procedure through instruction, encourage; and supply adaptive devices/programs, if needed, and necessary materials and support

Table 19.1

Recreational Objectives Observational Form
Music- Cognitive skills

Patient	Dependent (Totally dependent)	High Assistance (25+ ability)	Moderate Assist. (50+ ability)	Mild Assistance (75+ability)	Independent (Totally independent)
See codes below Use optional codes if appropriate	1	2	3	4	5
	3 cue/ 2-3 physical	2-3 cues/ 2 physical	2-3 cues/ 1 physical	1-2 cues	Encouragemen t

97530- Therapeutic activities or	**Skill**	**Goal**	**Objectives** ____times per ____	**Method**	**Outcome Date**			
97532 Cognitive skills	Orientation							
97532 Cognitive skills	Attention							
97532 Cognitive skills	Memory							
97532 Cognitive skills	Problem-Solving							
97532 Cognitive skills	Complete a Task							
97139 Speech Therapy 97532 Cognitive skills	Language							
97533	Sensory Stimulation/ Cognitive Stimulation							
97532	Perceptual Awareness							

97532-Development of cognitive skills to improve attention, memory, problem-solving, includes compensatory training and/or sensory integrative activities, direct (one-on-one) patient contact by the provider, each 15 minutes; **97530-Therapeutic activities**, direct (one-on-one) patient contact by the provider (use of dynamic activities to improve functional performance), each 15 minutes; **97533-Sensory integration techniques** to enhance sensory processing and promote adaptive responses to environmental demands, direct (one-on-one) patient contact by the provider, each 15 minutes; **97150-Therapeutic procedure(s)**, group (2 or more individuals); **97139-Unlisted therapeutic procedure** (specify) minutes; **97003- occupational therapy evaluation**; **97004- re-evaluation**	Staff Initial				
	Add total score here -Maximum Score 40 pt. each form per activity				
	See scale below or use own/facilities optional score system				

(Score 1-8)=1 (9-16) =2 (17-24) =3 (25-32) =4 (33-40) =5 If w/device add d if wish, ex: 1d, 2d, or If using 1-7 scale: (41-48) =6 (49-56)

Music
Physical Goals, Objectives, and Methods

Skill Basic music Instrument/or just music and clapping etc.	Goal	Objectives Sample	Method Sample
Fine Motor Skills	Increase fine motor skills, meaningful/fulfilling activities	-will pick up instruments, manipulate instruments	-Staff will give residents basic music instruments to play and explore
Hand-Eye Coordination	Increase hand-eye coordination	-will place the fingers on proper holes, keys, etc. to play instrument	Staff will instruct residents to put their hands, fingers, etc. on the instruments
Gross Motor Skills	Increase large motor skills, meaningful/fulfilling activities	-will walk to table or walk to table with device (independent if they do it on own w/device)	Staff will engage residents in a mild submaxial warm up before sitting and playing musical instruments
Perceptual Speed and Motor Function	Increase speed and motor ability for function, safety, meaningful /fulfilling activities	-will react and place fingers, on basic music instruments and increase speed of reaction and playing instrument.	Staff will decrease the amount of time waited between music sets and musical rhythm formats

Table 19.2

Recreational Objectives Observational Form
Music- Physical Skills

PATIENT		Dependent (Totally dependent)	High Assistance (25+ ability)	Moderate Assist. (50+ ability)	Mild Assistance (75+ability)	Independent (Totally independent)			
		1	2	3	4	5			
SEE CODES BELOW USE OPTIONAL CODES IF APPROPRIATE		3 cue/ 2-3 physical	2-3 cues/ 2 physical	2-3 cues/ 1 physical	1-2 cues	Encouragement			
97530- Therapeutic activities or	**SKILL**	**GOAL**	**OBJECTIVES** ____times per ____		**METHOD**	**OUTCOME DATE**			
Therapeutic Activity 97530	FINE MOTOR SKILLS								
97530	EYE-HAND COORDINATION								
97110/ 97530	GROSS MOTOR SKILLS								
97530 If under cognitive code 97532	PERCEPTUAL SPEED/MOTOR FUNCTION								
97530 Therapeutic activities, direct (one on one) patient contact by the provider (use of dynamic activities to improve functional performance),each 15 minutes; **97110 Therapeutic procedure, one or more areas**, each 15 minutes; therapeutic exercises to develop strength and endurance, range of motion and flexibility; ; **97150 Therapeutic procedure(s), group (2 or more individuals**; **97535-Self care/home management training** (e.g., activities of daily living and compensatory training, meal preparation, safety procedures, and instructions in use of adaptive equipment), direct (one-on-one) contact by provider, each 15 minutes; **Physical therapy 97001 evaluation, 97002 Re-evaluation. occupational therapy evaluation 97003, re-evaluation. 97004**					Staff Initials				
					Add total score here Maximum Score 20 pt. each form per activity				
					See scale below or use own/facilities optional score system				

(Score 1-4)=1 (5-8) =2 (9-12) =3 (13-16) =4 (17-20) =5 If w/device add d if wish, ex: 1d, 2d, or If using 1-7 scale: (21-24) =6 (25-28) =7

Music
Socio-emotional Goals, Objectives, and Methods

Skill	Goal	Objectives Sample	Method Sample
Socialization/Community Integration	Increase social interactions, meaningful/fulfilling activities	-will interact with peers, will engage in community integration experiences (for community adaptation and social skills), will use manners, share, practice social skills	Staff will offer a musical activity to support/encourage residents to socialize through community integration and being w/groups
Team Playing/Sharing	Increase teamwork/sharing, meaningful/fulfilling activities	-will join in on a singing activity with others and share, wait turn, support peers _____ time(s) this week.	Staff will encourage residents to play, share music tastes form teams, strategize/make music songs together
Initiative and Motivation	Increase initiative and motivation/wellness, and quality of life	-will choose if they wish to sing, will try a new song, will sing on own, will increase singing	Staff will support encourage the resident to prepare for music class in a timely fashion for their own personal gains of attending music classes -Staff will offer new techniques, music, themes to motivate
Emotional Gratification	Increase emotional gratification/wellness, and quality of life	-will state that singing is a gratifying experience, or will show pleasure by smiling, laughing, deep focus on songs, singing	Staff will ask residents if they enjoyed the music class and what they liked through verbal discussion, group discussions
Sense of Accomplishment	Increase feelings of self-worth, pride, productivity, dignity/wellness, and quality of life	-will use gestures to express pride in self, will talk about their accomplishments of singing	Staff will post a chart showing resident's music tastes/ produced music. The chart will be available for residents to see their personal choices and musical compositions (*Can submit songs for copyrights if wish to do activity)
Self-esteem/self-identity	Increase self-esteem, feelings of belonging, dignity, self-worth, integrity, self-identity/wellness, and quality of life	-will state/communicate positive feelings about self, will join singing to take an active role in health though exercising, will join singing based on own choices	Staff will educate residents on the value of music/exercise for muscle/stimulant benefits, and encourage to join classes
Sensory Integration/Tolerating Stimulation	Increase sensory processing and enhance awareness of sensations and toleration/adaptation of sensory stimulations and demands	-will adjust to the lights, sounds, and etc. _____ time this week.	-Staff will offer music classes, and residents will be exposed to sensory stimulating experiences of sound -Staff will support residents as they adjust to the stimulus one step at a time
Fostering Appropriate Behaviors	Increase social interaction, social opportunities and adjustment, safety, using appropriate behaviors during an activity for a calm environment/wellness, and quality of life	-will join in on singing class, listen, and follow instructions, will use appropriate behavior for the setting, will wait turn, stand in line quietly; will quiet down when asked	Before class begins, staff will discuss the rules, appropriate behaviors, respect of property, safety, and respect of fellow singers while singing/attending musical

Table 19.3

Recreational Objectives Observational Form
Music- Socio-emotional Skills

Patient		Dependent (Totally dependent)	High Assistance (25+ ability)	Moderate Assist. (50+ ability)	Mild Assistance (75+ability)	Independent (Totally independent.)			
See codes below Use optional codes if appropriate		1	2	3	4	5			
		3 cue/ 2-3 physical	2-3 cues/ 2 physical	2-3 cues/ 1 physical	1-2 cues	Encouragement			
97530- Therapeutic activities or	**Skill**	**Goal**	**Objectives** ____times per ____		**Method**	**Outcome Date**			
97537 Or 97535	Socialization/ Community Integration								
97537 Or 97535	Team Playing /Sharing								
97537 Or 97535	Initiative and Motivation								
97537 Or 97535	Emotional Gratification								
97537 Or 97535	Sense of Accomplishm ent								
97537 Or 97535	Self-esteem/ Self-identity								
97537 Or 97535	Fostering Appropriate Behaviors								
97533	Sensory Integration/ Tolerating								

97537-Community/work reintegration training (e.g., shopping, transportation, money management, avocational activities and/or work environment/modification analysis, work task analysis), direct (one-on-one) contact by provider, each 15 minutes; **97535-Self care/home management training** (e.g., activities of daily living and compensatory training, meal preparation, safety procedures, and instructions in use of adaptive equipment), direct (one-on-one) contact by provider, each 15 minutes; **97530-Therapeutic activities, direct (one-on-one)** patient contact by the provider (use of dynamic activities to improve functional performance), each 15 minutes; **97150-Therapeutic procedure(s), group (2 or more individuals); 97533-Sensory integration techniques** to enhance sensory processing and promote adaptive responses to environmental demands, direct (one-on-one) patient contact by the provider, each 15 minutes; **occupational therapy evaluation 97003, re-evaluation . 97004**	Staff Initial				
	Add total score here-Maximum Score 40 pt. each form per activity				
	See scale below or use own/facilities optional score system				

(Score 1-8)=1 (9-16) =2 (17-24) =3 (25-32) =4 (33-40) =5 If w/device add d if wish, ex: 1d, 2d, or If using 1-7 scale: (41-48) =6 (49-56) Current Procedural Terminology © 2005 American Medical Association. All rights reserved. Recreational Objectives Observational form© 2005. All rights reserved. Patent pending.

Musical Instruments

Objectives and benefits:

Cognitive Challenges: attention, memory, language, orientation, following patterns, keeping rhythm, cognitive stimulation

Physical Needs: fine motor skills, gross mot-or skills, hand-eye coordination, perc-eptual speed and motor function, breathing, vocal/larynx stimulation, muscle stimulation

Socio-emotional Needs: socialization, community integration, initiative and mo-tivation, self-expression, emotional gratifi-cation, sense of accomplishment, tolerating stimulation, fostering appropriate behaviors

Supplies: Keyboard or any instrument a staff member can play bells, tambourine, drums, etc. Usually you can purchase a kit with an array of musical instruments.

Time: As long as desired

Staff/older adult ratio: As assessed per needs of individuals or group

Instructions: Have residents come to a circle. Have staff members play instruments with the residents. It is a good idea to stress the beat of the music so that the older adults learn to understand the rhythm. It will help to have a staff member clap their hands to the beat of the music to give older adults an idea of the rhythm; they can then play instruments to the beat. If the staff sings, older adults will be comfortable and more likely to join in with singing and playing instruments. This activity can be a rewarding experience for many. Even the hearing impaired may be able to feel the vibration of the music.

Research has shown activities that help cognition of sensory/motor and speed processing will be geared towards help in visual and motor memory, discrimination, comparison, and categorizing areas. Reminiscing activities may help improve memory skills. Long-term studies (Arbuckle and others, 1998) have consistently showed that stimulating the brain with activities helps cognitive function in a similar way exercise helps muscle function. Staying productive and involved in stimulating activities has been shown to enhance socio-emotional wellness

Musical Instruments
Cognitive Goals, Objectives, and Methods

Skill	Goal	Objectives Sample	Method Sample
Orientation	Show increased awareness of, time/"timeframe," people, circumstances, and past experiences vs. present experiences, to engage in present-time activities, or for a reminiscing intended question	-will respond with correct answer to two choice questions (Ex: "Are you at the mall or at the activity center?") Or yes/no answer, will state where they are, time of day, present company of people on own and with the correct answer	Staff will ask residents a series of questions to stimulate focus to the present setting (Ex: "Do you know what kind of music kids listen to today? Are you at the opera or on the unit?") Or past if reminiscing exercise (Ex: "What where the most influential instruments in your time? Saxophone or piano?") (memory and orientation exercise)
Attention	Show increased attention span, task for function, and to engage in meaningful, recreational/fulfilling activities	-will make eye-contact with staff for _____ sec., will verbalize with staff and instructor, will read/listen to rules, say yes/no to show they understand or do the action	Staff will address or stand in front of resident, make eye-contact, ask questions, or use others methods to get resident's attention (Ex: "What kind of music are we going to play?")
Memory	Show increased memory skills of recall, recognition, retention of information, working memory	-will repeat/recall the music, will repeat/recall how to play the instrument, will remember music later or at next class	Staff will ask residents to name popular music from different time frames; or teach a new song and include using instruments, then ask residents to repeat it
Language	Show increased ability to communicate use of words, phrases, sentence structure, comprehension, interpretation	-will be asked a question and answer yes /no, will be asked to sing/say the words to the show, interact, will sing with peers, staff; will interpret instructor's request and follow	Staff will ask questions to stimulate communication (Ex: "What are the words to that song?") Interpretation/Lang. skills
Cognitive Stimulation (awareness, seeks information in)	Increased stimulus/exposure for visual/ motor memory, cognitive experiences/awareness and brain stimulation to enhance (function, pragmatics, neuroplasticity)	-will look around the room, will be engaged in game w/peers, will interact, will listen/seek cognitive stimulation, will accept challenge of input information and engage/interact in musical activity	Staff will set up a music tape and have residents listen to the song and explore music with musical instruments
Perceptual Awareness	Show increased abilities of depth perception, visio-spatial awareness, and acuity (for discrimination, comparison, and categorizing), safety	-will sing when music instructor/staff points to group they are in, as staff raises arms they can raise voice; will hit drum, tap bells, etc.	Staff will offer a setting where the residents will need to observe proportion of space to others and room for their instrument
Problem-solving (goes beyond thinking/stimulus and initiates thinking process)	Increase problem-solving ability, processing of information, thinking, reasoning, and use of good judgment and decision-making	-will follow rhythm and tones of music and play instrument in rhythm, will read words and sing songs, will read music if possible, will play instrument (bells, tangerine, etc.)	-A musical tape with a steady rhythm will be placed in the tape player. -Staff will show the resident the step-by-step words to the song, the pattern to hit/ring instruments, and ask residents to sing the whole song -Resident will sing/play instrument to the music rhythm
Complete a Task	Increase ability to complete a task	-will recall/retain and sort/gather information, problem-solve, and complete activity	Staff will support resident's ability to follow procedure through instruction, encourage; and supply adaptive devices/programs, if needed, and necessary materials and support

TABLE 20.1

Recreational Objectives Observational Form
Musical Instruments- Cognitive skills

PATIENT	Dependent (Totally dependent)	High Assistance (25+ ability)	Moderate Assist. (50+ ability)	Mild Assistance (75+ability)	Independent (Totally independent)
SEE CODES BELOW USE OPTIONAL CODES IF APPROPRIATE	1	2	3	4	5
	3 cue/ 2-3 physical	2-3 cues/ 2 physical	2-3 cues/ 1 physical	1-2 cues	Encouragement

97530-Therapeutic activities or	SKILL	GOAL	OBJECTIVES ____times per ____	METHOD	OUTCOME DATE			
97532 Cognitive skills	ORIENTATION							
97532 Cognitive skills	ATTENTION							
97532 Cognitive skills	MEMORY							
97532 Cognitive skills	PROBLEM-SOLVING							
97532 Cognitive skills	COMPLETE A TASK							
97139 Speech Therapy 97532 Cognitive skills	LANGUAGE							
97533	SENSORY STIMULATION/ COGNITIVE STIMULATION							
97532	PERCEPTUAL AWARENESS							

97532-Development of cognitive skills to improve attention, memory, problem-solving, includes compensatory training and/or sensory integrative activities, direct (one-on-one) patient contact by the provider, each 15 minutes; **97530-Therapeutic activities**, direct (one-on-one) patient contact by the provider (use of dynamic activities to improve functional performance), each 15 minutes**; 97533-Sensory integration techniques** to enhance sensory processing and promote adaptive responses to environmental demands, direct (one-on-one) patient contact by the provider, each 15 minutes; **97150-Therapeutic procedure(s)**, group (2 or more individuals); **97139-Unlisted therapeutic procedure** (specify) minutes; **97003- occupational therapy evaluation**; **97004- re-evaluation**	Staff Initial				
	Add total score here -Maximum Score 40 pt. each form per activity				
	See scale below or use own/facilities optional score system				

(Score 1-8)=1 (9-16) =2 (17-24) =3 (25-32) =4 (33-40) =5 If w/device add d if wish, ex: 1d, 2d, or If using 1-7 scale: (41-48) =6 (49-56)

Musical Instruments
Physical Goals, Objectives, and Methods

Skill	Goal	Objectives Sample	Method Sample
Fine Motor Skills	Increase fine motor skills, meaningful/fulfilling activities	-will pick up instruments, manipulate instruments	-Staff will give residents instruments to play and explore
Hand-Eye Coordination	Increase hand-eye coordination	-will place the fingers on proper holes, keys, etc. to play instrument	Staff will instruct residents to put their hands, fingers, etc. on the instruments
Gross Motor Skills	Increase large motor skills, meaningful/fulfilling activities	-will walk to table or walk to table with device (independent if they do it on own w/device)	Staff will engage residents in a mild submaxial warm up before sitting and playing musical instruments
Perceptual Speed and Motor Function	Increase speed and motor ability for function, safety, meaningful /fulfilling activities	-will react and place fingers, etc. on keys and increase speed of reaction and playing instrument.	Staff will decrease the amount of time waited between music sets and musical rhythm formats

TABLE 20.2

Recreational Objectives Observational Form
Musical Instruments- Physical Skills

PATIENT		Dependent (Totally dependent)	High Assistance (25+ ability)	Moderate Assist. (50+ ability)	Mild Assistance (75+ability)	Independent (Totally independent)
		1	2	3	4	5
SEE CODES BELOW USE OPTIONAL CODES IF APPROPRIATE		3 cue/ 2-3 physical	2-3 cues/ 2 physical	2-3 cues/ 1 physical	1-2 cues	Encouragement
97530- Therapeutic activities or	**SKILL**	**GOAL**	**OBJECTIVES** ____times per ____		**METHOD**	**OUTCOME DATE**
Therapeutic Activity 97530	FINE MOTOR SKILLS					
97530	EYE-HAND COORDINATION					
97110/ 97530	GROSS MOTOR SKILLS					
97530 If under cognitive code 97532	PERCEPTUAL SPEED/MOTOR FUNCTION					

97530 Therapeutic activities, direct (one on one) patient contact by the provider (use of dynamic activities to improve functional performance),each 15 minutes; **97110 Therapeutic procedure, one or more areas**, each 15 minutes; therapeutic exercises to develop strength and endurance, range of motion and flexibility; ; **97150 Therapeutic procedure(s), group (2 or more individuals**; **97535-Self care/home management training** (e.g., activities of daily living and compensatory training, meal preparation, safety procedures, and instructions in use of adaptive equipment), direct (one-on-one) contact by provider, each 15 minutes; **Physical therapy 97001 evaluation, 97002 Re-evaluation. occupational therapy evaluation 97003, re-evaluation. 97004**	Staff Initials
	Add total score here Maximum Score 20 pt. each form per activity
	See scale below or use own/facilities optional score system

(Score 1-4)=1 (5-8) =2 (9-12) =3 (13-16) =4 (17-20) =5 If w/device add d if wish, ex: 1d, 2d, or If using 1-7 scale: (21-24) =6 (25-28) =7

Music
Socio-emotional Goals, Objectives and Methods

Skill	Goal	Objectives	Method
Socialization/ Community Integration	Increase social interactions, meaningful /fulfilling activities	-will interact with peers, will engage in a community integration experiences (for community adaptation) (for social skills)–will use manners, share, practices social skills	Staff will offer a musical activity to support/encourage residents to socialize, through community integration and being w/ groups
Team playing/Sharing	Increase teamwork/sharing, meaningful /fulfilling activities	-will, join in on a singing activity and playing instruments with others and share, wait turn, support peers _____ time(s) this week.	Staff will encourage residents to play, share music tastes, share instrument times, form bands strategize/ make music songs together
Initiative and motivation	Increase initiative and motivation	-will choose if wishes to sing/play instrument, will try a new song and instrument, will sing /play instrument on own, will increase singing and playing of instruments	Will support /encourage the resident to prepare for music class in a timely fashion for their own personal gains of attending music classes -offer new techniques/music /themes /instruments to motivate
Emotional Gratification	Increase emotional gratification /wellness, fulfillment and quality of life	-will state that singing/playing instrument is a gratifying experiences or will show pleasure by smiling ,laughing , deep focus on songs, playing the instrument,	Will be asked if they enjoyed the musical instrumental class and what they liked through verbal discussion,, group discussions
Sense of Accomplishment	Increase feelings of self worth, pride, feelings of productivity, dignity	-will use gestures to express pride in self, will talk about their accomplishments of singing and ability to play instrument	A chart showing residents musical instrument abilities. will be available for residents to see their personal choices/ musical instrument talents/ abilities/ compositions * can submit songs for copyrights if wish to do activity
Self-esteem/self Identity	Increase self –esteem, feelings of belonging, dignity, self-worth, integrity Increase self-identity,	-will state/communicate positive feelings about self, will join singing /playing instruments to take an active role in maintaining health though exercising -will join singing based on own choices	Will be educated on the value of using music and musical instruments for brain muscle/stimulant benefits and encouraged to join classes
Tolerating Stimulation	Increase awareness of sensations and toleration/adaptation of sensory stimulation/demands	-will adjust to the lights, sounds etc. ____time(s) this week.	Staff will offer music classes/ musical instruments and residents will be exposed to sensory stimulating experiences of sound, textures of items, sights, Staff will support residence as they adjust to the stimulus
Fostering appropriate Behaviors	Increase awareness of social adaptation, safety , self-esteem, calm environment for all	-will join in on singing class, playing instrument, listen and follow instructions, use appropriate behavior for the setting, will wait turn, stand in line	Before class begins, staff will discuss the rules, appropriate behaviors, respect of property, safety, and respect of fellow swimmers while activity.

TABLE 20.3

Recreational Objectives Observational Form
Musical Instruments- Socio-emotional Skills

PATIENT	Dependent (Totally dependent)	High Assistance (25+ ability)	Moderate Assist. (50+ ability)	Mild Assistance (75+ability)	Independent (Totally independent.)
SEE CODES BELOW USE OPTIONAL CODES IF APPROPRIATE	1	2	3	4	5
	3 cue/ 2-3 physical	2-3 cues/ 2 physical	2-3 cues/ 1 physical	1-2 cues	Encouragement

97530- Therapeutic activities or	SKILL	GOAL	OBJECTIVES ____times per ____	METHOD	OUTCOME DATE			
97537 Or 97535	SOCIALIZATION/ COMMUNITY INTEGRATION							
97537 Or 97535	TEAM PLAYING /SHARING							
97537 Or 97535	INITIATIVE AND MOTIVATION							
97537 Or 97535	EMOTIONAL GRATIFICATION							
97537 Or 97535	SENSE OF ACCOMPLISHM ENT							
97537 Or 97535	SELF-ESTEEM/ SELF-IDENTITY							
97537 Or 97535	FOSTERING APPROPRIATE BEHAVIORS							
97533	SENSORY INTEGRATION/ TOLERATING							

97537-Community/work reintegration training (e.g., shopping, transportation, money management, avocational activities and/or work environment/modification analysis, work task analysis), direct (one-on-one) contact by provider, each 15 minutes; **97535-Self care/home management training** (e.g., activities of daily living and compensatory training, meal preparation, safety procedures, and instructions in use of adaptive equipment), direct (one-on-one) contact by provider, each 15 minutes; **97530-Therapeutic activities, direct (one-on-one)** patient contact by the provider (use of dynamic activities to improve functional performance), each 15 minutes; **97150-Therapeutic procedure(s), group (2 or more individuals); 97533-Sensory integration techniques** to enhance sensory processing and promote adaptive responses to environmental demands, direct (one-on-one) patient contact by the provider, each 15 minutes; **occupational therapy evaluation 97003, re-evaluation . 97004**	Staff Initial				
	Add total score here-Maximum Score 40 pt. each form per activity				
	See scale below or use own/facilities optional score system				

(Score 1-8)=1 (9-16) =2 (17-24) =3 (25-32) =4 (33-40) =5 If w/device add d if wish, ex: 1d, 2d, or If using 1-7 scale: (41-48) =6 (49-56)

Sharing Talents

Objectives and benefits:

Cognitive Challenges: attention, memory, language, orientation, following patterns, keeping rhythm, cognitive stimulation

Physical Needs: fine motor skills, gross motor skills, hand-eye coordination, perceptual speed and motor function, muscle stimulation

Socio-emotional Needs: socialization, community integration, initiative and motivation, self-expression, emotional gratification, sense of accomplishment, tolerating stimulation, fostering appropriate behaviors

Supplies: Will vary according to the talent and project the older adults choose to share. The older adult will have to let you know ahead of time what talent they will be sharing and supplies they will need.

Time: 30–45 minutes

Staff/older adult ratio: As assessed per needs of individuals or group

Instructions: Allow all older adults the opportunity to share a talent. They may need some encouragement and support, but with enthusiasm you can get older adults to share their talents. The talent does not need to be elaborate. It can range from complex, hands on work to something as simple as an interesting. The other older adults can either try to learn the talent, or just observe and enjoy the event.

Research has shown activities that help cognition of sensory/motor and speed processing will be geared towards help in visual and motor memory, discrimination, comparison, and categorizing areas. Reminiscing activities may help improve memory skills. Long-term studies (Arbuckle and others, 1998) have consistently showed that stimulating the brain with activities helps cognitive function in a similar way exercise helps muscle function. Staying productive and involved in stimulating activities has been shown to enhance socio-emotional wellness

Sharing Talents
Cognitive Goals, Objectives, and Methods

Skill	Goal	Objectives Sample	Method Sample
Orientation	Show increased awareness of, time/"timeframe," people, circumstances, and past experiences vs. present experiences, to engage in present-time activities, or for a reminiscing intended question	-will respond with correct answer to two choice questions (Ex: "Are you at the mall or at the activity center?") Or yes/no answer; will state where they are, time of day, present company of people on own and with the correct answer	Staff will ask residents a series of questions to stimulate focus to the present setting (Ex: "What talents are you going to share? Have you had this talent a long time?")
Attention	Show increased attention span, task for function, and to engage in meaningful, recreational/fulfilling activities	-will make eye-contact with staff for _____ sec., will verbalize with staff and instructor, will verbally share talents	Staff will address or stand in front of resident, make eye-contact, ask questions, or use others methods to get resident's attention (Ex: "What are you going to share?")
Memory	Show increased memory skills of recall, recognition, retention of information, working memory	-will recall talents learned though life, or new activity	Staff will show steps on how to follow recipe, and residents will add ingredients, etc.
Language	Show increased ability to communicate use of words, phrases, sentence structure, comprehension, interpretation	-will be asked a question and answer yes /no, will be asked what is included in recipe, poems, etc.; will state talents, will interact with peers, staff; will interpret instructor's request to share and follows through with sharing	Staff will ask questions to stimulate a communication (Ex: "Where did you learn this talent?") Interpretation/Lang. skills (Ex: "Can you try Bill's talent?")
Cognitive Stimulation (awareness, seeks information in)	Increased stimulus/exposure for visual/ motor memory, cognitive experiences/awareness and brain stimulation to enhance (function, pragmatics, neuroplasticity)	-will interact with peers, will listen/seek cognitive stimulation, will accept challenge of input information and engage/interact; will engage in sharing a talent or learning about one	Staff will ask residents to bring materials to the activity
Perceptual Awareness	Show increased abilities of depth perception, visio-spatical awareness, and acuity (for discrimination, comparison, and categorizing), safety	-will use perceptual awareness while showing, sharing , viewing, touching items; will discriminate, compare, categorize; will maneuver around the area, will put items away in proper containers associated with proper area	Staff will have residents pick up items, work with items, put items away, maneuver around items
Problem-solving (goes beyond thinking/stimulus and initiates thinking process)	Increase problem-solving ability, processing of information, thinking, reasoning, and use of good judgment and decision-making	-will follow protocol, will judge amount of water to use	-Staff will encourage residents to share their talents with their peers -Staff will show the resident the step-by-step actions to complete the task -Staff will support making decisions
Complete a Task	Increase ability to complete a task	-will recall/retain and sort/gather information, problem-solve, and complete activity	Staff will support resident's ability to follow procedure of project through instruction, encourage; supply adaptive devices/programs ,if needed, and necessary materials and support

TABLE 21.1

Recreational Objectives Observational Form
Sharing Talents- Cognitive skills

PATIENT		Dependent (Totally dependent)	High Assistance (25+ ability)	Moderate Assist. (50+ ability)	Mild Assistance (75+ability)	Independent (Totally independent)			
SEE CODES BELOW USE OPTIONAL CODES IF APPROPRIATE		1	2	3	4	5			
		3 cue/ 2-3 physical	2-3 cues/ 2 physical	2-3 cues/ 1 physical	1-2 cues	Encouragement			
97530- Therapeutic activities or	**SKILL**	**GOAL**	**OBJECTIVES** ____times per ____		**METHOD**	**OUTCOME DATE**			
97532 Cognitive skills	ORIENTATION								
97532 Cognitive skills	ATTENTION								
97532 Cognitive skills	MEMORY								
97532 Cognitive skills	PROBLEM-SOLVING								
97532 Cognitive skills	COMPLETE A TASK								
97139 Speech Therapy 97532 Cognitive skills	LANGUAGE								
97533	SENSORY STIMULATION/ COGNITIVE STIMULATION								
97532	PERCEPTUAL AWARENESS								

97532-Development of cognitive skills to improve attention, memory, problem-solving, includes compensatory training and/or sensory integrative activities, direct (one-on-one) patient contact by the provider, each 15 minutes; **97530-Therapeutic activities**, direct (one-on-one) patient contact by the provider (use of dynamic activities to improve functional performance), each 15 minutes; **97533-Sensory integration techniques** to enhance sensory processing and promote adaptive responses to environmental demands, direct (one-on-one) patient contact by the provider, each 15 minutes; **97150-Therapeutic procedure(s)**, group (2 or more individuals); **97139-Unlisted therapeutic procedure** (specify) minutes; **97003-occupational therapy evaluation**; **97004- re-evaluation**	Staff Initial				
	Add total score here -Maximum Score 40 pt. each form per activity				
	See scale below or use own/facilities optional score system				

(Score 1-8)=1 (9-16) =2 (17-24) =3 (25-32) =4 (33-40) =5 If w/device add d if wish, ex: 1d, 2d, or If using 1-7 scale: (41-48) =6 (49-56)

Sharing Talents
Physical Goals, Objectives, and Methods

Skill	Goal	Objectives Sample	Method Sample
Fine Motor Skills	Increase fine motor skills, meaningful/fulfilling activities	-will pick up items, use fingers, dexterity, etc.	Staff will encourage residents to pick up and manipulate materials
Hand-Eye Coordination	Increase hand-eye coordination		Staff will encourage residents to lift items using gross motor skills
Gross Motor Skills	Increase large motor skills, meaningful/fulfilling activities	-will lift larger item, bend, etc.	Staff will encourage residents to do the activity and decrease reaction times by shortening amount of time allotted or observation of resident ability increasing on own
Perceptual Speed and Motor Function	Increase speed and motor ability for function, safety, meaningful /fulfilling activities	-will increase speed of actions	Staff will encourage residents to place items using hand-eye fine motor abilities, detailed fine motor activities

TABLE 21.2

Recreational Objectives Observational Form
Sharing Talents- Physical Skills

PATIENT	Dependent (Totally dependent)	High Assistance (25+ ability)	Moderate Assist. (50+ ability)	Mild Assistance (75+ability)	Independent (Totally independent)
	1	2	3	4	5
SEE CODES BELOW USE OPTIONAL CODES IF APPROPRIATE	3 cue/ 2-3 physical	2-3 cues/ 2 physical	2-3 cues/ 1 physical	1-2 cues	Encouragement

97530- Therapeutic activities or	**SKILL**	**GOAL**	**OBJECTIVES** ____times per ____	**METHOD**	**OUTCOME DATE**			
Therapeutic Activity 97530	FINE MOTOR SKILLS							
97530	EYE-HAND COORDINATION							
97110/ 97530	GROSS MOTOR SKILLS							
97530 If under cognitive code 97532	PERCEPTUAL SPEED/MOTOR FUNCTION							

97530 Therapeutic activities, direct (one on one) patient contact by the provider (use of dynamic activities to improve functional performance),each 15 minutes; **97110 Therapeutic procedure, one or more areas**, each 15 minutes; therapeutic exercises to develop strength and endurance, range of motion and flexibility; ; **97150 Therapeutic procedure(s), group (2 or more individuals**; **97535-Self care/home management training** (e.g., activities of daily living and compensatory training, meal preparation, safety procedures, and instructions in use of adaptive equipment), direct (one-on-one) contact by provider, each 15 minutes; **Physical therapy 97001 evaluation, 97002 Re-evaluation. occupational therapy evaluation 97003, re-evaluation. 97004**	Staff Initials				
	Add total score here Maximum Score 20 pt. each form per activity				
	See scale below or use own/facilities optional score system				

(Score 1-4)=1 (5-8) =2 (9-12) =3 (13-16) =4 (17-20) =5 If w/device add d if wish, ex: 1d, 2d, or If using 1-7 scale: (21-24) =6 (25-28) =7

Sharing Talents
Socio-emotional Goals, Objectives, and Methods

Skill	Goal	Objectives Sample	Method Sample
Socialization/Community Integration	Increase social interactions, meaningful/fulfilling activities	-will interact with peers, will engage in community integration experiences (for community adaptation and social skills), will use manners, share, practice social skills	Staff will offer activities to support/encourage residents to socialize through community integration and being w/groups
Team Playing/Sharing	Increase teamwork/sharing, meaningful/fulfilling activities	-will join in and share talents, will listen as others share talents, will wait turn, support peers _____ time(s) this week.	Staff will encourage residents to create items, share, work as a team, support/use patience, show compassion to other residents
Initiative and Motivation	Increase initiative and motivation/wellness, and quality of life	-will choose if wishes to share, will try games or other types of activities as presented	-Staff will support/encourage the resident to prepare for planting/gardening activities in a timely fashion for their own personal gains of attending activity, -Staff will offer new techniques/season flowers to motivate
Emotional Gratification	Increase emotional gratification/wellness, and quality of life	-will state that sharing talents or learning new talents is a gratifying experience, or will show pleasure by smiling, laughing, deep focus on activities	Staff will ask residents if they enjoyed the activity and what they liked through verbal discussion, group discussions
Sense of Accomplishment	Increase feelings of self-worth, pride, productivity, dignity/wellness, and quality of life	-will use gestures to express pride in self, will talk about their accomplishments	Staff will offer activities as a way to support resident's desire to use creativity, imagination, etc.
Self-esteem/self-identity	Increase self-esteem, feelings of belonging, dignity, self-worth, integrity, self-identity/wellness, and quality of life	-will state/communicate positive feelings about self, will join class to take an active role in maintaining health though exercising, will join the creative activities/class based on own choices	Staff will educate residents on the value of doing crafts/ learning talents for brain muscle/stimulant benefits, and healing qualities, and encourage residents to join classes/share garden plants for unit
Sensory Integration/Tolerating Stimulation	Increase sensory processing and enhance awareness of sensations and toleration/adaptation of sensory stimulations and demands	-will adjust to the smells, lights, sounds, etc. of shared talents; will taste new meals, other's cooking, other activities _____ time(s) this week.	-Staff will offer activities, and residents will be exposed to sensory stimulating experiences of tactile stimulation, sights, hearing, communication, and possibly smell sensory stimulations -Residents will be supported as they adjust to the stimulus one step at a time
Fostering Appropriate Behaviors	Increase social interaction, social opportunities and adjustment, safety, using appropriate behaviors during an activity for a calm environment/wellness, and quality of life	-will join in on class, share cooking and tools, listen and follow instructions, use appropriate behavior for the setting; will wait turn, stand in line quietly; will quiet down when asked	Before class begins, staff will discuss the rules, appropriate behaviors, respect of property, safety, and respect of fellow peers/staff

TABLE 21.3

Recreational Objectives Observational Form
Sharing Talents- Socio-emotional Skills

PATIENT		Dependent (Totally dependent)	High Assistance (25+ ability)	Moderate Assist. (50+ ability)	Mild Assistance (75+ability)	Independent (Totally independent.)
SEE CODES BELOW USE OPTIONAL CODES IF APPROPRIATE		1	2	3	4	5
		3 cue/ 2-3 physical	2-3 cues/ 2 physical	2-3 cues/ 1 physical	1-2 cues	Encouragement
97530- Therapeutic activities or	**SKILL**	**GOAL**	**OBJECTIVES** ____times per ____		**METHOD**	**OUTCOME DATE**
97537 Or 97535	SOCIALIZATION/ COMMUNITY INTEGRATION					
97537 Or 97535	TEAM PLAYING /SHARING					
97537 Or 97535	INITIATIVE AND MOTIVATION					
97537 Or 97535	EMOTIONAL GRATIFICATION					
97537 Or 97535	SENSE OF ACCOMPLISHM ENT					
97537 Or 97535	SELF-ESTEEM/ SELF-IDENTITY					
97537 Or 97535	FOSTERING APPROPRIATE BEHAVIORS					
97533	SENSORY INTEGRATION/ TOLERATING					

97537-Community/work reintegration training (e.g., shopping, transportation, money management, avocational activities and/or work environment/modification analysis, work task analysis), direct (one-on-one) contact by provider, each 15 minutes; **97535-Self care/home management training** (e.g., activities of daily living and compensatory training, meal preparation, safety procedures, and instructions in use of adaptive equipment), direct (one-on-one) contact by provider, each 15 minutes; **97530-Therapeutic activities, direct (one-on-one)** patient contact by the provider (use of dynamic activities to improve functional performance), each 15 minutes; **97150-Therapeutic procedure(s), group (2 or more individuals); 97533-Sensory integration techniques** to enhance sensory processing and promote adaptive responses to environmental demands, direct (one-on-one) patient contact by the provider, each 15 minutes; **occupational therapy evaluation 97003, re-evaluation . 97004**	Staff Initial Add total score here-Maximum Score 40 pt. each form per activity See scale below or use own/facilities optional score system

(Score 1-8)=1 (9-16) =2 (17-24) =3 (25-32) =4 (33-40) =5 If w/device add d if wish, ex: 1d, 2d, or If using 1-7 scale: (41-48) =6 (49-56) Current Procedural Terminology © 2005 American Medical Association. All rights reserved. Recreational Objectives Observational form© 2005. All rights reserved. Patent pending.

Tangible Creative Art Activities

(High Cognitive, Physical and Socio-emotional Stimulation)
Reminiscing Qualities, Healing Qualities

Research has shown activities that help cognition of sensory/motor and speed processing will be geared towards help in visual and motor memory, discrimination, comparison, and categorizing areas. Reminiscing activities may help improve memory skills. Long-term studies (Arbuckle and others, 1998) have consistently showed that stimulating the brain with activities helps cognitive function in a similar way exercise helps muscle function. Staying productive has been shown to enhance socio-emotional wellness

Baking

Objectives and benefits:

Cognitive Challenges: attention, memory, language, orientation, following patterns, following directions, productivity, mastering a task

Physical Needs: fine motor skills, gross motor skills, hand-eye coordination, perceptual speed and motor function, manipulation of materials, dexterity

Socio-emotional Needs: socialization, community integration, initiative and motivation, emotional gratification, sense of accomplishment, fostering appropriate behaviors, nurturing, * Reminiscing Qualities, Healing Qualities

Supplies: Recipe and food supplies, measuring cups, spoons, bowls, whisks

Time: 30 minutes

Staff/older adult ratio: 1:6

Instructions: Have ingredients and supplies set out on the table. Decide which skills individual residents have and let them help according to their strengths or needs. Let residents rotate adding ingredients to the recipe mix. Let some measure out the dry mix, some add wet mix, and some stir the mixture. This activity can be repeated making cookies or any special recipes they would like to share. Sharing a recipe from their heritage can be very gratifying to residents. It is important to be extremely cautious and attentive when working with older adults who will be handling hot items

Research has shown activities that help cognition of sensory/motor and speed processing will be geared towards help in visual and motor memory, discrimination, comparison, and categorizing areas. Reminiscing activities may help improve memory skills. Long-term studies (Arbuckle and others, 1998) have consistently showed that stimulating the brain with activities helps cognitive function in a similar way exercise helps muscle function. Staying productive has been shown to enhance socio-emotional wellness

Baking
Cognitive Goals, Objectives, and Methods

Skill	Goal	Objectives Sample	Method Sample
Orientation	Show increased awareness of, time/"timeframe," people, circumstances, and past experiences vs. present experiences, to engage in present-time activities, or for a reminiscing intended question	-will respond with correct answer to two choice questions (Ex: "Are you at the mall or at the baking class?") Or yes/no answer: will state where they are, time of day, present company of people on own and with the correct answer	-Staff will ask residents a series of questions to stimulate focus to the present setting (Ex: "These cookies are for our snack. Did you already have lunch?") -Staff will state amount of time to bake and ask residents if item baking time is up. or past if reminiscing exercise (Ex: "What were your favorite baking activities growing up?")
Attention	Show increased attention span, task for function, and to engage in meaningful, recreational/fulfilling activities	-will make eye-contact with staff for _____ sec., will verbalize with staff and instructor, will read/listen to rules, will say yes/no to show they understand or do the action	Staff will address or stand in front of resident, make eye-contact, ask questions, or use others forms to get resident's attention (Ex: "What are we baking?")
Memory	Show increased memory skills of recall, recognition, retention of information, working memory	-will repeat/recall how to mix ingredients, will repeat/recall how to bake an item, will remember lesson at next class	Staff will show steps on how to follow recipe, and residents will add ingredients, etc.
Language	Show increased ability to communicate use of words, phrases, sentence structure, comprehension, interpretation	-will be asked a question and answer yes/no, will be asked what is included in recipe, will state ingredients, will interact with peers, staff; will interpret instructor's request and follow	Staff will ask questions to stimulate a communication (Ex: 'What flavor frosting will we add to the cookies?") for Interpretation/Lang. skills
Cognitive Stimulation (awareness, seeks information in)	Increased stimulus/exposure for visual/ motor memory, cognitive experiences/awareness and brain stimulation to enhance (function, pragmatics, neuroplasticity)	-will look around the room, will interact with peers, will look around the room, be engaged in game w/peers, will listen/seek cognitive stimulation, will accept challenge of input information and engage/interact in current baking activity	Staff will set up materials, including measuring cups, various bowls, ingredients baking
Perceptual Awareness	Show increased abilities of depth perception, visio-spatical awareness, and acuity (for discrimination, comparison, and categorizing), safety	-will pour ingredients in bowl, will discriminate, compare; will maneuver around kitchen area, will put baking items away in proper containers associated with proper area (milk in refrigerator)	Staff will have residents pick up items, place items in pans, put items away in proper areas
Problem-solving (goes beyond thinking/stimulus and initiates thinking process)	Increase problem-solving ability, processing of information, thinking, reasoning, and use of good judgment and decision-making	-will add ingredients, will mix ingredients, will bake item, will problem solve, think, reason and process information regarding use of comparisons; will discriminate, categorize, question regarding baking, will follow recipe protocol, including awareness of baking time	Staff will set up materials, including measuring cups, various bowls of ingredients, for baking and procedures to bake
Complete a Task	Increase ability to complete a task	will recall/retain and sort/gather information, problem-solve, and complete activity	Staff will support resident's ability to follow procedure through instruction, encourage; and supply adaptive devices/programs ,if needed, and necessary materials and support

TABLE 22.1

Recreational Objectives Observational Form
Baking- Cognitive skills

PATIENT		Dependent (Totally dependent)	High Assistance (25+ ability)	Moderate Assist. (50+ ability)	Mild Assistance (75+ability)	Independent (Totally independent)
SEE CODES BELOW USE OPTIONAL CODES IF APPROPRIATE		1	2	3	4	5
		3 cue/ 2-3 physical	2-3 cues/ 2 physical	2-3 cues/ 1 physical	1-2 cues	Encouragement
97530- Therapeutic activities or	**SKILL**	**GOAL**	**OBJECTIVES** ____times per ____		**METHOD**	**OUTCOME DATE**
97532 Cognitive skills	Orientation					
97532 Cognitive skills	Attention					
97532 Cognitive skills	Memory					
97532 Cognitive skills	Problem-Solving					
97532 Cognitive skills	Complete a Task					
97139 Speech Therapy 97532 Cognitive skills	Language					
97533	Sensory Stimulation/ Cognitive Stimulation					
97532	Perceptual Awareness					

97532-Development of cognitive skills to improve attention, memory, problem-solving, includes compensatory training and/or sensory integrative activities, direct (one-on-one) patient contact by the provider, each 15 minutes; **97530-Therapeutic activities**, direct (one-on-one) patient contact by the provider (use of dynamic activities to improve functional performance), each 15 minutes; **97533-Sensory integration techniques** to enhance sensory processing and promote adaptive responses to environmental demands, direct (one-on-one) patient contact by the provider, each 15 minutes; **97150-Therapeutic procedure(s)**, group (2 or more individuals); **97139-Unlisted therapeutic procedure** (specify) minutes; **97003- occupational therapy evaluation**; **97004- re-evaluation**	Staff Initial				
	Add total score here -Maximum Score 40 pt. each form per activity				
	See scale below or use own/facilities optional score system				

(Score 1-8)=1 (9-16) =2 (17-24) =3 (25-32) =4 (33-40) =5 If w/device add d if wish, ex: 1d, 2d, or If using 1-7 scale: (41-48) =6 (49-56)

Baking
Physical Goals, Objectives, and Methods

Skill	Goal	Objectives Sample	Method Sample
Fine motor skills	Increase fine motor skills, meaningful/fulfilling activities	-will mix, pour, sift ingredients	Staff will give residents baking items (rollers, cups, etc.) to manipulate the items using fine motor skills
Gross motor skills	Increase large motor skills, meaningful/fulfilling activities	-will lift pan and place in oven (bend, lift, etc.)	Staff will give residents baking items (floor bags, pans) to lift /manipulate the items using gross motor skills
Perceptual speed and motor function	Increase speed and motor ability for function, safety, meaningful/fulfilling activities	-will increase speed of actions by using skills to bake a cake (with Dr. approval)	Staff will have residents stir mixes, add eggs, place baking item in the oven, and decrease time "allowed" to increase reaction times; may add a second baking item within same time allotment
Following step patterns/backwards forward movement	Increase strength, balance, endurance, meaningful /fulfilling activities	-will walk to front of refrigerator, move back to open using awareness skills	Staff will have residents working in an area where they need to walk forwards and backwards to maneuver around the room

Table 22.2

Recreational Objectives Observational Form
Baking- Physical Skills

PATIENT	Dependent (Totally dependent)	High Assistance (25+ ability)	Moderate Assist. (50+ ability)	Mild Assistance (75+ability)	Independent (Totally independent)
	1	2	3	4	5
SEE CODES BELOW USE OPTIONAL CODES IF APPROPRIATE	3 cue/ 2-3 physical	2-3 cues/ 2 physical	2-3 cues/ 1 physical	1-2 cues	Encouragement

97530- Therapeutic activities or	SKILL	GOAL	OBJECTIVES ____times per ____	METHOD	OUTCOME DATE			
Therapeutic Activity 97530	FINE MOTOR SKILLS							
97530	EYE-HAND COORDINATION							
97110/ 97530	GROSS MOTOR SKILLS							
97530 If under cognitive code 97532	PERCEPTUAL SPEED/MOTOR FUNCTION							

97530 Therapeutic activities, direct (one on one) patient contact by the provider (use of dynamic activities to improve functional performance),each 15 minutes; **97110 Therapeutic procedure, one or more areas**, each 15 minutes; therapeutic exercises to develop strength and endurance, range of motion and flexibility; ; **97150 Therapeutic procedure(s), group (2 or more individuals**; **97535-Self care/home management training** (e.g., activities of daily living and compensatory training, meal preparation, safety procedures, and instructions in use of adaptive equipment), direct (one-on-one) contact by provider, each 15 minutes; **Physical therapy 97001 evaluation, 97002 Re-evaluation. occupational therapy evaluation 97003, re-evaluation. 97004**

Staff Initials				
Add total score here Maximum Score 20 pt. each form per activity				
See scale below or use own/facilities optional score system				

(Score 1-4)=1 (5-8) =2 (9-12) =3 (13-16) =4 (17-20) =5 If w/device add d if wish, ex: 1d, 2d, or If using 1-7 scale: (21-24) =6 (25-28) =7

Baking
Socio-emotional Goals, Objectives, and Methods

Skill	Goal	Objectives Sample	Method Sample
Socialization/Community Integration	Increase social interactions, meaningful/fulfilling activities	-will interact with peers, will engage in community integration experiences for community adaptation and social skills, will use manners, share, practice social skills	Staff will offer baking activities to support/encourage residents to socialize through community integration and being in paired w/groups
Team Playing/Sharing	Increase teamwork/sharing, meaningful/fulfilling activities	-will join in on a baking activity with others and share, wait turn, support peers ____ time(s) this week	Staff will offer recipe ideas or ask residents to offer recipes/themes for baking class
Initiative and Motivation	Increase initiative and motivation/wellness, and quality of life	-will choose if wishes to bake, will try new recipes, will bake on own or with assistance, will increase baking	Staff will support/encourage the resident to prepare to share baking recipes, etc. at the activity time for their own personal gains of sharing interesting recipes, such as ethnic recipes
Emotional Gratification	Increase emotional gratification/wellness, and quality of life	-will state that baking is a gratifying experience, or will show pleasure by smiling, laughing, deep focus on baking activities	Staff will ask residents if they enjoy baking activities and what they liked through verbal discussion, group discussions
Sense of Accomplishment	Increase feelings of self-worth, pride, productivity, dignity/wellness, and quality of life	-will use gestures to express pride in self, will talk about their accomplishments of baking cakes, pies, meals	Staff will post recipes the residents share and place the recipes on the bulletin board
Self-esteem/self-identity	Increase self-esteem, feelings of belonging, dignity, self-worth, integrity, self-identity/wellness, and quality of life	-will state/communicate positive feelings about self, will join bake class to take an active role in maintaining health though exercising, will join the baking/cooking class based on own choices	Staff will educate residents on the value of sharing ethnic heritage, baked goods, and learning new recipes, and encourage to continue to share recipes to be posted on the bulletin board
Sensory Integration/Tolerating Stimulation	Increase sensory processing and enhance awareness of sensations and toleration/adaptation of sensory stimulations and demands	-will adjust to the smells, lights, sounds, etc. in kitchen; will taste new meals and other's cooking	-Staff will ask for residents to share recipes and be exposed to sensory stimulating tastes, smells, food textures (be careful of allergies, swallowing limitations!) -Staff will support residents as they adjust to the stimulus one step at a time
Fostering Appropriate Behaviors	Increase social interaction, social opportunities and adjustment, safety, using appropriate behaviors during an activity for a calm environment/wellness, and quality of life	-will join in on baking class, share cooking and tools, listen and follow instructions, use appropriate behavior for the setting, wait turn, stand in line quietly; will quiet down when asked	Before activity begins, staff will discuss the rules, appropriate behaviors, respect of property, safety, and respect of fellow peers/instructor

Table 22.3

Recreational Objectives Observational Form
Baking- Socio-emotional Skills

PATIENT		Dependent (Totally dependent)	High Assistance (25+ ability)	Moderate Assist. (50+ ability)	Mild Assistance (75+ability)	Independent (Totally independent.)			
SEE CODES BELOW USE OPTIONAL CODES IF APPROPRIATE		1	2	3	4	5			
		3 cue/ 2-3 physical	2-3 cues/ 2 physical	2-3 cues/ 1 physical	1-2 cues	Encouragement			
97530- Therapeutic activities or	SKILL	GOAL	OBJECTIVES ____times per ____		METHOD	OUTCOME DATE			
97537 Or 97535	SOCIALIZATION/ COMMUNITY INTEGRATION								
97537 Or 97535	TEAM PLAYING /SHARING								
97537 Or 97535	INITIATIVE AND MOTIVATION								
97537 Or 97535	EMOTIONAL GRATIFICATION								
97537 Or 97535	SENSE OF ACCOMPLISHM ENT								
97537 Or 97535	SELF-ESTEEM/ SELF-IDENTITY								
97537 Or 97535	FOSTERING APPROPRIATE BEHAVIORS								
97533	SENSORY INTEGRATION/ TOLERATING								

97537-Community/work reintegration training (e.g., shopping, transportation, money management, avocational activities and/or work environment/modification analysis, work task analysis), direct (one-on-one) contact by provider, each 15 minutes; **97535-Self care/home management training** (e.g., activities of daily living and compensatory training, meal preparation, safety procedures, and instructions in use of adaptive equipment), direct (one-on-one) contact by provider, each 15 minutes; **97530-Therapeutic activities, direct (one-on-one)** patient contact by the provider (use of dynamic activities to improve functional performance), each 15 minutes; **97150-Therapeutic procedure(s), group (2 or more individuals); 97533-Sensory integration techniques** to enhance sensory processing and promote adaptive responses to environmental demands, direct (one-on-one) patient contact by the provider, each 15 minutes; **occupational therapy evaluation 97003, re-evaluation . 97004**	Staff Initial				
	Add total score here-Maximum Score 40 pt. each form per activity				
	See scale below or use own/facilities optional score system				

(Score 1-8)=1 (9-16) =2 (17-24) =3 (25-32) =4 (33-40) =5 If w/device add d if wish, ex: 1d, 2d, or If using 1-7 scale: (41-48) =6 (49-56)

Bookmarks

Objectives and benefits:

Cognitive Challenges: attention, memory, language, orientation, following patterns, following directions, productivity, mastering a task

Physical Needs: fine motor skills, gross motor skills, hand-eye coordination, perceptual speed and motor function, manipulation of materials, dexterity

Socio-emotional Needs: socialization, community integration, initiative and motivation, emotional gratification, sense of accomplishment, fostering appropriate behaviors, nurturing, * Reminiscing Qualities, Healing Qualities

Supplies: Markers, crayons, watercolors, magazines, yarn, glitter, dried flowers, decorating items, newspaper, construction paper, laminating sheets, hole punch

Time: 30 minutes

Staff/older adult ratio: 1:6 or as assessed per needs of individuals or group. All levels of function may do this activity.

Instructions: Have newspaper set out at each setting for easy clean up. Have different color poster board cut out in shape of bookmarks. Have baskets of decorating items around the table. Explain to the older adults they are free to make a bookmark designed however they would like; they can make a simple bookmark from crayons and paints, or they can use any other items to make a more decorative bookmark. Be sure to have glue available. You may use hot glue guns or Elmer's glue. When they are done, laminate the bookmarks. This activity can also be used when they would like to make a gift for family. This activity can also be used to donate to area libraries or schools. They will really enjoy making these for themselves and others.

Research has shown activities that help cognition of sensory/motor and speed processing will be geared towards help in visual and motor memory, discrimination, comparison, and categorizing areas. Reminiscing activities may help improve memory skills. Long-term studies (Arbuckle and others, 1998) have consistently showed that stimulating the brain with activities helps cognitive function in a similar way exercise helps muscle function. Staying productive has been shown to enhance socio-emotional wellness

Bookmarks
Cognitive Goals, Objectives, and Methods

Skill	Goal	Objectives Sample	Method Sample
Orientation	Show increased awareness of, time/"timeframe," people, circumstances, and past experiences vs. present experiences, to engage in present-time activities, or for a reminiscing intended question	-will respond with correct answer to two choice questions Or yes/no answer, will state where they are, time of day, present company of people on own and with the correct answer	Staff will ask residents a series of questions to stimulate focus to the present setting (Ex: "What talents are you going to share? Have you made bookmarks before?")
Attention	Show increased attention span, task for function, and to engage in meaningful, recreational/fulfilling activities	-will make eye-contact with staff for _____ sec., will verbalize with staff and instructor; will read/listen to rules, will say yes/no to show they understand or do the action	Staff will address or stand in front of resident, make eye-contact, ask questions, or use others forms to get resident's attention
Memory	Show increased memory skills of recall, recognition, retention of information, working memory	-will repeat/recall how to make project, will remember lesson at next class	Staff will show steps on how to make bookmarks, and residents will repeat the action using short-term memory/recall, working memory
Language	Show increased ability to communicate use of words, phrases, sentence structure, comprehension, interpretation	-will be asked a question and answer yes/no, will be asked what is included in project, will state ingredients, methods, items; will interact with peers, staff; will interpret instructor's request and follow	Staff will ask questions to stimulate a communication (Ex: "What materials are you using to make your bookmarks?") Interpretation/Lang. skills (Ex: "You need to add tacky glue to make it stick well.") and then note resident's actions to show they understood
Cognitive Stimulation (awareness, seeks information in)	Increased stimulus/exposure for visual/ motor memory, cognitive experiences/awareness and brain stimulation to enhance (function, pragmatics, neuroplasticity)	-will look around the room, will listen/seek cognitive stimulation, will accept challenge of input information and engage/interact in, will engage in a bookmark activity	Staff will set up crafts and put out a wide variety of art sand craft materials to encourage creativity, discrimination, comparison, categorizing, etc.
Perceptual Awareness	Show increased abilities of depth perception, visio-spatical awareness, and acuity (for discrimination, comparison, and categorizing), safety	-will use ingredients/items, will discriminate, compare; will maneuver around work area, will put items away in proper containers associated with proper area (buttons with buttons, glitter with glitter)	Staff will engage residents in an activity that requires use of acuity, discrimination, comparison, and categorizing for visio-spatical awareness (Ex: placing items on the bookmark using visual acuity, etc.)
Problem-solving (goes beyond thinking/stimulus and initiates thinking process)	Increase problem-solving ability, processing of information, thinking, reasoning, and use of good judgment and decision-making	-will think up a story, use creativity, or comprehend and process the information; will judge appropriate materials	-Staff will engage residents in a creative project and decision-making regarding whom to send the bookmarks to -Staff will show the resident the step-by-step actions to make a bookmark to stimulate working memory
Complete a Task	Increase ability to complete a task	-will recall/retain and sort/gather information, problem-solve, and complete activity	Staff will support resident's ability to follow the project through instruction, encourage; and supply adaptive devices/programs, if needed, and necessary materials and support

TABLE 23.1

Recreational Objectives Observational Form
Bookmarks- Cognitive skills

PATIENT	Dependent (Totally dependent)	High Assistance (25+ ability)	Moderate Assist. (50+ ability)	Mild Assistance (75+ability)	Independent (Totally independent)
SEE CODES BELOW USE OPTIONAL CODES IF APPROPRIATE	1	2	3	4	5
	3 cue/ 2-3 physical	2-3 cues/ 2 physical	2-3 cues/ 1 physical	1-2 cues	Encouragement

97530- Therapeutic activities or	SKILL	GOAL	OBJECTIVES ____times per ____	METHOD	OUTCOME DATE			
97532 Cognitive skills	ORIENTATION							
97532 Cognitive skills	ATTENTION							
97532 Cognitive skills	MEMORY							
97532 Cognitive skills	PROBLEM-SOLVING							
97532 Cognitive skills	COMPLETE A TASK							
97139 Speech Therapy 97532 Cognitive skills	LANGUAGE							
97533	SENSORY STIMULATION/ COGNITIVE STIMULATION							
97532	PERCEPTUAL AWARENESS							

97532-Development of cognitive skills to improve attention, memory, problem-solving, includes compensatory training and/or sensory integrative activities, direct (one-on-one) patient contact by the provider, each 15 minutes; **97530-Therapeutic activities**, direct (one-on-one) patient contact by the provider (use of dynamic activities to improve functional performance), each 15 minutes; **97533-Sensory integration techniques** to enhance sensory processing and promote adaptive responses to environmental demands, direct (one-on-one) patient contact by the provider, each 15 minutes; **97150-Therapeutic procedure(s)**, group (2 or more individuals); **97139-Unlisted therapeutic procedure** (specify) minutes; **97003-occupational therapy evaluation**; **97004- re-evaluation**	Staff Initial				
	Add total score here -Maximum Score 40 pt. each form per activity				
	See scale below or use own/facilities optional score system				

(Score 1-8)=1 (9-16) =2 (17-24) =3 (25-32) =4 (33-40) =5 If w/device add d if wish, ex: 1d, 2d, or If using 1-7 scale: (41-48) =6 (49-56)

Bookmarks
Physical Goals, Objectives, and Methods

Skill	Goal	Objectives Sample	Method Sample
Fine Motor Skills	Increase fine motor skills, meaningful/fulfilling activities	-will glue, paste, mix and pour items; will pick up small items, manipulate materials	Staff will encourage residents to pick up and manipulate materials
Gross Motor Skills	Increase large motor skills, meaningful/fulfilling activities	-will lift items using large motor skills, walk to group (with device or support)	Staff will encourage residents to lift items using gross motor skills
Perceptual Speed and Motor Function	Increase speed and motor ability for function, safety, meaningful/fulfilling activities	-will increase speed of actions by using skills (with Dr. approval)	Staff will encourage residents to do the activity and decrease reaction times by shortening amount of time allotted, or observation of resident ability increasing on own
Hand-Eye Coordination	Increase hand-eye coordination	-will paste items on craft	Staff will encourage residents to place items using hand-eye fine motor abilities, detailed fine motor activities

Table 23.2

Recreational Objectives Observational Form
Bookmarks - Physical Skills

PATIENT		Dependent (Totally dependent)	High Assistance (25+ ability)	Moderate Assist. (50+ ability)	Mild Assistance (75+ability)	Independent (Totally independent)
		1	2	3	4	5
SEE CODES BELOW USE OPTIONAL CODES IF APPROPRIATE		3 cue/ 2-3 physical	2-3 cues/ 2 physical	2-3 cues/ 1 physical	1-2 cues	Encouragement
97530- Therapeutic activities or	**SKILL**	**GOAL**	**OBJECTIVES** ____times per ____		**METHOD**	**OUTCOME DATE**
Therapeutic Activity 97530	FINE MOTOR SKILLS					
97530	EYE-HAND COORDINATION					
97110/ 97530	GROSS MOTOR SKILLS					
97530 If under cognitive code 97532	PERCEPTUAL SPEED/MOTOR FUNCTION					

97530 Therapeutic activities, direct (one on one) patient contact by the provider (use of dynamic activities to improve functional performance),each 15 minutes; **97110 Therapeutic procedure, one or more areas**, each 15 minutes; therapeutic exercises to develop strength and endurance, range of motion and flexibility; ; **97150 Therapeutic procedure(s), group (2 or more individuals**; **97535-Self care/home management training** (e.g., activities of daily living and compensatory training, meal preparation, safety procedures, and instructions in use of adaptive equipment), direct (one-on-one) contact by provider, each 15 minutes**; Physical therapy 97001 evaluation, 97002 Re-evaluation. occupational therapy evaluation 97003, re-evaluation. 97004**	Staff Initials	
	Add total score here Maximum Score 20 pt. each form per activity	
	See scale below or use own/facilities optional score system	

(Score 1-4)=1 (5-8) =2 (9-12) =3 (13-16) =4 (17-20) =5 If w/device add d if wish, ex: 1d, 2d, or If using 1-7 scale: (21-24) =6 (25-28) =7

Bookmarks
Socio-emotional Goals, Objectives and Methods

Skill	Goal	Objectives Sample	Method Sample
Socialization/Community Integration	Increase social interactions, meaningful/fulfilling activities	-will interact with peers, will engage in community integration experiences (for community adaptation and social skills), will use manners, share, practice social skills	Staff will offer activities that support/encourage residents to socialize through community integration and being w/groups
Team Playing/Sharing	Increase teamwork/sharing, meaningful/fulfilling activities	-will join in on a craft/ activity with others and share, wait turn, support peers _____ time(s) this week.	Staff will encourage residents to create items, share, work as a team, support/use patience, show compassion to other residents
Initiative and Motivation	Increase initiative and motivation/wellness, and quality of life	-will choose if wishes to do craft, will try new crafts, will increase amount of crafts done _____ times a week	Staff will support/encourage the resident to prepare for craft activities in a timely fashion for their own personal gains of attending activity, offer new techniques/creative materials to motivate residents to make a creative craft
Emotional Gratification	Increase emotional gratification/wellness, and quality of life	-will state that making crafts is a gratifying experience or will show pleasure by smiling, laughing, deep focus on activities	Staff will be residents if they enjoyed the activity and what they liked through verbal discussion, group discussions
Sense of Accomplishment	Increase feelings of self-worth, pride, productivity, dignity/wellness, and quality of life	-will use gestures to express pride in self, will show crafts to others	Staff will offer activities as a way to support resident's desire to use creativity, imagination, and produce items
Self-esteem/self-identity	Increase self-esteem, feelings of belonging, dignity, self-worth, integrity, self-identity/wellness, and quality of life	-will state/communicate positive feelings about self, will join craft class to take an active role in maintaining health though arts/crafts, volunteer work; will join the craft class based on own choices	Staff will educate residents on the value of doing crafts/ learning talents for brain muscle/stimulant benefits, healing qualities, and encourage residents to join classes/share crafts
Sensory Integration/Tolerating Stimulation	Increase sensory processing and enhance awareness of sensations and toleration/adaptation of sensory stimulations and demands	-will adjust to the smells, lights, sounds, etc. in environment	-Staff will offer activities, and residents will be exposed to sensory stimulating experiences of tactile stimulation, sights, hearing, communication, and possibly smell sensory stimulations -Residents will be supported as they adjust to the stimulus one step at a time
Fostering Appropriate Behaviors	Increase social interaction, social opportunities and adjustment, safety, using appropriate behaviors during an activity for a calm environment/wellness, and quality of life	-will join in on class, share items/tools, listen and follow instructions, use appropriate behavior for the setting; will wait turn, stand in line quietly; will quiet down when asked	Before class begins, staff will discuss the rules, appropriate behaviors, respect of property, safety, and respect of fellow peers/staff

TABLE 23.3

Recreational Objectives Observational Form

BOOKMARKS -SOCIO-EMOTIONALS SKILLS

PATIENT	Dependent (Totally dependent)	High Assistance (25+ ability)	Moderate Assist. (50+ ability)	Mild Assistance (75+ability)	Independent (Totally independent.)
SEE CODES BELOW USE OPTIONAL CODES IF APPROPRIATE	1	2	3	4	5
	3 cue/ 2-3 physical	2-3 cues/ 2 physical	2-3 cues/ 1 physical	1-2 cues	Encouragement

97530-Therapeutic activities or	SKILL	GOAL	OBJECTIVES ____times per ____	METHOD	OUTCOME DATE			
97537 Or 97535	SOCIALIZATION/ COMMUNITY INTEGRATION							
97537 Or 97535	TEAM PLAYING /SHARING							
97537 Or 97535	INITIATIVE AND MOTIVATION							
97537 Or 97535	EMOTIONAL GRATIFICATION							
97537 Or 97535	SENSE OF ACCOMPLISHM ENT							
97537 Or 97535	SELF-ESTEEM/ SELF-IDENTITY							
97537 Or 97535	FOSTERING APPROPRIATE BEHAVIORS							
97533	SENSORY INTEGRATION/ TOLERATING							
97537-Community/work reintegration training (e.g., shopping, transportation, money management, avocational activities and/or work environment/modification analysis, work task analysis), direct (one-on-one) contact by provider, each 15 minutes; **97535-Self care/home management training** (e.g., activities of daily living and compensatory training, meal preparation, safety procedures, and instructions in use of adaptive equipment), direct (one-on-one) contact by provider, each 15 minutes; **97530-Therapeutic activities, direct (one-on-one)** patient contact by the provider (use of dynamic activities to improve functional performance), each 15 minutes; **97150-Therapeutic procedure(s), group (2 or more individuals); 97533-Sensory integration techniques** to enhance sensory processing and promote adaptive responses to environmental demands, direct (one-on-one) patient contact by the provider, each 15 minutes; **occupational therapy evaluation 97003, re-evaluation . 97004**				Staff Initial				
				Add total score here-Maximum Score 40 pt. each form per activity				
				See scale below or use own/facilities optional score system				

(Score 1-8)=1 (9-16) =2 (17-24) =3 (25-32) =4 (33-40) =5 If w/device add d if wish, ex: 1d, 2d, or If using 1-7 scale: (41-48) =6 (49-56)

Flower Baskets

Objectives and benefits:

Cognitive Challenges: attention, memory, language, orientation, following patterns, following directions, productivity, mastering a task

Physical Needs: fine motor skills, gross motor skills, hand-eye coordination, perceptual speed and motor function, manipulation of materials, dexterity

Socio-emotional Needs: socialization, community integration, initiative and motivation, emotional gratification, sense of accomplishment, fostering appropriate behaviors, nurturing, * Reminiscing Qualities, Healing Qualities

Supplies: Flower baskets, green foam to insert flowers inside basket, artificial flowers, artificial stems, and other types of material used for floral baskets. You may even include trinkets for a theme in a floral basket. You may need a glue gun as well as ribbon and pins.

Time: 30 minutes

Staff/older adult ratio: 1:3 or as assessed per needs of individuals or group

Instructions: Have residents sit at a table with supplies set up. If they each make their own basket, be sure to have a basket and green foam at each table setting. If they all make one basket, then you can put the green foam into one large basket. Let them each pick flowers they would like to include. Have them decorate the baskets. If these baskets are for a cause, have them do a theme. You could also do this activity for cemetery plots.

> Research has shown activities that help cognition of sensory/motor and speed processing will be geared towards help in visual and motor memory, discrimination, comparison, and categorizing areas. Reminiscing activities may help improve memory skills. Long-term studies (Arbuckle and others, 1998) have consistently showed that stimulating the brain with activities helps cognitive function in a similar way exercise helps muscle function. Staying productive has been shown to enhance socio-emotional wellness

Flower Baskets Cognitive Goals, Objectives and Methods

Skill	Goal	Objectives Sample	Method Sample
Orientation	Show increased awareness of, time/"timeframe," people, circumstances, and past experiences vs. present experiences, to engage in present-time activities, or for a reminiscing intended question	-will respond with correct answer to two choice questions Or yes/no answer, will state where they are, time of day, present company of people on own and with the correct answer	Staff will ask residents a series of questions to stimulate focus to the present setting (Ex: "What talents are you going to share? Have you made flower baskets before?")
Attention	Show increased attention span, task for function, and to engage in meaningful, recreational/fulfilling activities	-will make eye-contact with staff for _____ sec., will verbalize with staff and instructor, will read/listen to rules, will say yes/no to show they understand or do the action	Staff will address or stand in front of resident, make eye-contact, ask questions, or use others methods to get resident's attention
Memory	Show increased memory skills of recall, recognition, retention of information, working memory	-will repeat/recall how to make project, will remember lesson at next class	Staff will show steps on how to make bookmarks, and residents will repeat the action using short-term memory/recall, working memory
Language	Show increased ability to communicate use of words, phrases, sentence structure, comprehension, interpretation	-will be asked a question and answer yes/no, will be asked what is included in project, will state ingredients, methods, items; will interact with peers, staff; will interpret instructor's request and follow	Staff will ask questions to stimulate a communication (Ex: "What materials are you using to make your flower basket?") Interpretation/Lang. skills (Ex: "You need to push down the flower stems into the green cone to make it stay in the basket."), and then note resident's actions to show they understood
Cognitive Stimulation (awareness, seeks information in)	Increased stimulus/exposure for visual/ motor memory, cognitive experiences/awareness and brain stimulation to enhance (function, pragmatics, neuroplasticity)	-will look around the room, will listen/seek cognitive stimulation, will accept challenge of input information and engage/interact in, will engage in a flower basket activity	Staff will set up crafts and put out a wide variety of arts and craft materials to encourage creativity, discrimination, comparison, categorizing, etc.
Perceptual Awareness	Show increased abilities of depth perception, visio-spatial awareness, and acuity (for discrimination, comparison, and categorizing), safety	-will use ingredients/items, will discriminate, compare; will maneuver around work area, will put items away in proper containers associated with proper area (buttons with buttons, glitter with glitter)	Staff will engage residents in an activity that requires use of acuity, discrimination, comparison, and categorizing for visio-spatial awareness (Ex: placing items in the basket using visual acuity, etc.)
Problem-solving (goes beyond thinking/stimulus and initiates thinking process)	Increase problem-solving ability, processing of information, thinking, reasoning, and use of good judgment and decision-making	-will think up a story, use creativity or comprehend and process the information; will judge appropriate materials and follow instructions	-Staff will engage residents in a creative project and decision-making regarding whom to send the flower baskets to. -Staff will show the resident the step-by-step actions to make a flower basket to stimulate working memory
Complete a Task	Increase ability to complete a task	-will recall/retain and sort/gather information, problem-solve, and complete activity	Staff will support resident's ability to follow the project through instruction, encourage; and supply adaptive devices/programs, if needed, and necessary materials and support

TABLE 24.1

Recreational Objectives Observational Form
Flower Baskets- Cognitive skills

PATIENT	Dependent (Totally dependent)	High Assistance (25+ ability)	Moderate Assist. (50+ ability)	Mild Assistance (75+ability)	Independent (Totally independent)
SEE CODES BELOW USE OPTIONAL CODES IF APPROPRIATE	1	2	3	4	5
	3 cue/ 2-3 physical	2-3 cues/ 2 physical	2-3 cues/ 1 physical	1-2 cues	Encouragement

97530- Therapeutic activities or	SKILL	GOAL	OBJECTIVES ____times per ____	METHOD	OUTCOME DATE			
97532 Cognitive skills	ORIENTATION							
97532 Cognitive skills	ATTENTION							
97532 Cognitive skills	MEMORY							
97532 Cognitive skills	PROBLEM-SOLVING							
97532 Cognitive skills	COMPLETE A TASK							
97139 Speech Therapy 97532 Cognitive skills	LANGUAGE							
97533	SENSORY STIMULATION/ COGNITIVE STIMULATION							
97532	PERCEPTUAL AWARENESS							

97532-Development of cognitive skills to improve attention, memory, problem-solving, includes compensatory training and/or sensory integrative activities, direct (one-on-one) patient contact by the provider, each 15 minutes; **97530-Therapeutic activities**, direct (one-on-one) patient contact by the provider (use of dynamic activities to improve functional performance), each 15 minutes; **97533-Sensory integration techniques** to enhance sensory processing and promote adaptive responses to environmental demands, direct (one-on-one) patient contact by the provider, each 15 minutes; **97150-Therapeutic procedure(s)**, group (2 or more individuals); **97139-Unlisted therapeutic procedure** (specify) minutes; **97003- occupational therapy evaluation**; **97004- re-evaluation**	Staff Initial				
	Add total score here -Maximum Score 40 pt. each form per activity				
	See scale below or use own/facilities optional score system				

(Score 1-8)=1 (9-16) =2 (17-24) =3 (25-32) =4 (33-40) =5 If w/device add d if wish, ex: 1d, 2d, or If using 1-7 scale: (41-48) =6 (49-56)

Flower Baskets
Physical Goals, Objectives, and Methods

Skill	Goal	Objectives Sample	Method Sample
Fine Motor Skills	Increase fine motor skills, meaningful/fulfilling activities	-will glue, paste, mix and pour items, will pick up small items, manipulate materials	Staff will encourage residents to pick up and manipulate materials using fine motor skills
Gross Motor Skills	Increase large motor skills, meaningful/fulfilling activities	-will lift items using large motor skills, walk to group (with device or support)	Staff will encourage residents to lift items using gross motor skills
Perceptual Speed and Motor Function	Increase speed and motor ability for function, safety, meaningful/fulfilling activities	-will increase speed of actions by using skills (with Dr. approval)	Staff will encourage residents to do the activity and decrease reaction times by shortening amount of time allotted, or observation of resident ability increasing on own
Hand-Eye Coordination	Increase hand-eye coordination	-will paste items on craft	Staff will encourage residents to place items using hand-eye fine motor abilities, detailed fine motor activities

Table 24.1

Recreational Objectives Observational Form
Flower Baskets- Physical Skills

PATIENT		Dependent (Totally dependent)	High Assistance (25+ ability)	Moderate Assist. (50+ ability)	Mild Assistance (75+ability)	Independent (Totally independent)
SEE CODES BELOW USE OPTIONAL CODES IF APPROPRIATE		1	2	3	4	5
		3 cue/ 2-3 physical	2-3 cues/ 2 physical	2-3 cues/ 1 physical	1-2 cues	Encouragement
97530- Therapeutic activities or	**SKILL**	**GOAL**	**OBJECTIVES** ____times per ____		**METHOD**	**OUTCOME DATE**
Therapeutic Activity 97530	FINE MOTOR SKILLS					
97530	EYE-HAND COORDINATION					
97110/ 97530	GROSS MOTOR SKILLS					
97530 If under cognitive code 97532	PERCEPTUAL SPEED/MOTOR FUNCTION					

97530 Therapeutic activities, direct (one on one) patient contact by the provider (use of dynamic activities to improve functional performance),each 15 minutes; **97110 Therapeutic procedure, one or more areas**, each 15 minutes; therapeutic exercises to develop strength and endurance, range of motion and flexibility; ; **97150 Therapeutic procedure(s), group (2 or more individuals**; **97535-Self care/home management training** (e.g., activities of daily living and compensatory training, meal preparation, safety procedures, and instructions in use of adaptive equipment), direct (one-on-one) contact by provider, each 15 minutes; **Physical therapy 97001 evaluation, 97002 Re-evaluation. occupational therapy evaluation 97003, re-evaluation. 97004**	Staff Initials
	Add total score here Maximum Score 20 pt. each form per activity
	See scale below or use own/facilities optional score system

(Score 1-4)=1 (5-8) =2 (9-12) =3 (13-16) =4 (17-20) =5 If w/device add d if wish, ex: 1d, 2d, or If using 1-7 scale: (21-24) =6 (25-28) =7Current Procedural Terminology © 2005 American Medical Association. All rights reserved. Recreational Objectives Observational forms© 2005. All rights reserved. Patent pending.

Flower Baskets
Socio-emotional Goals, Objectives, and Methods

Skill	Goal	Objectives Sample	Method Sample
Socialization/Community Integration	Increase social interactions, meaningful/fulfilling activities	-will interact with peers, will engage in a community integration experiences (for community adaptation) (for social skills)will use manners, share, practices social skills	Staff will offer activities that support/encourage residents to socialize, through community integration and being w/ groups
Team Playing/Sharing	Increase teamwork/sharing, meaningful/fulfilling activities	-will, join in on a craft/ activity, with others and share, wait turn, support peers _____ time(s) this week.	Staff will encourage residents to create items, share, work as a team, support/use patience ,show compassion to other residents
Initiative and Motivation	Increase initiative and motivation/wellness, and quality of life	-will choose if wishes do craft, will try a new crafts, will increase amount of crafts done --- times a week	Staff will support/encourage the resident to prepare for craft activities in a timely fashion for their own personal gains of attending activity , offer new techniques/creative materials to motivate residents to make a creative craft
Emotional Gratification	Increase emotional gratification/wellness, and quality of life	-will state that making crafts is a gratifying experiences or will show pleasure by smiling, laughing , deep focus on activities	Staff will be ask residents if they enjoyed the activity and what they liked through verbal discussion, group discussions
Sense of Accomplishment	Increase feelings of self-worth, pride, productivity, dignity/wellness, and quality of life	-will use gestures to express pride in self, will show crafts to others	Staff will offer activities as a way to support residents desire to use creativity, imagination and produce items
Self-esteem/self-identity	Increase self-esteem, feelings of belonging, dignity, self-worth, integrity, self-identity/wellness, and quality of life	-will state/communicate positive feelings about self, will join craft class to take an active role in maintaining health though arts/crafts, volunteer work,; will join the craft class based on own choices	Staff will educate residents on the value of doing crafts/ learning talents for brain muscle/stimulant benefits, healing qualities, and encourage residents to join classes/share crafts
Sensory Integration/Tolerating Stimulation	Increase sensory processing and enhance awareness of sensations and toleration/adaptation of sensory stimulations and demands	-will adjust to the smells, lights, sounds, etc. in environment	-Staff will offer activities and residents will be exposed to sensory stimulating experiences of tactile stimulation, sights, hearing, communication, and possibly smell sensory stimulations -Residents will be supported as they adjust to the stimulus one step at a time
Fostering Appropriate Behaviors	Increase social interaction, social opportunities and adjustment, safety, using appropriate behaviors during an activity for a calm environment/wellness, and quality of life	-will join in on class, share items/tools, listen and follow instructions, use appropriate behavior for the setting; will wait turn, stand in line quietly; will quiet down when asked	Before class begins, staff will discuss the rules, appropriate behaviors, respect of property, safety, and respect of fellow peers/staff

TABLE 24.3

Recreational Objectives Observational Form
Flower Baskets- Socio-emotional Skills

PATIENT		Dependent (Totally dependent)	High Assistance (25+ ability)	Moderate Assist. (50+ ability)	Mild Assistance (75+ability)	Independent (Totally independent.)
SEE CODES BELOW USE OPTIONAL CODES IF APPROPRIATE		1	2	3	4	5
		3 cue/ 2-3 physical	2-3 cues/ 2 physical	2-3 cues/ 1 physical	1-2 cues	Encouragement
97530- Therapeutic activities or	SKILL	GOAL	OBJECTIVES ____times per ____		METHOD	OUTCOME DATE
97537 Or 97535	SOCIALIZATION/ COMMUNITY INTEGRATION					
97537 Or 97535	TEAM PLAYING /SHARING					
97537 Or 97535	INITIATIVE AND MOTIVATION					
97537 Or 97535	EMOTIONAL GRATIFICATION					
97537 Or 97535	SENSE OF ACCOMPLISHM ENT					
97537 Or 97535	SELF-ESTEEM/ SELF-IDENTITY					
97537 Or 97535	FOSTERING APPROPRIATE BEHAVIORS					
97533	SENSORY INTEGRATION/ TOLERATING					

97537-Community/work reintegration training (e.g., shopping, transportation, money management, avocational activities and/or work environment/modification analysis, work task analysis), direct (one-on-one) contact by provider, each 15 minutes; **97535-Self care/home management training** (e.g., activities of daily living and compensatory training, meal preparation, safety procedures, and instructions in use of adaptive equipment), direct (one-on-one) contact by provider, each 15 minutes; **97530-Therapeutic activities, direct (one-on-one)** patient contact by the provider (use of dynamic activities to improve functional performance), each 15 minutes; **97150-Therapeutic procedure(s), group (2 or more individuals); 97533-Sensory integration techniques** to enhance sensory processing and promote adaptive responses to environmental demands, direct (one-on-one) patient contact by the provider, each 15 minutes; **occupational therapy evaluation 97003, re-evaluation . 97004**	Staff Initial
	Add total score here-Maximum Score 40 pt. each form per activity
	See scale below or use own/facilities optional score system

(Score 1-8)=1 (9-16) =2 (17-24) =3 (25-32) =4 (33-40) =5 If w/device add d if wish, ex: 1d, 2d, or If using 1-7 scale: (41-48) =6 (49-56)

Making Soaps

Objectives and benefits:

Cognitive Challenges: attention, memory, language, orientation, following patterns, following directions, productivity, mastering a task

Physical Needs: fine motor skills, gross motor skills, hand-eye coordination, perceptual speed and motor function, manipulation of materials, dexterity

Socio-emotional Needs: socialization, community integration, initiative and motivation, emotional gratification, sense of accomplishment, fostering appropriate behaviors, nurturing, * Reminiscing Qualities, Healing Qualities

Supplies: Soap molds, blocks of soap, booklet of soap making ideas, glass measuring cup, microwave or hot plate, soap fragrances, soap coloring

Time: 30 minutes

Staff/older adult ratio: 1:2 or as assessed per needs of individuals or group

Instructions: Place supplies on table. Have older adults chose soap molds or follow a theme. For example, holiday soaps in the shapes of stars, trees, or dreidels. Have blocks of soap already cut into small cubes. Have the older adults put the small cubes of soap into the measuring cup. Have staff melt the soap at medium heat. It only takes about forty-five seconds to melt soap. Have the older adults pour the soap into the molds. Let them sit and dry for approximately one half hour, then remove the soap from the molds. They can use the soap in their traditional fashion or simply for decoration. These are also great holiday gifts. Let the older adults experiment with adding different kinds of items in the soap such as dried flowers. To do this, make half of the soap in a mold, let the soap harden just a bit, add the items over this half of the soap, add the remaining warm soap to the mold, let it dry, and remove it from the mold.

Be extremely cautious when handling warmed soaps. It may be safer for the staff to pour the warm soap into the molds. Never allow the older adult to handle the container of soap either in the measuring cup or in the mold without a member of the staff to hold the container securely.

> Research has shown activities that help cognition of sensory/motor and speed processing will be geared towards help in visual and motor memory, discrimination, comparison, and categorizing areas. Reminiscing activities may help improve memory skills. Long-term studies (Arbuckle and others, 1998) have consistently showed that stimulating the brain with activities helps cognitive function in a similar way exercise helps muscle function. Staying productive has been shown to enhance socio-emotional wellness

Making Soaps Cognitive Goals, Objectives and Methods

Skill	Goal	Objectives Sample	Method Sample
Orientation	Show increased awareness of, time/"timeframe," people, circumstances, and past experiences vs. present experiences, to engage in present-time activities, or for a reminiscing intended question	-will respond with correct answer to two choice questions Or yes/no answer, will state where they are, time of day, present company of people on own and with the correct answer	Staff will ask residents a series of questions to stimulate focus to the present setting (Ex: "What talents are you going to share? Have you made soaps before?")
Attention	Show increased attention span, task for function, and to engage in meaningful, recreational/fulfilling activities	-will make eye-contact with staff for _____ sec., will verbalize with staff and instructor, will read/listen to rules, will say yes/no to show they understand, or do the action	Staff will address or stand in front of resident, make eye-contact, ask questions, or use others methods to get resident's attention
Memory	Show increased memory skills of recall, recognition, retention of information, working memory	-will repeat/recall how to make project, will remember lesson at next class	Staff will show steps on how to make soaps, and residents will repeat the action using short-term memory/recall, working memory
Language	Show increased ability to communicate use of words, phrases, sentence structure, comprehension, interpretation	-will be asked a question and answer yes/no, will be asked what is included in project, will state ingredients, methods., and items; will interact with peers, staff; will interpret instructor's request and follow	Staff will ask questions to stimulate a communication (Ex: "What materials are you using to make your soaps?") Interpretation/Lang. skills (Ex: "You need to pour the warm soap into the mold.") and then note resident's actions to show they understood
Cognitive Stimulation (awareness, seeks information in)	Increased stimulus/exposure for visual/ motor memory, cognitive experiences/awareness and brain stimulation to enhance (function, pragmatics, neuroplasticity)	-will look around the room, will listen/seek cognitive stimulation, will accept challenge of input information and engage/interact in, will engage in a bookmark activity	Staff will set up crafts and put out a wide variety of art and craft materials to encourage creativity, discrimination, comparison, categorizing, etc.
Perceptual Awareness	Show increased abilities of depth perception, visio-spatical awareness, and acuity (for discrimination, comparison, and categorizing), safety	-will use ingredients/items, will discriminate, compare; will maneuver around work area, will put items away in proper containers associated with proper area (buttons with buttons, glitter with glitter, etc.)	Staff will engage residents in an activity that requires use of acuity, discrimination, comparison, and categorizing for visio-spatical awareness (Ex: placing items in the soap molds using visual acuity, etc.)
Problem-solving (goes beyond thinking/stimulus and initiates thinking process)	Increase problem-solving ability, processing of information, thinking, reasoning, and use of good judgment and decision-making	-will process the information, will judge appropriate materials, mix ingredients, measure, pour into molds	-Staff will engage residents in a creative project and decision-making regarding whom to send the soaps to -Staff will show the resident the step-by-step actions to make soap to stimulate working memory
Complete a Task	Increase ability to complete a task	will recall/retain and sort/gather information, problem-solve, and complete activity	Staff will support resident's ability to follow the project through instruction, encourage, supply adaptive devices/programs, if needed, and necessary materials and support

TABLE 25.1

RECREATIONAL OBJECTIVES OBSERVATIONAL FORM

MAKING SOAPS- COGNITIVE SKILLS

PATIENT	Dependent (Totally dependent)	High Assistance (25+ ability)	Moderate Assist. (50+ ability)	Mild Assistance (75+ability)	Independent (Totally independent)
SEE CODES BELOW USE OPTIONAL CODES IF APPROPRIATE	1	2	3	4	5
	3 cue/ 2-3 physical	2-3 cues/ 2 physical	2-3 cues/ 1 physical	1-2 cues	Encouragement

97530- Therapeutic activities or	SKILL	GOAL	OBJECTIVES ____times per ____	METHOD	OUTCOME DATE			
97532 Cognitive skills	ORIENTATION							
97532 Cognitive skills	ATTENTION							
97532 Cognitive skills	MEMORY							
97532 Cognitive skills	PROBLEM-SOLVING							
97532 Cognitive skills	COMPLETE A TASK							
97139 Speech Therapy 97532 Cognitive skills	LANGUAGE							
97533	SENSORY STIMULATION/ COGNITIVE STIMULATION							
97532	PERCEPTUAL AWARENESS							

97532-Development of cognitive skills to improve attention, memory, problem-solving, includes compensatory training and/or sensory integrative activities, direct (one-on-one) patient contact by the provider, each 15 minutes; **97530-Therapeutic activities**, direct (one-on-one) patient contact by the provider (use of dynamic activities to improve functional performance), each 15 minutes**; 97533-Sensory integration techniques** to enhance sensory processing and promote adaptive responses to environmental demands, direct (one-on-one) patient contact by the provider, each 15 minutes; **97150-Therapeutic procedure(s)**, group (2 or more individuals); **97139-Unlisted therapeutic procedure** (specify) minutes; **97003-occupational therapy evaluation**; **97004- re-evaluation**	Staff Initial				
	Add total score here -Maximum Score 40 pt. each form per activity				
	See scale below or use own/facilities optional score system				

(Score 1-8)=1 (9-16) =2 (17-24) =3 (25-32) =4 (33-40) =5 If w/device add d if wish, ex: 1d, 2d, or If using 1-7 scale: (41-48) =6 (49-56)

Making Soaps
Physical Goals, Objectives, and Methods

Skill	Goal	Objectives Sample	Method Sample
Fine Motor Skills	Increase fine motor skills, meaningful/fulfilling activities	-will glue, paste, mix and pour items, will pick up small items, manipulate materials	Staff will encourage residents to pick up and manipulate materials
Gross Motor Skills	Increase large motor skills, meaningful/fulfilling activities	-will lift items using large motor skills, walk to group (with device or support)	Staff will encourage residents to lift items using gross motor skills
Perceptual Speed and Motor Function	Increase speed and motor ability for function, safety, meaningful/fulfilling activities	-will increase speed of actions by using skills (with Dr. approval)	Staff will encourage residents to do the activity and decrease reaction times by shortening amount of time allotted, or observation of resident ability increasing on own
Hand-Eye Coordination	Increase hand-eye coordination	-will paste items on craft	Staff will encourage residents to place items using hand-eye fine motor abilities, detailed fine motor activities

TABLE 25.2

Recreational Objectives Observational Form
Making Soaps- Physical Skills

PATIENT		Dependent (Totally dependent)	High Assistance (25+ ability)	Moderate Assist. (50+ ability)	Mild Assistance (75+ability)	Independent (Totally independent)
		1	2	3	4	5
SEE CODES BELOW USE OPTIONAL CODES IF APPROPRIATE		3 cue/ 2-3 physical	2-3 cues/ 2 physical	2-3 cues/ 1 physical	1-2 cues	Encouragement
97530- Therapeutic activities or	**SKILL**	**GOAL**	**OBJECTIVES** ____times per ____		**METHOD**	**OUTCOME DATE**
Therapeutic Activity 97530	FINE MOTOR SKILLS					
97530	EYE-HAND COORDINATION					
97110/ 97530	GROSS MOTOR SKILLS					
97530 If under cognitive code 97532	PERCEPTUAL SPEED/MOTOR FUNCTION					

97530 Therapeutic activities, direct (one on one) patient contact by the provider (use of dynamic activities to improve functional performance),each 15 minutes; **97110 Therapeutic procedure, one or more areas**, each 15 minutes; therapeutic exercises to develop strength and endurance, range of motion and flexibility; ; **97150 Therapeutic procedure(s), group (2 or more individuals**; **97535-Self care/home management training** (e.g., activities of daily living and compensatory training, meal preparation, safety procedures, and instructions in use of adaptive equipment), direct (one-on-one) contact by provider, each 15 minutes; **Physical therapy 97001 evaluation, 97002 Re-evaluation. occupational therapy evaluation 97003, re-evaluation. 97004**

Staff Initials				
Add total score here Maximum Score 20 pt. each form per activity				
See scale below or use own/facilities optional score system				

(Score 1-4)=1 (5-8) =2 (9-12) =3 (13-16) =4 (17-20) =5 If w/device add d if wish, ex: 1d, 2d, or If using 1-7 scale: (21-24) =6 (25-28) =7

Making Soaps
Socio-emotional Goals, Objectives, and Methods

Skill	Goal	Objectives Sample	Method Sample
Socialization/Community Integration	Increase social interactions, meaningful/fulfilling activities	-will interact with peers, will engage in community integration experiences (for community adaptation and social skills), will use manners, share, practice social skills	Staff will offer activities that support/encourage residents to socialize through community integration and being w/groups
Team Playing/Sharing	Increase teamwork/sharing, meaningful/fulfilling activities	-will join in on a craft/ activity with others, and share, wait turn, support peers _____ time(s) this week.	Staff will encourage residents to create items, share, work as a team, support/use patience, show compassion to other residents
Initiative and Motivation	Increase initiative and motivation/wellness, and quality of life	-will choose if wishes to do craft, will try new crafts, will increase amount of crafts done _____ times a week	-Staff will support/encourage the resident to prepare for craft activities in a timely fashion for their own personal gains of attending activity -Staff will offer new techniques/creative materials to motivate residents to make a creative craft
Emotional Gratification	Increase emotional gratification/wellness, and quality of life	-will state that making crafts is a gratifying experience, or will show pleasure by smiling, laughing, deep focus on activities	Staff will ask residents if they enjoyed the activity and what they liked through verbal discussion, group discussions
Sense of Accomplishment	Increase feelings of self-worth, pride, productivity, dignity/wellness, and quality of life	-will use gestures to express pride in self, will show crafts to others	Staff will offer activities as a way to support resident's desire to use creativity, imagination, and produce items
Self-esteem/self-identity	Increase self-esteem, feelings of belonging, dignity, self-worth, integrity, self-identity/wellness, and quality of life	-will state/communicate positive feelings about self, will join craft class to take an active role in maintaining health though arts/crafts, volunteer work; will join the craft class based on own choices	Staff will be educate residents on the value of doing crafts/ learning talents for brain muscle/stimulant benefits, and healing qualities, and encourage residents to join classes/share crafts
Sensory Integration/Tolerating Stimulation	Increase sensory processing and enhance awareness of sensations and toleration/adaptation of sensory stimulations and demands	-will adjust to the smells, lights, sounds, etc. in environment	-Staff will offer activities, and residents will be exposed to sensory stimulating experiences of tactile stimulation, sights, hearing, communication, and possibly smell sensory stimulations -Residents will be supported as they adjust to the stimulus one step at a time
Fostering Appropriate Behaviors	Increase social interaction, social opportunities and adjustment, safety, using appropriate behaviors during an activity for a calm environment/wellness, and quality of life	-will join in on class, share items/tools, listen and follow instructions, use appropriate behavior for the setting; will wait turn, stand in line quietly; will quiet down when asked	Before class begins, staff will discuss the rules, appropriate behaviors, respect of property, safety, and respect of fellow peers/staff

TABLE 25.3

Recreational Objectives Observational Form
Making Soaps- Socio-emotional Skills

PATIENT	Dependent (Totally dependent)	High Assistance (25+ ability)	Moderate Assist. (50+ ability)	Mild Assistance (75+ability)	Independent (Totally independent.)
SEE CODES BELOW USE OPTIONAL CODES IF APPROPRIATE	1	2	3	4	5
	3 cue/ 2-3 physical	2-3 cues/ 2 physical	2-3 cues/ 1 physical	1-2 cues	Encouragement

97530- Therapeutic activities or	SKILL	GOAL	OBJECTIVES ____times per ____	METHOD	OUTCOME DATE			
97537 Or 97535	SOCIALIZATION/ COMMUNITY INTEGRATION							
97537 Or 97535	TEAM PLAYING /SHARING							
97537 Or 97535	INITIATIVE AND MOTIVATION							
97537 Or 97535	EMOTIONAL GRATIFICATION							
97537 Or 97535	SENSE OF ACCOMPLISHM ENT							
97537 Or 97535	SELF-ESTEEM/ SELF-IDENTITY							
97537 Or 97535	FOSTERING APPROPRIATE BEHAVIORS							
97533	SENSORY INTEGRATION/ TOLERATING							

Staff Initial				
Add total score here-Maximum Score 40 pt. each form per activity				
See scale below or use own/facilities optional score system				

97537-Community/work reintegration training (e.g., shopping, transportation, money management, avocational activities and/or work environment/modification analysis, work task analysis), direct (one-on-one) contact by provider, each 15 minutes; **97535-Self care/home management training** (e.g., activities of daily living and compensatory training, meal preparation, safety procedures, and instructions in use of adaptive equipment), direct (one-on-one) contact by provider, each 15 minutes; **97530-Therapeutic activities, direct (one-on-one)** patient contact by the provider (use of dynamic activities to improve functional performance), each 15 minutes; **97150-Therapeutic procedure(s), group (2 or more individuals); 97533-Sensory integration techniques** to enhance sensory processing and promote adaptive responses to environmental demands, direct (one-on-one) patient contact by the provider, each 15 minutes; **occupational therapy evaluation 97003, re-evaluation . 97004**

(Score 1-8)=1 (9-16) =2 (17-24) =3 (25-32) =4 (33-40) =5 If w/device add d if wish, ex: 1d, 2d, or If using 1-7 scale: (41-48) =6 (49-56)

Painting

Objectives and benefits:

Cognitive Challenges: attention, memory, language, orientation, following patterns, following directions, productivity, mastering a task

Physical Needs: fine motor skills, gross motor skills, hand-eye coordination, perceptual speed and motor function, manipulation of materials, dexterity

Socio-emotional Needs: socialization, community integration, initiative and motivation, emotional gratification, sense of accomplishment, fostering appropriate behaviors, nurturing, * Reminiscing Qualities, Healing Qualities

Supplies: Various mediums of paints, art materials

Time: 30–45 minutes

Staff/older adult ratio: As assessed per needs of individuals or group

Instructions: Provide an array of art activities using an assortment of mediums. Set up the supplies. Include newspaper for easy cleanup. Sometimes it is hard for the elderly to initiate their own picture. In this case, offering a bowl of fruit or an already completed picture may be helpful. This activity is okay when working with the blind or those with vision problems. They can create pictures using a variation of tactile items. Using a picture with borders heightened can help them paint in a way similar to the idea of paint-by-number. Just use fabric paint in patterns consistent to the picture. It will stiffen up and they will be able to paint within the lines.

Each week, offer a variety of art mediums. Here are a few suggestions:

Painting w/ oil-based paint
Painting w/ watercolors
Drawing w/ charcoal
Painting w/ music
Painting w/ pre-printed themes
Painting w/ bubbles, sponges, seashells, tactile items (sand, stones).

Research has shown activities that help cognition of sensory/motor and speed processing will be geared towards help in visual and motor memory, discrimination, comparison, and categorizing areas. Reminiscing activities may help improve memory skills. Long-term studies (Arbuckle and others, 1998) have consistently showed that stimulating the brain with activities helps cognitive function in a similar way exercise helps muscle function. Staying productive has been shown to enhance socio-emotional wellness

Painting
Cognitive Goals, Objectives, and Methods

Skill	Goal	Objectives Sample	Method Sample
Orientation	Show increased awareness of, time/"timeframe," people, circumstances, and past experiences vs. present experiences, to engage in present-time activities, or for a reminiscing intended question	-will respond with correct answer to two choice questions, will state where they are, time of day, present company of people on own and with the correct answer	Staff will ask residents a series of questions to stimulate focus to the present setting (Ex: "It's Friday. Do we do art on Fridays or do we do Bingo?") Or past if reminiscing exercise (Ex: "What where the most influential artists in your time?") (memory and orientation exercise)
Attention	Show increased attention span, task for function, and to engage in meaningful, recreational/fulfilling activities	-will make eye-contact with staff for _____ sec., will verbalize with staff, instructor, will read/listen to rules-say yes/no to show they understand or do the action	Staff will address or stand in front of resident, make eye-contact, ask questions, or use others forms to get resident's attention (Ex: "What kind of art are we going to work with today? Are we going to use clay or paints?")
Memory	Show increased memory skills of recall, recognition, retention of information, working memory	-will retain repeat/recall how to draw the asked art drawing and how to use tools, etc.	-Staff will ask residents to name popular art methods (clay, oils, etc.) -Staff will offer art supplies to stimulate memories
Language	Show increased ability to communicate use of words, phrases, sentence structure, comprehension, interpretation	-will be asked a question and answer yes/no, will be asked to describe the art they produced	Staff will ask questions to stimulate a communication (Ex: "Tell me about your Drawing.") Interpretation/Lang. skills (Ex: " Can you draw a square in front of that grass scene to add to our collective house painting?")
Cognitive Stimulation (awareness, seeks information in)	Increased stimulus/exposure for visual/ motor memory, cognitive experiences/awareness and brain stimulation to enhance (function, pragmatics, neuroplasticity)	-will look around the room, be engaged in game w/ peers will interact, listen/seek cognitive stimulation, will accept challenge of input information and engage/interact in painting activity	Staff will expose residents to photo or designs using various media and materials
Perceptual Awareness	Show increased abilities of depth perception, visio-spatical awareness, and acuity (for discrimination, comparison, and categorizing), safety	-will draw a variety of pictures or use other forms of art materials and include perceptual modes and "looks" ex: dimensional paintings	Staff will offer a painting activity that requires residents to use visual acuity, spatial relationships, etc. (Ex: "Can you draw a square in front of that grass scene to add to our collective house painting?")
Problem-solving (goes beyond thinking/stimulus and initiates thinking process)	Increase problem-solving ability, processing of information, thinking, reasoning, and use of good judgment and decision-making	-will follow directions on how to make a 3-d picture, will problem-solve while building a clay structure	Staff will engage resident in painting activity and ask resident to copy a picture of fruits in a bowl (have picture available to copy)
Complete a Task	Increase ability to complete a task	will recall/retain and sort/gather information, problem-solve, and complete activity	Staff will support resident's ability to follow procedure of project through instruction, encourage residents, and supply adaptive devices/programs ,if needed, and necessary materials and support

Table 26.1

Recreational Objectives Observational Form
Painting- Cognitive skills

PATIENT		Dependent (Totally dependent)	High Assistance (25+ ability)	Moderate Assist. (50+ ability)	Mild Assistance (75+ability)	Independent (Totally independent)
SEE CODES BELOW USE OPTIONAL CODES IF APPROPRIATE		1	2	3	4	5
		3 cue/ 2-3 physical	2-3 cues/ 2 physical	2-3 cues/ 1 physical	1-2 cues	Encouragement

97530- Therapeutic activities or	SKILL	GOAL	OBJECTIVES ____times per ____	METHOD	OUTCOME DATE
97532 Cognitive skills	ORIENTATION				
97532 Cognitive skills	ATTENTION				
97532 Cognitive skills	MEMORY				
97532 Cognitive skills	PROBLEM-SOLVING				
97532 Cognitive skills	COMPLETE A TASK				
97139 Speech Therapy 97532 Cognitive skills	LANGUAGE				
97533	SENSORY STIMULATION/ COGNITIVE STIMULATION				
97532	PERCEPTUAL AWARENESS				

97532-Development of cognitive skills to improve attention, memory, problem-solving, includes compensatory training and/or sensory integrative activities, direct (one-on-one) patient contact by the provider, each 15 minutes; **97530-Therapeutic activities**, direct (one-on-one) patient contact by the provider (use of dynamic activities to improve functional performance), each 15 minutes**; 97533-Sensory integration techniques** to enhance sensory processing and promote adaptive responses to environmental demands, direct (one-on-one) patient contact by the provider, each 15 minutes; **97150-Therapeutic procedure(s)**, group (2 or more individuals); **97139-Unlisted therapeutic procedure** (specify) minutes; **97003- occupational therapy evaluation**; **97004- re-evaluation**	Staff Initial Add total score here -Maximum Score 40 pt. each form per activity See scale below or use own/facilities optional score system

(Score 1-8)=1 (9-16) =2 (17-24) =3 (25-32) =4 (33-40) =5 If w/device add d if wish, ex: 1d, 2d, or If using 1-7 scale: (41-48) =6 (49-56)

Painting
Physical Goals, Objectives, and Methods

Skill	Goal	Objectives Sample	Method Sample
Fine Motor Skills	Increase fine motor skills, meaningful/fulfilling activities	-will glue, paste, mix and pour items, will pick up small items, manipulate materials	Staff will encourage residents to pick up and manipulate materials
Gross Motor Skills	Increase large motor skills, meaningful/fulfilling activities	-will lift items using large motor skills, walk to group (with device or support)	Staff will encourage residents to lift items using gross motor skills
Perceptual Speed and Motor Function	Increase speed and motor ability for function, safety, meaningful/fulfilling activities	-will increase speed of actions by using skills	Staff will encourage residents to do the activity and decrease reaction times by shortening amount of time allotted, or observation of resident ability increasing on own
Hand-Eye Coordination	Increase hand-eye coordination	-will use drawing tools, use detailed fine motor skills	Staff will encourage residents to place items using hand-eye fine motor abilities, detailed fine motor activities

TABLE 26.2

Recreational Objectives Observational Form
Painting- Physical Skills

PATIENT		Dependent (Totally dependent)	High Assistance (25+ ability)	Moderate Assist. (50+ ability)	Mild Assistance (75+ability)	Independent (Totally independent)
		1	2	3	4	5
SEE CODES BELOW USE OPTIONAL CODES IF APPROPRIATE		3 cue/ 2-3 physical	2-3 cues/ 2 physical	2-3 cues/ 1 physical	1-2 cues	Encouragement
97530- Therapeutic activities or	**SKILL**	**GOAL**	**OBJECTIVES** ____times per ____		**METHOD**	**OUTCOME DATE**
Therapeutic Activity 97530	FINE MOTOR SKILLS					
97530	EYE-HAND COORDINATION					
97110/ 97530	GROSS MOTOR SKILLS					
97530 If under cognitive code 97532	PERCEPTUAL SPEED/MOTOR FUNCTION					

97530 Therapeutic activities, direct (one on one) patient contact by the provider (use of dynamic activities to improve functional performance),each 15 minutes; **97110 Therapeutic procedure, one or more areas**, each 15 minutes; therapeutic exercises to develop strength and endurance, range of motion and flexibility; ; **97150 Therapeutic procedure(s), group (2 or more individuals**; **97535-Self care/home management training** (e.g., activities of daily living and compensatory training, meal preparation, safety procedures, and instructions in use of adaptive equipment), direct (one-on-one) contact by provider, each 15 minutes; **Physical therapy 97001 evaluation, 97002 Re-evaluation. occupational therapy evaluation 97003, re-evaluation. 97004**	Staff Initials
	Add total score here Maximum Score 20 pt. each form per activity
	See scale below or use own/facilities optional score system

(Score 1-4)=1 (5-8) =2 (9-12) =3 (13-16) =4 (17-20) =5 If w/device add d if wish, ex: 1d, 2d, or If using 1-7 scale: (21-24) =6 (25-28) =7

Painting
Socio-emotional Goals, Objectives, and Methods

Skill	Goal	Objectives Sample	Method Sample
Socialization/Community Integration	Increase social interactions, meaningful/fulfilling activities	-will interact with peers, will engage in community integration experiences (for community adaptation and social skills), will use manners, share, practice social skills	Staff will offer art classes to support/encourage residents to socialize through community integration and being w/groups
Team Playing/Sharing	Increase teamwork/sharing, meaningful/fulfilling activities	-will join in on an art activity with others and share; will wait turn, support peers _____ time(s) this week	Residents will be encouraged to draw, paint, create art pieces
Initiative and Motivation	Increase initiative and motivation/wellness, and quality of life	-will choose if wishes to paint, will try an art form on own, will increase number of art pieces they produce	-Staff will support/encourage the resident to prepare for art class in a timely fashion for their own personal gains of attending art/painting classes -Staff will offer new techniques, music, themes, instruments to motivate
Emotional Gratification	Increase emotional gratification/wellness, and quality of life	-will state that creating art is a gratifying experiences, or will show pleasure by smiling, laughing, deep focus on art activity	Staff will ask residents if they enjoyed the art class and what they liked by way of verbal discussion, group discussions
Sense of Accomplishment	Increase feelings of self-worth, pride, productivity, dignity/wellness, and quality of life	-will use gestures to express pride in self , will talk about their accomplishments of drawing and ability to create art pieces	-Staff will exhibit resident's art works on the wall at tables and awards will be handed out for best art in categories, etc.
Self-esteem/self-identity	Increase self-esteem, feelings of belonging, dignity, self-worth, integrity, self-identity/wellness, and quality of life	-will state/communicate positive feelings about self, will join art class, draw, paint to take an active role in health though art exercises; will join art class based on own choices	Staff will educate residents on the value of using art for brain muscle/stimulant benefits, healing qualities, and will encourage residents to join classes/share works
Sensory Integration/Tolerating Stimulation	Increase sensory processing and enhance awareness of sensations and toleration/adaptation of sensory stimulations and demands	-will adjust to the lights, sounds, and etc. _____ time this week.	-Staff will offer art classes using various mediums, and residents will be exposed to sensory stimulating experiences of sound, textures of items, sights, smells -Staff will support residents as they adjust to the stimulus one step at a time
Fostering Appropriate Behaviors	Increase social interaction, social opportunities and adjustment, safety, using appropriate behaviors during an activity for a calm environment/wellness, and quality of life	-will join in on art class, using art materials and tools, will listen and follow instructions, use appropriate behavior for the setting; will wait turn, stand in line quietly; will quiet down when asked	Before class begins, staff will discuss the rules, appropriate behaviors, respect of property, safety, and respect of peers/instructor

TABLE 26.3

Recreational Objectives Observational Form
Painting - Socio-emotional Skills

PATIENT		Dependent (Totally dependent)	High Assistance (25+ ability)	Moderate Assist. (50+ ability)	Mild Assistance (75+ability)	Independent (Totally independent.)
SEE CODES BELOW USE OPTIONAL CODES IF APPROPRIATE		1	2	3	4	5
		3 cue/ 2-3 physical	2-3 cues/ 2 physical	2-3 cues/ 1 physical	1-2 cues	Encouragement
97530- Therapeutic activities or	**SKILL**	**GOAL**	**OBJECTIVES** ____times per ____		**METHOD**	**OUTCOME DATE**
97537 Or 97535	SOCIALIZATION/ COMMUNITY INTEGRATION					
97537 Or 97535	TEAM PLAYING /SHARING					
97537 Or 97535	INITIATIVE AND MOTIVATION					
97537 Or 97535	EMOTIONAL GRATIFICATION					
97537 Or 97535	SENSE OF ACCOMPLISHMENT					
97537 Or 97535	SELF-ESTEEM/ SELF-IDENTITY					
97537 Or 97535	FOSTERING APPROPRIATE BEHAVIORS					
97533	SENSORY INTEGRATION/ TOLERATING					

97537-Community/work reintegration training (e.g., shopping, transportation, money management, avocational activities and/or work environment/modification analysis, work task analysis), direct (one-on-one) contact by provider, each 15 minutes; **97535-Self care/home management training** (e.g., activities of daily living and compensatory training, meal preparation, safety procedures, and instructions in use of adaptive equipment), direct (one-on-one) contact by provider, each 15 minutes; **97530-Therapeutic activities, direct (one-on-one)** patient contact by the provider (use of dynamic activities to improve functional performance), each 15 minutes; **97150-Therapeutic procedure(s), group (2 or more individuals); 97533-Sensory integration techniques** to enhance sensory processing and promote adaptive responses to environmental demands, direct (one-on-one) patient contact by the provider, each 15 minutes; **occupational therapy evaluation 97003, re-evaluation . 97004**	Staff Initial	
	Add total score here-Maximum Score 40 pt. each form per activity	
	See scale below or use own/facilities optional score system	

(Score 1-8)=1 (9-16) =2 (17-24) =3 (25-32) =4 (33-40) =5 If w/device add d if wish, ex: 1d, 2d, or If using 1-7 scale: (41-48) =6 (49-56)

Picture Frames

Objectives and benefits:

Cognitive Challenges: attention, memory, language, orientation, following patterns, following directions, productivity, mastering a task

Physical Needs: fine motor skills, gross motor skills, hand-eye coordination, perceptual speed and motor function, manipulation of materials, dexterity

Socio-emotional Needs: socialization, community integration, initiative and motivation, emotional gratification, sense of accomplishment, fostering appropriate behaviors, nurturing, * Reminiscing Qualities, Healing Qualities

Supplies: Cardboard squares with area for picture already cut out, cardboard back, glue or glue gun, variety of art materials (sea shells, stars, glitter, feathers, etc.), piece of glass or Plexiglas

Time: 30–45 minutes

Staff/older adult ratio: 1:3 or as assessed per needs of individuals or group

Instructions: Make a sample frame so the residents see what they will be making. Have the front and back cardboard pieces set at a place for each resident. Have them take a favorite picture they would like to frame. Be sure the picture measurements are correct for the frame area. Let them place the picture in between both pieces of cardboard. After the glue dries, let them decorate the outside of their frames. Be sure to offer art supplies that are geared for the older adult.

Research has shown activities that help cognition of sensory/motor and speed processing will be geared towards help in visual and motor memory, discrimination, comparison, and categorizing areas. Reminiscing activities may help improve memory skills. Long-term studies (Arbuckle and others, 1998) have consistently showed that stimulating the brain with activities helps cognitive function in a similar way exercise helps muscle function. Staying productive has been shown to enhance socio-emotional wellness

Picture Frames
Cognitive Goals, Objectives, and Methods

Skill	Goal	Objectives Sample	Method Sample
Orientation	Show increased awareness of, time/"timeframe," people, circumstances, and past experiences vs. present experiences, to engage in present-time activities, or for a reminiscing intended question	-will respond with correct answer to two choice questions Or yes/no answer, will state where they are, time of day, present company of people on own and with the correct answer	Staff will ask residents a series of questions to stimulate focus to the present setting (Ex: "What talents are you going to share? Have you made picture frames before? Who are the people in your pictures? Are these old friends or new acquaintances?")
Attention	Show increased attention span, task for function, and to engage in meaningful, recreational/fulfilling activities	-will make eye-contact with staff for ______ sec., will verbalize with staff and instructor, will read/listen to rules, will say yes/no to show they understand or do the action	Staff will address or stand in front of resident, make eye-contact, ask questions, or use others methods to get resident's attention
Memory	Show increased memory skills of recall, recognition, retention of information, working memory	-will repeat/recall how to make project, will remember lesson at next class	Staff will show steps and actions on how to make picture frames, and residents will repeat the action using short-term memory/recall, working memory
Language	Show increased ability to communicate use of words, phrases, sentence structure, comprehension, interpretation	-will be asked a question and answer yes/no, will be asked what is included in the project, will state ingredients, methods, items; will interact with peers and staff, will interpret instructor's request and follow	-Staff will ask questions to stimulate a communication (Ex: "What materials are you using for your picture frame?") -Interpretation/Lang. skills (Ex: "You need to add tacky glue to make it stick well.") and then note resident's actions to show they understood
Cognitive Stimulation (awareness, seeks information in)	Increased stimulus/exposure for visual/ motor memory, cognitive experiences/awareness and brain stimulation to enhance (function, pragmatics, neuron-plasticity)	-will look around the room, will listen/seek cognitive stimulation, will accept challenge of input information and engage/interact in, will engage in a picture-frame activity	Staff will set up crafts and put out a wide variety of arts and craft materials to encourage creativity, discrimination, comparison, categorizing, etc.
Perceptual Awareness	Show increased abilities of depth perception, visio-spatial awareness, and acuity (for discrimination, comparison, and categorizing), safety	-will use ingredients /items, will discriminate, compare; will maneuver around work area, will put items away in proper containers associated with proper area	Staff will engage residents in an activity that requires use of acuity, discrimination, comparison, and categorizing for visio-spatial awareness (Ex: placing items on the bookmark using visual acuity, etc.)
Problem-solving (goes beyond thinking/stimulus and initiates thinking process)	Increase problem-solving ability, processing of information, thinking, reasoning, and use of good judgment and decision-making	-will use creativity or comprehend and process the information, will judge appropriate materials, temperatures, consistency	-Staff will engage residents in a creative project and decision-making regarding materials that will work well in the middle of the picture frame -Staff will show the resident the step-by-step actions to make picture frames to stimulate working memory
Complete a Task	Increase ability to complete a task	-will recall/retain and sort/gather information, problem-solve, and complete activity	Staff will support resident's ability to follow the project through instruction, encourage, and supply adaptive devices/programs if needed, and necessary materials and support

TABLE 27.1

Recreational Objectives Observational Form
Picture Frames- Cognitive skills

PATIENT		Dependent (Totally dependent)	High Assistance (25+ ability)	Moderate Assist. (50+ ability)	Mild Assistance (75+ability)	Independent (Totally independent)
SEE CODES BELOW USE OPTIONAL CODES IF APPROPRIATE		1	2	3	4	5
		3 cue/ 2-3 physical	2-3 cues/ 2 physical	2-3 cues/ 1 physical	1-2 cues	Encourageme nt
97530- Therapeutic activities or	**SKILL**	**GOAL**	**OBJECTIVES** ____times per ____		**METHOD**	**OUTCOME DATE**
97532 Cognitive skills	ORIENTATION					
97532 Cognitive skills	ATTENTION					
97532 Cognitive skills	MEMORY					
97532 Cognitive skills	PROBLEM-SOLVING					
97532 Cognitive skills	COMPLETE A TASK					
97139 Speech Therapy 97532 Cognitive skills	LANGUAGE					
97533	SENSORY STIMULATION/ COGNITIVE STIMULATION					
97532	PERCEPTUAL AWARENESS					

97532-Development of cognitive skills to improve attention, memory, problem-solving, includes compensatory training and/or sensory integrative activities, direct (one-on-one) patient contact by the provider, each 15 minutes; **97530-Therapeutic activities**, direct (one-on-one) patient contact by the provider (use of dynamic activities to improve functional performance), each 15 minutes; **97533-Sensory integration techniques** to enhance sensory processing and promote adaptive responses to environmental demands, direct (one-on-one) patient contact by the provider, each 15 minutes; **97150-Therapeutic procedure(s)**, group (2 or more individuals); **97139-Unlisted therapeutic procedure** (specify) minutes; **97003- occupational therapy evaluation**; **97004- re-evaluation**	Staff Initial Add total score here -Maximum Score 40 pt. each form per activity See scale below or use own/facilities optional score system

(Score 1-8)=1 (9-16) =2 (17-24) =3 (25-32) =4 (33-40) =5 If w/device add d if wish, ex: 1d, 2d, or If using 1-7 scale: (41-48) =6 (49-56)

Picture Frames
Physical Goals, Objectives, and Methods

Skill	Goal	Objectives Sample	Method Sample
Fine Motor Skills	Increase fine motor skills, meaningful/fulfilling activities	-will glue, paste, mix, and pour items -will pick up small items and manipulate materials	Staff will encourage residents to pick up and manipulate materials
Gross Motor Skills	Increase large motor skills, meaningful/fulfilling activities	-will lift items using large motor skills, will walk to group (with device or support)	Staff will encourage residents to lift items using gross motor skills
Perceptual Speed and Motor Function	Increase speed and motor ability for function, safety, meaningful/fulfilling activities	-will increase speed of actions by using skills (with Dr. approval)	Staff will encourage residents to do the activity and decrease reaction times by shortening amount of time allotted, or observation of resident ability increasing on own
Hand-Eye Coordination	Increase hand-eye coordination	-will paste items on craft	Staff will encourage residents to place items using hand-eye fine motor abilities, detailed fine motor activities

TABLE 27.2

Recreational Objectives Observational Form
Picture Frames - Physical Skills

PATIENT		Dependent (Totally dependent)	High Assistance (25+ ability)	Moderate Assist. (50+ ability)	Mild Assistance (75+ability)	Independent (Totally independent)			
		1	2	3	4	5			
SEE CODES BELOW USE OPTIONAL CODES IF APPROPRIATE		3 cue/ 2-3 physical	2-3 cues/ 2 physical	2-3 cues/ 1 physical	1-2 cues	Encouragement			
97530- Therapeutic activities or	**SKILL**	**GOAL**	**OBJECTIVES** ____times per ____		**METHOD**	**OUTCOME DATE**			
Therapeutic Activity 97530	FINE MOTOR SKILLS								
97530	EYE-HAND COORDINATION								
97110/ 97530	GROSS MOTOR SKILLS								
97530 If under cognitive code 97532	PERCEPTUAL SPEED/MOTOR FUNCTION								
97530 Therapeutic activities, direct (one on one) patient contact by the provider (use of dynamic activities to improve functional performance),each 15 minutes; **97110 Therapeutic procedure, one or more areas**, each 15 minutes; therapeutic exercises to develop strength and endurance, range of motion and flexibility; ; **97150 Therapeutic procedure(s), group (2 or more individuals**; **97535-Self care/home management training** (e.g., activities of daily living and compensatory training, meal preparation, safety procedures, and instructions in use of adaptive equipment), direct (one-on-one) contact by provider, each 15 minutes; **Physical therapy 97001 evaluation, 97002 Re-evaluation. occupational therapy evaluation 97003, re-evaluation. 97004**					Staff Initials				
					Add total score here Maximum Score 20 pt. each form per activity				
					See scale below or use own/facilities optional score system				

(Score 1-4)=1 (5-8) =2 (9-12) =3 (13-16) =4 (17-20) =5 If w/device add d if wish, ex: 1d, 2d, or If using 1-7 scale: (21-24) =6 (25-28) =7

Picture Frames
Socio-emotional Goals, Objectives, and Methods

Skill	Goal	Objectives Sample	Method Sample
Socialization/ Community Integration	Increase social interactions, meaningful/fulfilling activities	-will interact with peers, will engage in community integration experiences (for community adaptation and social skills), will use manners, share, practice social skills	Staff will offer activities that support/encourage residents to socialize through community integration and being w/groups
Team Playing/Sharing	Increase teamwork/sharing, meaningful/fulfilling activities	-will join in on a craft/ activity with others and share, wait turn, support peers _____ time(s) this week.	Staff will encourage residents to create items, share, work as a team, support/use patience, show compassion to other residents
Initiative and Motivation	Increase initiative and motivation/wellness, and quality of life	-will choose if wishes to do craft, will try new crafts, will increase amount of crafts done _____ times a week	-Staff will support/encourage the resident to prepare for craft activities in a timely fashion for their own personal gains of attending activity -Staff will offer new techniques/creative materials to motivate residents to make a creative craft
Emotional Gratification	Increase emotional gratification/wellness, and quality of life	-will state that making crafts is a gratifying experience or will show pleasure by smiling, laughing, deep focus on activities	Staff will ask residents if they enjoyed the activity and what they liked through verbal discussion, group discussions
Sense of Accomplishment	Increase feelings of self-worth, pride, productivity, dignity/wellness, and quality of life	-will use gestures to express pride in self, will show crafts to others	Staff will offer activities as a way to support resident's desires to use creativity, imagination, and produce items
Self-esteem/ Self-identity	Increase self-esteem, feelings of belonging, dignity, self-worth, integrity, self-identity/wellness, and quality of life	-will state/communicate positive feelings about self, will join craft class to take an active role in maintaining health though arts/crafts, volunteer work; will join the craft class based on own choices	Staff will educate residents on the value of doing crafts/ learning talents for brain muscle/stimulant benefits, healing qualities, and will encourage residents to join classes/share crafts
Sensory Integration/Tolerating Stimulation	Increase sensory processing and enhance awareness of sensations and toleration/adaptation of sensory stimulations and demands	-will adjust to the smells, lights, sounds, etc. in environment	-Staff will offer activities, and residents will be exposed to sensory stimulating experiences of tactile stimulation, sights, hearing, communication, and possibly smell sensory stimulations -Residents will be supported as they adjust to the stimulus one step at a time
Fostering Appropriate Behaviors	Increase social interaction, social opportunities and adjustment, safety, using appropriate behaviors during an activity for a calm environment/wellness, and quality of life	-will join in on class, share items/tools, listen and follow instructions, use appropriate behavior for the setting; will wait turn, stand in line, quietly, will quiet down when asked	Before class begins, staff will discuss the rules, appropriate behaviors, respect of property, safety, and respect of fellow peers/staff

Table 27.3

Recreational Objectives Observational Form

Picture Frames- Socio-emotional Skills

PATIENT	Dependent (Totally dependent)	High Assistance (25+ ability)	Moderate Assist. (50+ ability)	Mild Assistance (75+ability)	Independent (Totally independent.)
SEE CODES BELOW USE OPTIONAL CODES IF APPROPRIATE	1	2	3	4	5
	3 cue/ 2-3 physical	2-3 cues/ 2 physical	2-3 cues/ 1 physical	1-2 cues	Encouragement

97530-Therapeutic activities or	**SKILL**	**GOAL**	**OBJECTIVES** ____times per ____	**METHOD**	**OUTCOME DATE**			
97537 Or 97535	SOCIALIZATION/ COMMUNITY INTEGRATION							
97537 Or 97535	TEAM PLAYING /SHARING							
97537 Or 97535	INITIATIVE AND MOTIVATION							
97537 Or 97535	EMOTIONAL GRATIFICATION							
97537 Or 97535	SENSE OF ACCOMPLISHM ENT							
97537 Or 97535	SELF-ESTEEM/ SELF-IDENTITY							
97537 Or 97535	FOSTERING APPROPRIATE BEHAVIORS							
97533	SENSORY INTEGRATION/ TOLERATING							

97537-Community/work reintegration training (e.g., shopping, transportation, money management, avocational activities and/or work environment/modification analysis, work task analysis), direct (one-on-one) contact by provider, each 15 minutes; **97535-Self care/home management training** (e.g., activities of daily living and compensatory training, meal preparation, safety procedures, and instructions in use of adaptive equipment), direct (one-on-one) contact by provider, each 15 minutes; **97530-Therapeutic activities, direct (one-on-one)** patient contact by the provider (use of dynamic activities to improve functional performance), each 15 minutes; **97150-Therapeutic procedure(s), group (2 or more individuals); 97533-Sensory integration techniques** to enhance sensory processing and promote adaptive responses to environmental demands, direct (one-on-one) patient contact by the provider, each 15 minutes; **occupational therapy evaluation 97003, re-evaluation . 97004**	Staff Initial			

Add total score here-Maximum Score 40 pt. each form per activity				
See scale below or use own/facilities optional score system				

(Score 1-8)=1 (9-16) =2 (17-24) =3 (25-32) =4 (33-40) =5 If w/device add d if wish, ex: 1d, 2d, or If using 1-7 scale: (41-48) =6 (49-56)

Potting Plants

Objectives and benefits:

***Cognitive Challenges*:** attention, memory, language, orientation, following patterns, following directions, productivity, mastering a task

***Physical Needs*:** fine motor skills, gross motor skills, hand-eye coordination, perceptual speed and motor function, manipulation of materials, dexterity

***Socio-emotional Needs*:** socialization, community integration, initiative and motivation, emotional gratification, sense of accomplishment, fostering appropriate behaviors, nurturing, * Reminiscing Qualities, Healing Qualities

Supplies: Plastic container, potting soil, seeds or already started plant, newspaper for table coverage, water.

Time: 30–45 minutes.

Staff/older adult ratio: 1:8 or as assessed per needs of individuals or group.

Instructions: Have the supplies ready at the table before residents are seated. Put down newspaper for easy cleanup. Have a bowl of potting soil for every three older adults. Offer packages of seeds or already growing plants. Let them choose their own flowers. Next, have them place dirt in the container and add the seedling or plant. Put one-fourth inch of dirt over the seeds. Let them add a small amount of water to the planter. Be sure the planter has a saucer for watering. Afterward, let them take the plant back to their rooms. Remind them to water their plant everyday. The older adult sometimes struggles with the issues of usefulness and purpose; a plant gives them something to care for, which can be very gratifying for them. A plant is also a nice addition to their room.

Research has shown activities that help cognition of sensory/motor and speed processing will be geared towards help in visual and motor memory, discrimination, comparison, and categorizing areas. Reminiscing activities may help improve memory skills. Long-term studies (Arbuckle and others, 1998) have consistently showed that stimulating the brain with activities helps cognitive function in a similar way exercise helps muscle function. Staying productive has been shown to enhance socio-emotional wellness

Potting Plants
Cognitive Goals, Objectives, and Methods

Skill	Goal	Objectives Sample	Method Sample
Orientation	Show increased awareness of, time/"timeframe," people, circumstances, and past experiences vs. present experiences, to engage in present-time activities, or for a reminiscing intended question	-will respond with correct answer to two choice questions Or yes/no answer, will state where they are, time of day, present company of people on own and with the correct answer	Staff will ask residents a series of questions to stimulate focus to the present setting (Ex: "Where are you? Are you at home or in the nursing home garden?") Or past if reminiscing exercise (Ex: "What kind of flowers did you plant?" (memory and orientation exercise))
Attention	Show increased attention span, task for function, and to engage in meaningful, recreational/fulfilling activities	-will make eye-contact with staff for ____ sec., will verbalize with staff and instructor, will read/listen to rules, will say yes/no to show they understand or do the action	Staff will address or stand in front of resident, make eye contact, ask questions or use others forms to get residents attention What supplies did I say we need?
Memory	Show increased memory skills of recall, recognition, retention of information, working memory	-will repeat/recall how to pot and seed plants, will repeat/recall how to care for plants, will remember lesson at next class	Staff will name the flowers the residents will be planting and ask residents to name flowers they will be planting 5-to-10 minutes later, etc.
Language	Show increased ability to communicate use of words, phrases, ntence structure, comprehension, interpretation	-will be asked a question and answer yes/no, will be asked what is included in maintaining plants and states ingredients (water, etc.), will interact with peers and staff, will interpret instructor's request and follow	Staff will ask questions to stimulate a communication (Ex:: "Which are your favorite flowers? Do you like roses or daffodils?" Interpretation/Lang. skills (Ex: "Can you please pour the water on the plant?")
Cognitive Stimulation (awareness, seeks information in)	Increased stimulus/exposure for visual/ motor memory, cognitive experiences/awareness and brain stimulation to enhance (function, pragmatics, neuroplasticity)	-will learn all they can about plants and growing plants, will interact with peers about plant care, will listen/seek cognitive stimulation, will accept challenge of input information and engage/interact in the potting of plants	Staff will teach residents about plants and plant care
Perceptual Awareness	Show increased abilities of depth perception, visio-spatical awareness, and acuity (for discrimination, comparison, and categorizing), safety	-will pour ingredients into the pot, will discriminate, compare; will maneuver around garden/room, will put plant items away in proper containers associated with proper area	-Staff will offer a planting activity that requires residents to use visual acuity, spatial relationships, etc. by judging pouring abilities, space between seeds, etc. -Staff will encourage resident to consider ways to care for their plant, add mulching foods to the potted plant
Problem-solving (goes beyond thinking/stimulus and initiates thinking process)	Increase problem-solving ability, processing of information, thinking, reasoning, and use of good judgment and decision-making	-will follow planting protocol, will judge amount of water to use	-Staff will engage resident in gardening activity and ask resident to plant seeds in the pot, add water, continue to care for plant -Staff will engage resident in planting procedures and care of the plant
Complete a Task	Increase ability to complete a task	-will add dirt to pot, will add seeds, will water plants as needed, will prune as needed	Staff will support resident's ability to follow procedure of project through instruction, encouragement, adaptive devices/programs if needed, and supply necessary materials and support

TABLE 28.1

Recreational Objectives Observational Form
Potting Plants- Cognitive skills

PATIENT		Dependent (Totally dependent)	High Assistance (25+ ability)	Moderate Assist. (50+ ability)	Mild Assistance (75+ability)	Independent (Totally independent)
SEE CODES BELOW USE OPTIONAL CODES IF APPROPRIATE		1	2	3	4	5
		3 cue/ 2-3 physical	2-3 cues/ 2 physical	2-3 cues/ 1 physical	1-2 cues	Encouragement
97530- Therapeutic activities or	**SKILL**	**GOAL**	**OBJECTIVES** ____times per ____		**METHOD**	**OUTCOME DATE**
97532 Cognitive skills	ORIENTATION					
97532 Cognitive skills	ATTENTION					
97532 Cognitive skills	MEMORY					
97532 Cognitive skills	PROBLEM-SOLVING					
97532 Cognitive skills	COMPLETE A TASK					
97139 Speech Therapy	LANGUAGE					
97533	SENSORY STIMULATION/ COGNITIVE STIMULATION					
97532	PERCEPTUAL AWARENESS					

97532-Development of cognitive skills to improve attention, memory, problem-solving, includes compensatory training and/or sensory integrative activities, direct (one-on-one) patient contact by the provider, each 15 minutes; **97530-Therapeutic activities**, direct (one-on-one) patient contact by the provider (use of dynamic activities to improve functional performance), each 15 minutes; **97533-Sensory integration techniques** to enhance sensory processing and promote adaptive responses to environmental demands, direct (one-on-one) patient contact by the provider, each 15 minutes; **97150-Therapeutic procedure(s)**, group (2 or more individuals); **97139-Unlisted therapeutic procedure** (specify) minutes; **97003- occupational therapy evaluation**; **97004- re-evaluation**	Staff Initial
	Add total score here - Maximum Score 40 pt. each form per activity
	See scale below or use own/facilities optional score system

(Score 1-8)=1 (9-16) =2 (17-24) =3 (25-32) =4 (33-40) =5 If w/device add d if wish, ex: 1d, 2d, or If using 1-7 scale: (41-48) =6 (49-56)

Potting Plants
Physical Goals, Objectives, and Methods

Skill	Goal	Objectives Sample	Method Sample
Fine Motor Skills	Increase fine motor skills, meaningful/fulfilling activities	-will mix, and pour items -will pick up small items and manipulate materials	Staff will encourage residents to pick up and manipulate materials
Gross Motor Skills	Increase large motor skills, meaningful/fulfilling activities	-will lift items using large motor skills, will walk to group (with device or support)	Staff will encourage residents to lift items using gross motor skills
Perceptual Speed and Motor Function	Increase speed and motor ability for function, safety, meaningful/fulfilling activities	-will increase speed of actions by using skills	Staff will encourage residents to do the activity and decrease reaction times by shortening amount of time allotted, or observation of resident ability increasing on own
Hand-Eye Coordination	Increase hand-eye coordination	-will paste items on craft	Staff will encourage residents to place items using hand-eye fine motor abilities, detailed fine motor activities

TABLE 28.2

Recreational Objectives Observational Form
Potting Plants- Physical Skills

PATIENT		Dependent (Totally dependent)	High Assistance (25+ ability)	Moderate Assist. (50+ ability)	Mild Assistance (75+ability)	Independent (Totally independent)
		1	2	3	4	5
SEE CODES BELOW USE OPTIONAL CODES IF APPROPRIATE		3 cue/ 2-3 physical	2-3 cues/ 2 physical	2-3 cues/ 1 physical	1-2 cues	Encouragement
97530- Therapeutic activities or	**SKILL**	**GOAL**	**OBJECTIVES** ____times per ____		**METHOD**	**OUTCOME DATE**
Therapeutic Activity 97530	FINE MOTOR SKILLS					
97530	EYE-HAND COORDINATION					
97110/ 97530	GROSS MOTOR SKILLS					
97530 If under cognitive code 97532	PERCEPTUAL SPEED/MOTOR FUNCTION					

97530 Therapeutic activities, direct (one on one) patient contact by the provider (use of dynamic activities to improve functional performance),each 15 minutes; **97110 Therapeutic procedure, one or more areas**, each 15 minutes; therapeutic exercises to develop strength and endurance, range of motion and flexibility; ; **97150 Therapeutic procedure(s), group (2 or more individuals**; **97535-Self care/home management training** (e.g., activities of daily living and compensatory training, meal preparation, safety procedures, and instructions in use of adaptive equipment), direct (one-on-one) contact by provider, each 15 minutes; **Physical therapy 97001 evaluation, 97002 Re-evaluation. occupational therapy evaluation 97003, re-evaluation. 97004**	Staff Initials
	Add total score here Maximum Score 20 pt. each form per activity
	See scale below or use own/facilities optional score system

(Score 1-4)=1 (5-8) =2 (9-12) =3 (13-16) =4 (17-20) =5 If w/device add d if wish, ex: 1d, 2d, or If using 1-7 scale: (21-24) =6 (25-28) =7

Potting Plants
Socio-emotional Goals, Objectives, and Methods

Skill	Goal	Objectives Sample	Method Sample
Socialization/Community Integration	Increase social interactions, meaningful/fulfilling activities	-will interact with peers, will engage in community integration experiences (for community adaptation and social skills), will use manners, share, practice social skills	Staff will offer gardening classes to support/encourage residents to socialize through community integration and being w/groups
Team Playing/Sharing	Increase teamwork/sharing, meaningful/fulfilling activities	-will join in on a planting activity with others and share, wait turn, support peers _____ time(s) this week.	Residents will be encouraged to plant, share seeds, water, work on a flower garden, make plants for the unit, as a team
Initiative and Motivation	Increase initiative and motivation/wellness, and quality of life	-will choose if wishes to plant, will plant on own (or with needed assistance), will continue to plant plants and put in room, etc.	-Staff will support and encourage the resident to prepare for planting/gardening activities in a timely fashion for their own personal gains of attending activity -Staff will offer new techniques/season flowers to motivate
Emotional Gratification	Increase emotional gratification/wellness, and quality of life	-will state that planting/gardening is a gratifying experience or will show pleasure by smiling, laughing, deep focus on planning activities	Staff will ask residents if they enjoyed the gardening/planting activity and what they liked through the use of verbal discussion, group discussions
Sense of Accomplishment	Increase feelings of self-worth, pride, productivity, dignity/wellness, and quality of life	-will use gestures to express pride in self, will talk about their accomplishments planting and types of flowers and plants	Staff will offer gardening/planting as a way to support resident's desire to garden, create, etc.
Self-esteem/ self-identity	Increase self-esteem, feelings of belonging, dignity, self-worth, integrity, self-identity/wellness, and quality of life	-will state/communicate positive feelings about self, will join in on gardening to take an active role in maintaining health through exercising, will join in gardening based on own choices	-Staff will educate residents on the value of gardening/planting for brain muscle/stimulant benefits, healing qualities -Staff will encourage residents to join classes/share garden plants for unit, nursing home setting
Sensory Integration/Tolerating Stimulation	Increase sensory processing and enhance awareness of sensations and toleration/adaptation of sensory stimulations and demands	-will adjust to the smells, lights, sounds, and etc. while gardening/planting _____ time this week.	-Staff will offer gardening /planting classes and residents will be exposed to sensory stimulating experiences of touching dirt, water, seeds, smells, sights -Residents will be supported as they adjust to the stimulus one step at a time
Fostering Appropriate Behaviors	Increase social interaction, social opportunities and adjustment, safety, using appropriate behaviors during an activity for a calm environment/wellness, and quality of life	-will join in on planting/gardening class, will share seeds, water pitcher, dirt etc.; will listen and follow instructions, use appropriate behavior for the setting, will wait turn, stand in line quietly, will quiet down when asked	Before class begins, staff will discuss the rules, appropriate behaviors, respect of property, safety, and respect of fellow gardeners, peers

TABLE 28.3
RECREATIONAL OBJECTIVES OBSERVATIONAL FORM
POTTING PLANTS- SOCIO-EMOTIONAL SKILLS

PATIENT	Dependent (Totally dependent)	High Assistance (25+ ability)	Moderate Assist. (50+ ability)	Mild Assistance (75+ability)	Independent (Totally independent.)
SEE CODES BELOW USE OPTIONAL CODES IF APPROPRIATE	1	2	3	4	5
	3 cue/ 2-3 physical	2-3 cues/ 2 physical	2-3 cues/ 1 physical	1-2 cues	Encouragement

97530- Therapeutic activities or	SKILL	GOAL	OBJECTIVES ____times per ____	METHOD	OUTCOME DATE			
97537 Or 97535	SOCIALIZATION/ COMMUNITY INTEGRATION							
97537 Or 97535	TEAM PLAYING /SHARING							
97537 Or 97535	INITIATIVE AND MOTIVATION							
97537 Or 97535	EMOTIONAL GRATIFICATION							
97537 Or 97535	SENSE OF ACCOMPLISHMENT							
97537 Or 97535	SELF-ESTEEM/ SELF-IDENTITY							
97537 Or 97535	FOSTERING APPROPRIATE BEHAVIORS							
97533	SENSORY INTEGRATION/ TOLERATING							

97537-Community/work reintegration training (e.g., shopping, transportation, money management, avocational activities and/or work environment/modification analysis, work task analysis), direct (one-on-one) contact by provider, each 15 minutes; **97535-Self care/home management training** (e.g., activities of daily living and compensatory training, meal preparation, safety procedures, and instructions in use of adaptive equipment), direct (one-on-one) contact by provider, each 15 minutes; **97530-Therapeutic activities, direct (one-on-one)** patient contact by the provider (use of dynamic activities to improve functional performance), each 15 minutes; **97150-Therapeutic procedure(s), group (2 or more individuals); 97533-Sensory integration techniques** to enhance sensory processing and promote adaptive responses to environmental demands, direct (one-on-one) patient contact by the provider, each 15 minutes; **occupational therapy evaluation 97003, re-evaluation . 97004**	Staff Initial				
	Add total score here-Maximum Score 40 pt. each form per activity				
	See scale below or use own/facilities optional score system				

(Score 1-8)=1 (9-16) =2 (17-24) =3 (25-32) =4 (33-40) =5 If w/device add d if wish, ex: 1d, 2d, or If using 1-7 scale: (41-48) =6 (49-56)

Safety Pin Art

Objectives and benefits:

Cognitive Challenges: attention, memory, language, orientation, following patterns, following directions, productivity, mastering a task

Physical Needs: fine motor skills, gross motor skills, hand-eye coordination, perceptual speed and motor function, manipulation of materials, dexterity

Socio-emotional Needs: socialization, community integration, initiative and motivation, emotional gratification, sense of accomplishment, fostering appropriate behaviors, nurturing, * Reminiscing Qualities, Healing Qualities

Supplies: Safety pins, seed beads, picture or pattern of object

Time: 60 minutes.

Staff/older adult ratio: 1:2 this activity may be done alone w/ resident or with a group.

Instructions: Have residents choose a design or have one design based on a theme. Take beads and arrange them in order of design. Put beads onto small safety pin. Close safety pin and, using pliers, squeeze top of pin closed. Continue this with each small safety pin until you have all the beadwork done in the order of the design pattern. Taking a larger pin, pry between the loops in the center of the large pin. Add the smaller safety pins onto the large pin. Continue to pull smaller pin completely around the loop of the larger pin until pin is on other side of the loop. After you have all your pins on the other side of the loop, you can take pliers and shut the loop. Your beaded jewelry is ready to be pinned on to shirt or any other way you would like to wear it. These also make nice gifts.

Research has shown activities that help cognition of sensory/motor and speed processing will be geared towards help in visual and motor memory, discrimination, comparison, and categorizing areas. Reminiscing activities may help improve memory skills. Long-term studies (Arbuckle and others, 1998) have consistently showed that stimulating the brain with activities helps cognitive function in a similar way exercise helps muscle function. Staying productive has been shown to enhance socio-emotional wellness

Safety Pin Art
Cognitive Goals, Objectives, and Methods

Skill	Goal	Objectives Sample	Method Sample
Orientation	Show increased awareness of, time/"timeframe," people, circumstances, and past experiences vs. present experiences, to engage in present-time activities, or for a reminiscing intended question	-will respond with correct answer to two choice questions Or yes/no answer, will state where they are, time of day, present company of people on own and with the correct answer	Staff will ask residents a series of questions to stimulate focus to the present setting (Ex: "What talents are you going to share? Have you made safety pin art before? What did you make? Did you make it recently or a long time ago"?)
Attention	Show increased attention span, task for function, and to engage in meaningful, recreational/fulfilling activities	-will make eye-contact with staff for _____ sec., will verbalize with staff and instructor, will read/listen to rules, say yes/no to show understand or do the action	Staff will address or stand in front of resident, make eye-contact, ask questions, or use others forms to get resident's attention
Memory	Show increased memory skills of recall, recognition, retention of information, working memory	-will repeat/recall how to make project, will remember lesson at next class	Staff will show step, actions on how to make bookmarks and residents will repeat the action using short term memory/recall, working memory
Language	Show increased ability to communicate use of words, phrases, sentence structure, comprehension, interpretation	-will be asked a question and answer yes/no, will be asked what is included in project states ingredients, methods, items; will interact with peers and staff; will interpret instructor's request and follow	Staff will ask questions to stimulate a communication (Ex: "What materials are you using to make your safety art pins?") Interpretation/Lang. skills (Ex: "You need to string that bead on the pin. Can you do it?") and then note resident's actions to show they understood
Cognitive Stimulation (awareness, seeks information in)	Increased stimulus/exposure for visual/ motor memory, cognitive experiences/awareness and brain stimulation to enhance (function, pragmatics, neuro-plasticity)	-will look around the room, will listen/seek cognitive stimulation, will accept challenge of input information and engage/interact in, will engage in a safety pin art activity	Staff will set up crafts and put out a wide variety of arts and craft materials to encourage creativity, discrimination, comparison, categorizing, etc.
Perceptual Awareness	Show increased abilities of depth perception, visio-spatical awareness, and acuity (for discrimination, comparison, and categorizing), safety	-will use ingredients /items, will discriminate, compare; will maneuver around work area, pins onto safety pin, will put items away in proper containers associated with proper area (Ex: place beads into containers)	Staff will engage residents in an activity that requires use of acuity, discrimination, comparison, and categorizing for visio-spatical awareness (Ex: placing items on the safety pin using visual acuity, etc.)
Problem-solving (goes beyond thinking/stimulus and initiates thinking process)	Increase problem-solving ability, processing of information, thinking, reasoning, and use of good judgment and decision-making	-will think up a story, use creativity, and/or comprehend and process the information; will judge appropriate materials	-Staff will engage residents in a creative project and decision-making regarding whom to send the safety pin art to. -Staff will show the resident the step-by-step actions to make safety pin art to stimulate working memory
Complete a Task	Increase ability to complete a task	-will recall/retain and sort/gather information, problem-solve, and complete activity	Staff will support resident's ability to follow the project through instruction, encourage, and supply adaptive devices/programs if needed, and necessary materials and support

TABLE 29.1

Recreational Objectives Observational Form
Safety Pin Art- Cognitive skills

PATIENT	Dependent (Totally dependent)	High Assistance (25+ ability)	Moderate Assist. (50+ ability)	Mild Assistance (75+ability)	Independent (Totally independent)
SEE CODES BELOW USE OPTIONAL CODES IF APPROPRIATE	1	2	3	4	5
	3 cue/ 2-3 physical	2-3 cues/ 2 physical	2-3 cues/ 1 physical	1-2 cues	Encouragement

97530-Therapeutic activities or	SKILL	GOAL	OBJECTIVES ____times per ____	METHOD	OUTCOME DATE			
97532 Cognitive skills	ORIENTATION							
97532 Cognitive skills	ATTENTION							
97532 Cognitive skills	MEMORY							
97532 Cognitive skills	PROBLEM-SOLVING							
97532 Cognitive skills	COMPLETE A TASK							
97139 Speech Therapy 97532 Cognitive skills	LANGUAGE							
97533	SENSORY STIMULATION/ COGNITIVE STIMULATION							
97532	PERCEPTUAL AWARENESS							

97532-Development of cognitive skills to improve attention, memory, problem-solving, includes compensatory training and/or sensory integrative activities, direct (one-on-one) patient contact by the provider, each 15 minutes; **97530-Therapeutic activities**, direct (one-on-one) patient contact by the provider (use of dynamic activities to improve functional performance), each 15 minutes; **97533-Sensory integration techniques** to enhance sensory processing and promote adaptive responses to environmental demands, direct (one-on-one) patient contact by the provider, each 15 minutes; **97150-Therapeutic procedure(s)**, group (2 or more individuals); **97139-Unlisted therapeutic procedure** (specify) minutes; **97003- occupational therapy evaluation**; **97004- re-evaluation**	Staff Initial				
	Add total score here -Maximum Score 40 pt. each form per activity				
	See scale below or use own/facilities optional score system				

(Score 1-8)=1 (9-16) =2 (17-24) =3 (25-32) =4 (33-40) =5 If w/device add d if wish, ex: 1d, 2d, or If using 1-7 scale: (41-48) =6 (49-56)

Safety Pin Art
Physical Goals, Objectives, and Methods

Skill	Goal	Objectives Sample	Method Sample
Fine Motor Skills	Increase fine motor skills, meaningful/fulfilling activities	-will glue, paste, mix and pour items, will pick up small items, manipulate materials	Staff will encourage residents to pick up and manipulate materials
Gross Motor Skills	Increase large motor skills, meaningful/fulfilling activities	-will lift items using large motor skills, walk to group (with device or support)	Staff will encourage residents to lift items using gross motor skills
Perceptual Speed and Motor Function	Increase speed and motor ability for function, safety, meaningful/fulfilling activities	-will increase speed of actions by using skills	Staff will encourage residents to do the activity and decrease reaction times by shortening amount of time allotted, or observation of resident ability increasing on own
Hand-Eye Coordination	Increase hand-eye coordination	-will paste items on craft	Staff will encourage residents to place items., using hand-eye fine motor abilities, detailed fine motor activities

TABLE 29.2

Recreational Objectives Observational Form

Safety Pin art - Physical Skills

PATIENT	Dependent (Totally dependent)	High Assistance (25+ ability)	Moderate Assist. (50+ ability)	Mild Assistance (75+ability)	Independent (Totally independent)
	1	2	3	4	5
SEE CODES BELOW USE OPTIONAL CODES IF APPROPRIATE	3 cue/ 2-3 physical	2-3 cues/ 2 physical	2-3 cues/ 1 physical	1-2 cues	Encouragement

97530- Therapeutic activities or	**SKILL**	**GOAL**	**OBJECTIVES** ____times per ____	**METHOD**	**OUTCOME DATE**			
Therapeutic Activity 97530	FINE MOTOR SKILLS							
97530	EYE-HAND COORDINATION							
97110/ 97530	GROSS MOTOR SKILLS							
97530 If under cognitive code 97532	PERCEPTUAL SPEED/MOTOR FUNCTION							

97530 Therapeutic activities, direct (one on one) patient contact by the provider (use of dynamic activities to improve functional performance),each 15 minutes**; 97110 Therapeutic procedure, one or more areas**, each 15 minutes; therapeutic exercises to develop strength and endurance, range of motion and flexibility; ; **97150 Therapeutic procedure(s), group (2 or more individuals**; **97535-Self care/home management training** (e.g., activities of daily living and compensatory training, meal preparation, safety procedures, and instructions in use of adaptive equipment), direct (one-on-one) contact by provider, each 15 minutes; **Physical therapy 97001 evaluation, 97002 Re-evaluation. occupational therapy evaluation 97003, re-evaluation. 97004**

Staff Initials				
Add total score here Maximum Score 20 pt. each form per activity				
See scale below or use own/facilities optional score system				

(Score 1-4)=1 (5-8) =2 (9-12) =3 (13-16) =4 (17-20) =5 If w/device add d if wish, ex: 1d, 2d, or If using 1-7 scale: (21-24) =6 (25-28) =7

Safety Pin Art
Socio-emotional Goals, Objectives, and Methods

Skill	Goal	Objectives Sample	Method Sample
Socialization/Community Integration	Increase social interactions, meaningful/fulfilling activities	-will interact with peers, will engage in community integration experiences (for community adaptation and social skills), will use manners, share, practice social skills	Staff will offer activities that support/encourage residents to socialize through community integration and being w/groups
Team Playing/Sharing	Increase teamwork/sharing, meaningful/fulfilling activities	-will, join in on a craft/activity with others and share, wait turn, support peers _____ time(s) this week.	Staff will encourage residents to create items, share, work as a team, support/use patience, show compassion to other residents
Initiative and Motivation	Increase initiative and motivation/wellness, and quality of life	-will choose if wishes to do craft, will try new crafts, will increase amount of crafts done _____ time(s) a week	Staff will support/encourage the resident to prepare for craft activities in a timely fashion for their own personal gains of attending activity -Staff will offer new techniques and creative materials to motivate residents to make a creative craft
Emotional Gratification	Increase emotional gratification/wellness, and quality of life	-will state that making crafts is a gratifying experience, or will show pleasure by smiling ,laughing, deep focus on activities	Staff will ask residents if they enjoyed the activity and what they liked through verbal discussion, group discussions
Sense of Accomplishment	Increase feelings of self-worth, pride, productivity, dignity/wellness, and quality of life	-will use gestures to express pride in self, will show crafts to others	Staff will offer activities as a way to support resident's desire to use creativity, imagination, and produce items
Self-esteem/self-identity	Increase self-esteem, feelings of belonging, dignity, self-worth, integrity, self-identity/wellness, and quality of life	-will state/communicate positive feelings about self, will join craft class to take an active role in maintaining health though arts/crafts, volunteer work; will join the craft class based on own choices	Staff will educate residents on the value of doing crafts/learning talents for brain muscle/stimulant benefits, healing qualities; and encourage residents to join classes/ share crafts
Sensory Integration/Tolerating Stimulation	Increase sensory processing and enhance awareness of sensations and toleration/adaptation of sensory stimulations and demands	-will adjust to the smells, lights, sounds, etc. in environment	-Staff will offer activities and residents will be exposed to sensory stimulating experiences of tactile stimulation, sights, hearing, communication, and possibly smell sensory stimulations -Staff will support residents as they adjust to the stimulus
Fostering Appropriate Behaviors	Increase social interaction, social opportunities and adjustment, safety, using appropriate behaviors during an activity for a calm environment/wellness, and quality of life	-will join in on class, share items/tools, listen, and follow instructions; will use appropriate behavior for the setting, will wait turn, stand in line quietly; will quiet down when asked	Before class begins, staff will discuss the rules, appropriate behaviors, respect of property, safety, and respect of fellow peers/staff

TABLE 29.3

Recreational Objectives Observational Form
Safety Pin Art- Socio-emotional Skills

PATIENT	Dependent (Totally dependent)	High Assistance (25+ ability)	Moderate Assist. (50+ ability)	Mild Assistance (75+ability)	Independent (Totally independent.)
SEE CODES BELOW USE OPTIONAL CODES IF APPROPRIATE	1	2	3	4	5
	3 cue/ 2-3 physical	2-3 cues/ 2 physical	2-3 cues/ 1 physical	1-2 cues	Encouragement

97530- Therapeutic activities or	**SKILL**	**GOAL**	**OBJECTIVES** ____times per ____	**METHOD**	**OUTCOME DATE**			
97537 Or 97535	SOCIALIZATION/ COMMUNITY INTEGRATION							
97537 Or 97535	TEAM PLAYING /SHARING							
97537 Or 97535	INITIATIVE AND MOTIVATION							
97537 Or 97535	EMOTIONAL GRATIFICATION							
97537 Or 97535	SENSE OF ACCOMPLISHMENT							
97537 Or 97535	SELF-ESTEEM/ SELF-IDENTITY							
97537 Or 97535	FOSTERING APPROPRIATE BEHAVIORS							
97533	SENSORY INTEGRATION/ TOLERATING							

97537-Community/work reintegration training (e.g., shopping, transportation, money management, avocational activities and/or work environment/modification analysis, work task analysis), direct (one-on-one) contact by provider, each 15 minutes; **97535-Self care/home management training** (e.g., activities of daily living and compensatory training, meal preparation, safety procedures, and instructions in use of adaptive equipment), direct (one-on-one) contact by provider, each 15 minutes; **97530-Therapeutic activities, direct (one-on-one)** patient contact by the provider (use of dynamic activities to improve functional performance), each 15 minutes; **97150-Therapeutic procedure(s), group (2 or more individuals); 97533-Sensory integration techniques** to enhance sensory processing and promote adaptive responses to environmental demands, direct (one-on-one) patient contact by the provider, each 15 minutes; **occupational therapy evaluation 97003, re-evaluation . 97004**	Staff Initial				
	Add total score here-Maximum Score 40 pt. each form per activity				
	See scale below or use own/facilities optional score system				

(Score 1-8)=1 (9-16) =2 (17-24) =3 (25-32) =4 (33-40) =5 If w/device add d if wish, ex: 1d, 2d, or If using 1-7 scale: (41-48) =6 (49-56)

Storytelling/Collage

Objectives and benefits:

Cognitive Challenges: attention, memory, language, orientation, following patterns, following directions, productivity, mastering a task

Physical Needs: fine motor skills, gross motor skills, hand-eye coordination, perceptual speed and motor function, manipulation of materials, dexterity

Socio-emotional Needs: socialization, community integration, initiative and motivation, emotional gratification, sense of accomplishment, fostering appropriate behaviors, nurturing, * Reminiscing Qualities, Healing Qualities

Supplies: Poster board, markers, magazines, glue, scissors.

Time: 30 minutes.

Staff/older adult ratio: 1:8 or as assessed per needs of individuals or group.

Instructions: Have magazine pages cut out and spread around tables in boxes. Tell the residents to find magazine pictures that represent them, whether it be what they like to do, what music they like, movie stars they like, or other interests they have. You can also include items that they might want to add, such as art supplies to make a favorite thing for the poster. Then let them take turns sharing their posters. They can tell a story about themselves or just share the poster.

Research has shown activities that help cognition of sensory/motor and speed processing will be geared towards help in visual and motor memory, discrimination, comparison, and categorizing areas. Reminiscing activities may help improve memory skills. Long-term studies (Arbuckle and others, 1998) have consistently showed that stimulating the brain with activities helps cognitive function in a similar way exercise helps muscle function. Staying productive has been shown to enhance socio-emotional wellness

Storytelling/College
Goals, Objectives, and Methods

Skill	Goal	Objectives Sample	Method Sample
Orientation	Show increased awareness of, time/"timeframe," people, circumstances, and past experiences vs. present experiences, to engage in present-time activities, or for a reminiscing intended question	-will respond with correct answer to two choice questions (Ex: shares sequence of stories in correct year), will state where they are, time of day, present company of people on own and with the correct answer	The resident will be asked a series of questions to stimulate focus to the present setting (Ex: "What talents are you going to share? Have you had this talent a long time?")
Attention	Show increased attention span, task for function, and to engage in meaningful, recreational/fulfilling activities	-will make eye-contact with staff for _____ sec., will verbalize with staff and instructor, will share stories, will say yes/no to show they understand or do the action	Staff will address or stand in front of resident, make eye-contact, ask questions or use others forms to get resident's attention (Ex: "What kind of story are you going to share?")
Memory	Show increased memory skills of recall, recognition, retention of information, working memory	-will repeat/recall how to make project, will remember lesson at next class	Staff will ask residents to think of a funny story, a poem they love, a story they know, or other form of storytelling Or staff will have a resident/visitor share storytelling.
Language	Show increased ability to communicate use of words, phrases, sentence structure, comprehension, interpretation	-will be asked a question and answer yes/no, will be asked what is included in project, will state ingredients, methods, items; will interact with peers and staff, will interpret instructor's request and follow	Staff will ask questions to stimulate a communication (Ex: "What did you learn from this story? What did it make you think of?") Interpretation/Lang. skills
Cognitive Stimulation (awareness, seeks information in)	Increased stimulus/exposure for visual/ motor memory, cognitive experiences/awareness and brain stimulation to enhance (function, pragmatics, neuroplasticity)	-will listen/seek cognitive stimulation, will accept challenge of input information and engage/interact, will engage in a storytelling event by listening or sharing	Residents will be asked to bring materials to the activity
Perceptual Awareness	Show increased abilities of depth perception, visio-spatical awareness, and acuity (for discrimination, comparison, and categorizing), safety	-will use ingredients/items will discriminate, compare; will maneuver around work area, will put items away in proper containers associated with proper area (glue with glues, the magazines back on the rack)	Staff will have residents pick up items, work with items, put items away, maneuver around items
Problem-solving (goes beyond thinking/stimulus and initiates thinking process)	Increase problem-solving ability, processing of information, thinking, reasoning, and use of good judgment and decision-making	-will follow think up a story, use creativity or comprehend and process the information, will judge appropriate materials	-Staff will encourage residents to share their talents with their peers -Staff will show the resident the step-by-step actions to complete the task and support making decisions
Complete a Task	Increase ability to complete a task	-will recall retain , sort/gather information , problem solve, and complete activity	Staff will support residents ability to follow do the project through instruction, encouragement, adaptive devices/programs if needed, and supply necessary materials and support

Table 30.1

Recreational Objectives Observational Form
Storytelling/Collage- Cognitive skills

PATIENT	Dependent (Totally dependent)	High Assistance (25+ ability)	Moderate Assist. (50+ ability)	Mild Assistance (75+ability)	Independent (Totally independent)
SEE CODES BELOW USE OPTIONAL CODES IF APPROPRIATE	1	2	3	4	5
	3 cue/ 2-3 physical	2-3 cues/ 2 physical	2-3 cues/ 1 physical	1-2 cues	Encouragement

97530-Therapeutic activities or	SKILL	GOAL	OBJECTIVES ____times per ____	METHOD	OUTCOME DATE			
97532 Cognitive skills	ORIENTATION							
97532 Cognitive skills	ATTENTION							
97532 Cognitive skills	MEMORY							
97532 Cognitive skills	PROBLEM-SOLVING							
97532 Cognitive skills	COMPLETE A TASK							
97139 Speech Therapy 97532 Cognitive skills	LANGUAGE							
97533	SENSORY STIMULATION/ COGNITIVE STIMULATION							
97532	PERCEPTUAL AWARENESS							

97532-Development of cognitive skills to improve attention, memory, problem-solving, includes compensatory training and/or sensory integrative activities, direct (one-on-one) patient contact by the provider, each 15 minutes; **97530-Therapeutic activities**, direct (one-on-one) patient contact by the provider (use of dynamic activities to improve functional performance), each 15 minutes**; 97533-Sensory integration techniques** to enhance sensory processing and promote adaptive responses to environmental demands, direct (one-on-one) patient contact by the provider, each 15 minutes; **97150-Therapeutic procedure(s)**, group (2 or more individuals); **97139-Unlisted therapeutic procedure** (specify) minutes; **97003- occupational therapy evaluation**; **97004- re-evaluation**	Staff Initial				
	Add total score here -Maximum Score 40 pt. each form per activity				
	See scale below or use own/facilities optional score system				

(Score 1-8)=1 (9-16) =2 (17-24) =3 (25-32) =4 (33-40) =5 If w/device add d if wish, ex: 1d, 2d, or If using 1-7 scale: (41-48) =6 (49-56)

Storytelling/Collage
Physical Goals, Objectives, and Methods

Skill	Goal	Objectives Sample	Method Sample
Fine Motor Skills	Increase fine motor skills, meaningful/fulfilling activities	-will glue, paste, mix and pour items; will pick up small items and manipulate materials	Staff will encourage residents to pick up and manipulate materials
Gross Motor Skills	Increase large motor skills, meaningful/fulfilling activities	-will lift items using large motor skills, will walk to group (with device or support)	Staff will encourage residents to lift items using gross motor skills
Perceptual Speed and Motor Function	Increase speed and motor ability for function, safety, meaningful/fulfilling activities	-will increase speed of actions by using skills	Staff will encourage residents to do the activity and decrease reaction times by shortening amount of time allotted, or observation of resident ability increasing on own
Hand-Eye Coordination	Increase hand-eye coordination	-will paste items on craft	Staff will encourage residents to place items using hand-eye fine motor abilities, detailed fine motor activities

TABLE 30.2

Recreational Objectives Observational Form
Storytelling/Collage- Physical Skills

PATIENT		Dependent (Totally dependent)	High Assistance (25+ ability)	Moderate Assist. (50+ ability)	Mild Assistance (75+ability)	Independent (Totally independent)
		1	2	3	4	5
SEE CODES BELOW USE OPTIONAL CODES IF APPROPRIATE		3 cue/ 2-3 physical	2-3 cues/ 2 physical	2-3 cues/ 1 physical	1-2 cues	Encouragement
97530- Therapeutic activities or	**SKILL**	**GOAL**	**OBJECTIVES** ____times per ____		**METHOD**	**OUTCOME DATE**
Therapeutic Activity 97530	FINE MOTOR SKILLS					
97530	EYE-HAND COORDINATION					
97110/ 97530	GROSS MOTOR SKILLS					
97530 If under cognitive code 97532	PERCEPTUAL SPEED/MOTOR FUNCTION					

97530 Therapeutic activities, direct (one on one) patient contact by the provider (use of dynamic activities to improve functional performance),each 15 minutes; **97110 Therapeutic procedure, one or more areas**, each 15 minutes; therapeutic exercises to develop strength and endurance, range of motion and flexibility; ; **97150 Therapeutic procedure(s), group (2 or more individuals**; **97535-Self care/home management training** (e.g., activities of daily living and compensatory training, meal preparation, safety procedures, and instructions in use of adaptive equipment), direct (one-on-one) contact by provider, each 15 minutes; **Physical therapy 97001 evaluation, 97002 Re-evaluation. occupational therapy evaluation 97003, re-evaluation. 97004**	Staff Initials
	Add total score here Maximum Score 20 pt. each form per activity
	See scale below or use own/facilities optional score system

(Score 1-4)=1 (5-8) =2 (9-12) =3 (13-16) =4 (17-20) =5 If w/device add d if wish, ex: 1d, 2d, or If using 1-7 scale: (21-24) =6 (25-28) =7

Storytelling/Collage
Socio-emotional Goals, Objectives, and Methods

Skill	Goal	Objectives Sample	Method Sample
Socialization/Community Integration	Increase social interactions, meaningful/fulfilling activities	-will interact with peers, will engage in community integration experiences (for community adaptation and social skills), will use manners, share, practice social skills	Staff will offer activities to support/encourage residents to socialize through community integration and being w/groups
Team Playing/Sharing	Increase teamwork/sharing, meaningful/fulfilling activities	-will join in on a craft/ activity with others and share, wait turn, support peers ______ time(s) this week.	Staff will encourage residents to create items, share, work as a team, support/use patience, show compassion to other residents
Initiative and Motivation	Increase initiative and motivation/wellness, and quality of life	-will choose if wishes to do craft, will try new crafts, will increase amount of crafts completed	-Staff will support/encourage the resident to prepare for planting/gardening activities in a timely fashion for their own personal gains of attending activity -Staff will offer new techniques/season flowers to motivate
Emotional Gratification	Increase emotional gratification/wellness, and quality of life	-will state that making crafts is a gratifying experience by sharing a story or show pleasure by smiling, laughing, deep focus on activities and storytelling	Staff will ask residents if they enjoyed the activity and what they liked through the use of verbal discussion, group discussions
Sense of Accomplishment	Increase feelings of self-worth, pride, productivity, dignity/wellness, and quality of life	-will use gestures to express pride in self, will show craft to others	Staff will offer activities as a way to support resident's desire to use creativity, imagination, etc.
Self-esteem/self-identity	Increase self-esteem, feelings of belonging, dignity, self-worth, integrity, self-identity/wellness, and quality of life	-will state/communicate positive feelings about self, will join a storytelling event/making collages, will take an active role in maintaining health and intelligence through creative stories, will join the class based on own choices	Staff will educate residents on the value of doing crafts/ learning talents for brain muscle/stimulant benefits, healing qualities, and will encourage residents to join classes/share storytelling talents
Sensory Integration/Tolerating Stimulation	Increase sensory processing and enhance awareness of sensations and toleration/adaptation of sensory stimulations and demands	-will adjust to the smells, lights, sounds, etc. in environment	-Staff will offer activities and residents will be exposed to sensory stimulating experiences of tactile stimulation, sights, hearing, communication, and possibly smell sensory stimulations- --Staff will be support residents as they adjust to the stimulus
Fostering Appropriate Behaviors	Increase social interaction, social opportunities and adjustment, safety, using appropriate behaviors during an activity for a calm environment/wellness, and quality of life	-will join in on class, share stories/ items/tools, listen and follow instructions, use appropriate behavior for the setting; will wait turn, stand in line quietly; will quiet down when asked	Before class begins, staff will discuss the rules, appropriate behaviors, respect of property, safety, and respect of fellow peers/staff

TABLE 30.3

Recreational Objectives Observational Form
Storytelling/ Collage- Socio-emotional Skills

PATIENT	Dependent (Totally dependent)	High Assistance (25+ ability)	Moderate Assist. (50+ ability)	Mild Assistance (75+ability)	Independent (Totally independent.)
SEE CODES BELOW USE OPTIONAL CODES IF APPROPRIATE	1	2	3	4	5
	3 cue/ 2-3 physical	2-3 cues/ 2 physical	2-3 cues/ 1 physical	1-2 cues	Encouragement

97530-Therapeutic activities or	SKILL	GOAL	OBJECTIVES ____times per ____	METHOD	OUTCOME DATE			
97537 Or 97535	SOCIALIZATION/ COMMUNITY INTEGRATION							
97537 Or 97535	TEAM PLAYING /SHARING							
97537 Or 97535	INITIATIVE AND MOTIVATION							
97537 Or 97535	EMOTIONAL GRATIFICATION							
97537 Or 97535	SENSE OF ACCOMPLISHMENT							
97537 Or 97535	SELF-ESTEEM/ SELF-IDENTITY							
97537 Or 97535	FOSTERING APPROPRIATE BEHAVIORS							
97533	SENSORY INTEGRATION/ TOLERATING							

97537-Community/work reintegration training (e.g., shopping, transportation, money management, avocational activities and/or work environment/modification analysis, work task analysis), direct (one-on-one) contact by provider, each 15 minutes; **97535-Self care/home management training** (e.g., activities of daily living and compensatory training, meal preparation, safety procedures, and instructions in use of adaptive equipment), direct (one-on-one) contact by provider, each 15 minutes; **97530-Therapeutic activities, direct (one-on-one)** patient contact by the provider (use of dynamic activities to improve functional performance), each 15 minutes; **97150-Therapeutic procedure(s), group (2 or more individuals); 97533-Sensory integration techniques** to enhance sensory processing and promote adaptive responses to environmental demands, direct (one-on-one) patient contact by the provider, each 15 minutes; **occupational therapy evaluation 97003, re-evaluation . 97004**	Staff Initial				
	Add total score here-Maximum Score 40 pt. each form per activity				
	See scale below or use own/facilities optional score system				

(Score 1-8)=1 (9-16) =2 (17-24) =3 (25-32) =4 (33-40) =5 If w/device add d if wish, ex: 1d, 2d, or If using 1-7 scale: (41-48) =6 (49-56)

Sun Catchers

Objectives and benefits:

Cognitive Challenges: attention, memory, language, orientation, following patterns, following directions, productivity, mastering a task

Physical Needs: fine motor skills, gross motor skills, hand-eye coordination, perceptual speed and motor function, manipulation of materials, dexterity

Socio-emotional Needs: socialization, community integration, initiative and motivation, emotional gratification, sense of accomplishment, fostering appropriate behaviors, nurturing, * Reminiscing Qualities, Healing Qualities

Supplies: A variety of colored transparent plastic wrapping paper, glue (hot glue gun or white glue), fabric paints or markers, tin foil, newspaper, hole punch, glitter.

Time: 30–45 minutes.

Staff/older adult ratio: 1:2 or as assessed per needs of individuals or group.

Instructions: Place newspaper at each setting for easy clean up. Have different colored transparent paper set up on the table. Have a model of a window sun catcher. This can be a good visual aid for the older adults to follow. Make a front piece of frame from tin foil. You can make one in the shape of a heart or a square, etc. Then choose a color of transparent paper and place behind the frame. Add hot glue to back of frame and glue the transparent colored paper to the frame. Then make a back frame in the same shape as the front frame. Add hot glue to the back frame. Attach back frame, being sure that the colored transparent paper is between both frames now. Be sure to have a wide enough area of transparent paper because this is where the sun will come through your finished picture. Decorate the inside of transparent paper as well as around the frame. Decorate with fabric makers or permanent marker. You can add a light amount of glitter if you like. Once it is all done and dry, punch a hole at the top of the frame. Put a piece of yarn through it and hang it by a window.

Research has shown activities that help cognition of sensory/motor and speed processing will be geared towards help in visual and motor memory, discrimination, comparison, and categorizing areas. Reminiscing activities may help improve memory skills. Long-term studies (Arbuckle and others, 1998) have consistently showed that stimulating the brain with activities helps cognitive function in a similar way exercise helps muscle function. Staying productive has been shown to enhance socio-emotional wellness

Sun Catcher
Cognitive Goals, Objectives, and Methods

Skill	Goal	Objectives Sample	Method Sample
Orientation	Show increased awareness of, time/"timeframe," people, circumstances, and past experiences vs. present experiences, to engage in present-time activities, or for a reminiscing intended question	-will respond with correct answer to two choice questions Or yes/no answer; will state where they are, time of day, present company of people on own and with the correct answer	Staff will ask residents a series of questions to stimulate focus to the present setting (Ex: "What talents are you going to share? Have you made sun catchers before? Do we get a lot of sun where we live or is this a rainy area?")
Attention	Show increased attention span, task for function, and to engage in meaningful, recreational/fulfilling activities	-will make eye-contact with staff for _____ sec., will verbalize with staff and instructor, will read and listen to rules, will say yes/no to show they understand or do the action	Staff will address or stand in front of resident, make eye-contact, ask questions, or use others forms of communication to get resident's attention
Memory	Show increased memory skills of recall, recognition, retention of information, working memory	-will repeat/recall how to make project, will remember lesson at next class	Staff will show step, actions on how to make sun catchers, and residents will repeat the action using short-term memory/recall, working memory
Language	Show increased ability to communicate use of words, phrases, sentence structure, comprehension, interpretation	-will be asked a question and answer yes/no, will be asked what is included in project, will state ingredients, methods, items; will interact with peers and staff, will interpret instructor's request and follow	Staff will ask questions to stimulate a communication (Ex: "What materials are you using to make your sun catchers?") Interpretation/Lang. skills (Ex: "You need to add tacky glue to make it stick well.") and then note resident's actions to show if they have understood.
Cognitive Stimulation (awareness, seeks information in)	Increased stimulus/exposure for visual/ motor memory, cognitive experiences/awareness and brain stimulation to enhance (function, pragmatics, neuron-plasticity)	-will look around the room, will listen/seek cognitive stimulation, will accept challenge of input information and engage/interact in craft activity	Staff will set up crafts and put out a wide variety of arts and craft materials to encourage creativity, discrimination, comparison, categorizing, etc.
Perceptual Awareness	Show increased abilities of depth perception, visual-spatial awareness, and acuity (for discrimination, comparison, and categorizing), safety	-will use ingredients; will discriminate, compare, will maneuver around work area, will put items away in proper containers associated with proper area (glitter with glitter etc.)	Staff will engage residents in an activity that requires use of acuity, discrimination, comparison, and categorizing for visual-spatial awareness (Ex: placing items on the bookmark using visual acuity, etc.)
Problem-solving (goes beyond thinking/stimulus and initiates thinking process)	Increase problem-solving ability, processing of information, thinking, reasoning, and use of good judgment and decision-making	-will use creativity or comprehend and process the information; will judge appropriate materials	-Staff will engage residents in a creative project and decision-making regarding where to place the sun catchers. -Staff will show the resident the step-by-step actions to make sun catchers to stimulate working memory
Complete a Task	Increase ability to complete a task	-will recall retain , sort/gather information , problem solve, and complete activity	Staff will support residents ability to follow do the project through instruction, encouragement, adaptive devices/programs if needed, and supply necessary materials and support

TABLE 31.1

Recreational Objectives Observational Form
Sun Catchers- Cognitive skills

PATIENT		Dependent (Totally dependent)	High Assistance (25+ ability)	Moderate Assist. (50+ ability)	Mild Assistance (75+ability)	Independent (Totally independent)
SEE CODES BELOW USE OPTIONAL CODES IF APPROPRIATE		1	2	3	4	5
		3 cue/ 2-3 physical	2-3 cues/ 2 physical	2-3 cues/ 1 physical	1-2 cues	Encouragement
97530- Therapeutic activities or	**SKILL**	**GOAL**	**OBJECTIVES** ____times per ____		**METHOD**	**OUTCOME DATE**
97532 Cognitive skills	ORIENTATION					
97532 Cognitive skills	ATTENTION					
97532 Cognitive skills	MEMORY					
97532 Cognitive skills	PROBLEM-SOLVING					
97532 Cognitive skills	COMPLETE A TASK					
97139 Speech Therapy 97532 Cognitive skills	LANGUAGE					
97533	SENSORY STIMULATION/ COGNITIVE STIMULATION					
97532	PERCEPTUAL AWARENESS					

97532-Development of cognitive skills to improve attention, memory, problem-solving, includes compensatory training and/or sensory integrative activities, direct (one-on-one) patient contact by the provider, each 15 minutes; **97530-Therapeutic activities**, direct (one-on-one) patient contact by the provider (use of dynamic activities to improve functional performance), each 15 minutes**; 97533-Sensory integration techniques** to enhance sensory processing and promote adaptive responses to environmental demands, direct (one-on-one) patient contact by the provider, each 15 minutes; **97150-Therapeutic procedure(s)**, group (2 or more individuals); **97139-Unlisted therapeutic procedure** (specify) minutes; **97003- occupational therapy evaluation**; **97004- re-evaluation**	Staff Initial
	Add total score here -Maximum Score 40 pt. each form per activity
	See scale below or use own/facilities optional score system

(Score 1-8)=1 (9-16) =2 (17-24) =3 (25-32) =4 (33-40) =5 If w/device add d if wish, ex: 1d, 2d, or If using 1-7 scale: (41-48) =6 (49-56)

Sun Catchers
Physical Goals, Objectives, and Methods

Skill	Goal	Objectives	Method
Fine Motor Skills	Increase fine motor skills, meaningful/fulfilling activities	-will glue, paste, mix, and pour items; will pick up small items, and manipulate materials	Staff will encourage residents to pick up and manipulate materials
Gross Motor Skills	Increase large motor skills, meaningful/fulfilling activities	-will lift items using large motor skills, walk to group (with device or support)	Staff will encourage residents to lift items using gross motor skills
Perceptual Speed and Motor Function	Increase speed and motor ability for function, safety, meaningful/fulfilling activities	-will increase speed of actions by using skills (with Dr. approval)	Staff will encourage to do the activity and decrease reaction times by shortening amount of time allotted or observation of resident ability increasing on own
Hand-Eye Coordination	Increase hand-eye coordination	-will paste items on craft	Staff will encourage residents to place items. using hand-eye fine motor abilities and detailed fine motor activities

TABLE 31.2

Recreational Objectives Observational Form
Sun Catchers- Physical Skills

PATIENT		Dependent (Totally dependent)	High Assistance (25+ ability)	Moderate Assist. (50+ ability)	Mild Assistance (75+ability)	Independent (Totally independent)
		1	2	3	4	5
SEE CODES BELOW USE OPTIONAL CODES IF APPROPRIATE		3 cue/ 2-3 physical	2-3 cues/ 2 physical	2-3 cues/ 1 physical	1-2 cues	Encouragement
97530- Therapeutic activities or	**SKILL**	**GOAL**	**OBJECTIVES** ____times per ____		**METHOD**	**OUTCOME DATE**
Therapeutic Activity 97530	FINE MOTOR SKILLS					
97530	EYE-HAND COORDINATION					
97110/ 97530	GROSS MOTOR SKILLS					
97530 If under cognitive code 97532	PERCEPTUAL SPEED/MOTOR FUNCTION					

97530 Therapeutic activities, direct (one on one) patient contact by the provider (use of dynamic activities to improve functional performance),each 15 minutes; **97110 Therapeutic procedure, one or more areas**, each 15 minutes; therapeutic exercises to develop strength and endurance, range of motion and flexibility; ; **97150 Therapeutic procedure(s), group (2 or more individuals**; **97535-Self care/home management training** (e.g., activities of daily living and compensatory training, meal preparation, safety procedures, and instructions in use of adaptive equipment), direct (one-on-one) contact by provider, each 15 minutes; **Physical therapy 97001 evaluation, 97002 Re-evaluation. occupational therapy evaluation 97003, re-evaluation. 97004**	Staff Initials
	Add total score here Maximum Score 20 pt. each form per activity
	See scale below or use own/facilities optional score system

(Score 1-4)=1 (5-8) =2 (9-12) =3 (13-16) =4 (17-20) =5 If w/device add d if wish, ex: 1d, 2d, or If using 1-7 scale: (21-24) =6 (25-28) =7

Sun Catchers
Socio-emotional Goals, Objectives, and Methods

Skill	Goal	Objectives Sample	Method Sample
Socialization/Community Integration	Increase social interactions, meaningful/fulfilling activities	-will interact with peers, will engage in community integration experiences (for community adaptation and social skills), will use manners, share, practice social skills	Staff will offer activities that support/encourage residents to socialize through community integration and being w/groups
Team Playing/Sharing	Increase teamwork/sharing, meaningful/fulfilling activities	-will, join in on a craft/ activity with others and share, wait turn, support peers _____ time(s) this week.	Staff will encourage residents to create items, share, work as a team, support/use patience, show compassion to other residents
Initiative and Motivation	Increase initiative and motivation/wellness, and quality of life	-will choose if wishes to do craft, will try new crafts, will increase amount of crafts done _____ times a week	Staff will support /encourage the resident to prepare for craft activities in a timely fashion for their own personal gains of attending activity -Staff will offer new techniques/creative materials to motivate residents to make a creative craft
Emotional Gratification	Increase emotional gratification/wellness, and quality of life	-will state that making crafts is a gratifying experience or will show pleasure by smiling, laughing, deep focus on activities	Staff will ask residents if they enjoyed the activity and what they liked through verbal discussion, group discussions
Sense of Accomplishment	Increase feelings of self-worth, pride, productivity, dignity/wellness, and quality of life	-will use gestures to express pride in self, will show crafts to others	Staff will offer activities as a way to support residents' desire to use creativity and imagination and produce items
Self-esteem/self-identity	Increase self-esteem, feelings of belonging, dignity, self-worth, integrity, self-identity/wellness, and quality of life	-will state/communicate positive feelings about self, will join craft class to take an active role in maintaining health though arts/crafts, volunteer work; will join the craft class based on own choices	Staff will educate residents on the value of doing crafts and learning talents for brain muscle/stimulant benefits, healing qualities, and encourage residents to join classes and share crafts
Sensory Integration/Tolerating Stimulation	Increase sensory processing and enhance awareness of sensations and toleration/adaptation of sensory stimulations and demands	-will adjust to the smells, lights, sounds, etc. in environment	-Staff will offer activities and residents will be exposed to sensory stimulating experiences of tactile stimulation, sights, hearing, communication, and possibly smell sensory stimulations -Staff will support residents as they adjust to the stimulus one step at a time
Fostering Appropriate Behaviors	Increase social interaction, social opportunities and adjustment, safety, using appropriate behaviors during an activity for a calm environment/wellness, and quality of life	-will join in on class, share items/tools; will listen and follow instructions, use appropriate behavior for the setting; will wait turn, stand in line quietly; will quiet down when asked	Before class begins, staff will discuss the rules, appropriate behaviors, respect of property, safety, and respect of fellow peers/staff

TABLE 31.3

Recreational Objectives Observational Form
Sun Catchers- Socio-emotional Skills

PATIENT	Dependent (Totally dependent)	High Assistance (25+ ability)	Moderate Assist. (50+ ability)	Mild Assistance (75+ability)	Independent (Totally independent.)
SEE CODES BELOW USE OPTIONAL CODES IF APPROPRIATE	1	2	3	4	5
	3 cue/ 2-3 physical	2-3 cues/ 2 physical	2-3 cues/ 1 physical	1-2 cues	Encouragement

97530- Therapeutic activities or	**SKILL**	**GOAL**	**OBJECTIVES** ____times per ____	**METHOD**	**OUTCOME DATE**			
97537 Or 97535	SOCIALIZATION/ COMMUNITY INTEGRATION							
97537 Or 97535	TEAM PLAYING /SHARING							
97537 Or 97535	INITIATIVE AND MOTIVATION							
97537 Or 97535	EMOTIONAL GRATIFICATION							
97537 Or 97535	SENSE OF ACCOMPLISHMENT							
97537 Or 97535	SELF-ESTEEM/ SELF-IDENTITY							
97537 Or 97535	FOSTERING APPROPRIATE BEHAVIORS							
97533	SENSORY INTEGRATION/ TOLERATING							

97537-Community/work reintegration training (e.g., shopping, transportation, money management, avocational activities and/or work environment/modification analysis, work task analysis), direct (one-on-one) contact by provider, each 15 minutes; **97535-Self care/home management training** (e.g., activities of daily living and compensatory training, meal preparation, safety procedures, and instructions in use of adaptive equipment), direct (one-on-one) contact by provider, each 15 minutes; **97530-Therapeutic activities, direct (one-on-one)** patient contact by the provider (use of dynamic activities to improve functional performance), each 15 minutes; **97150-Therapeutic procedure(s), group (2 or more individuals); 97533-Sensory integration techniques** to enhance sensory processing and promote adaptive responses to environmental demands, direct (one-on-one) patient contact by the provider, each 15 minutes; **occupational therapy evaluation 97003, re-evaluation . 97004**

Staff Initial				
Add total score here-Maximum Score 40 pt. each form per activity				
See scale below or use own/facilities optional score system				

(Score 1-8)=1 (9-16) =2 (17-24) =3 (25-32) =4 (33-40) =5 If w/device add d if wish, ex: 1d, 2d, or If using 1-7 scale: (41-48) =6 (49-56)

Theme Baskets

Objectives and benefits:

Cognitive Challenges: attention, memory, language, orientation, following patterns, following directions, productivity, mastering a task

Physical Needs: fine motor skills, gross motor skills, hand-eye coordination, perceptual speed and motor function, manipulation of materials, dexterity

Socio-emotional Needs: socialization, community integration, initiative and motivation, emotional gratification, sense of accomplishment, fostering appropriate behaviors, nurturing, * Reminiscing Qualities, Healing Qualities

Supplies: Items that fit in a certain theme, green foam squares.

Time: 30 minutes

Staff/older adult ratio: 1:4 or as assessed per needs of individuals or group

Instructions: Have the supplies set up on a table. At each setting have a basket with green foam. Let the residents choose items to put in their baskets. Let them design their basket as they wish. They can then add bows, ribbons, etc. After the baskets are done, you can offer wrapping for them to cover their baskets. They can make them for family, events, or as decoration for their rooms.

> Research has shown activities that help cognition of sensory/motor and speed processing will be geared towards help in visual and motor memory, discrimination, comparison, and categorizing areas. Reminiscing activities may help improve memory skills. Long-term studies (Arbuckle and others, 1998) have consistently showed that stimulating the brain with activities helps cognitive function in a similar way exercise helps muscle function. Staying productive has been shown to enhance socio-emotional wellness

Theme Baskets
Cognitive Goals, Objectives, and Methods

Skill	Goal	Objectives Sample	Method Sample
Orientation	Show increased awareness of, time/"timeframe," people, circumstances, and past experiences vs. present experiences, to engage in present-time activities, or for a reminiscing intended question	-will respond with correct answer to two choice questions Or yes/no answer, will state where they are, time of day, present company of people on own and with the correct answer	Staff will ask residents a series of questions to stimulate focus to the present setting (Ex: "What talents are you going to share? Have you made theme baskets before? Who did you make them with?")
Attention	Show increased attention span, task for function, and to engage in meaningful, recreational/fulfilling activities	-will make eye-contact with staff for _____ sec., will verbalize with staff and instructor, will read/listen to rules and say yes/no to show understand or do the action	Staff will address or stand in front of resident, make eye contact, ask questions or use others forms to get residents attention
Memory	Show increased memory skills of recall, recognition, retention of information, working memory	-will repeat/recall how to make project, will remember will lesson at next class	Staff will show steps/actions on how to make theme baskets, and residents will repeat the action using short-term memory/recall, working memory
Language	Show increased ability to communicate use of words, phrases, sentence structure, comprehension, interpretation	-will be asked a question and answer yes/no, will be asked what is included in project, will state ingredients, methods, items; will interact with peers and staff; will interpret instructor's request and follow	Staff will ask questions to stimulate a communication (Ex: "What materials are you using to make your theme basket?") Interpretation/Lang. skills (Ex: "You need to add tacky glue to make it stick well.") and then note resident's actions to show understood
Cognitive Stimulation (awareness, seeks information in)	Increased stimulus/exposure for visual/ motor memory, cognitive experiences/awareness and brain stimulation to enhance (function, pragmatics, neuron-plasticity)	-will look around the room, will listen/seek cognitive stimulation, will accept challenge of input information and engage/interact in, will engage in a bookmark activity	Staff will set up crafts and put out a wide variety of arts and craft materials to encourage creativity, discrimination, comparison, categorizing, etc.
Perceptual Awareness	Show increased abilities of depth perception, visual-spatial awareness, and acuity (for discrimination, comparison, and categorizing), safety	-will use ingredients/items, will discriminate, compare; will maneuver around work area, will put items away in proper containers associated with proper area (birthday theme baskets, etc.)	Staff will engage residents in an activity that requires use of acuity, discrimination, comparison, and categorizing for visual-spatial awareness (Ex: placing items in baskets)
Problem-solving (goes beyond thinking/stimulus and initiates thinking process)	Increase problem-solving ability, processing of information, thinking, reasoning, and use of good judgment and decision-making	-will recall/retain and sort/gather information, will problem-solve by deciding what belongs in the baskets and placements of articles	-Staff will engage residents in a creative project and decision-making regarding whom to send the theme baskets to. -Staff will show the resident the step-by-step actions to make a bookmark to stimulate working memory
Complete a Task	Increase ability to complete a task	will recall/retain and sort/gather information, will problem-solve and complete activity	Staff will support resident's ability to follow and do the project through instruction, encourage, and supply adaptive devices/programs if needed, and necessary materials and support

TABLE 32.1

Recreational Objectives Observational Form
Theme Baskets-Cognitive skills

PATIENT		Dependent (Totally dependent)	High Assistance (25+ ability)	Moderate Assist. (50+ ability)	Mild Assistance (75+ability)	Independent (Totally independent)
SEE CODES BELOW USE OPTIONAL CODES IF APPROPRIATE		1	2	3	4	5
		3 cue/ 2-3 physical	2-3 cues/ 2 physical	2-3 cues/ 1 physical	1-2 cues	Encouragement
97530-Therapeutic activities or	SKILL	GOAL	OBJECTIVES ____times per ____		METHOD	OUTCOME DATE
97532 Cognitive skills	ORIENTATION					
97532 Cognitive skills	ATTENTION					
97532 Cognitive skills	MEMORY					
97532 Cognitive skills	PROBLEM-SOLVING					
97532 Cognitive skills	COMPLETE A TASK					
97139 Speech Therapy 97532 Cognitive skills	LANGUAGE					
97533	SENSORY STIMULATION/ COGNITIVE STIMULATION					
97532	PERCEPTUAL AWARENESS					

97532-Development of cognitive skills to improve attention, memory, problem-solving, includes compensatory training and/or sensory integrative activities, direct (one-on-one) patient contact by the provider, each 15 minutes; **97530-Therapeutic activities**, direct (one-on-one) patient contact by the provider (use of dynamic activities to improve functional performance), each 15 minutes; **97533-Sensory integration techniques** to enhance sensory processing and promote adaptive responses to environmental demands, direct (one-on-one) patient contact by the provider, each 15 minutes; **97150-Therapeutic procedure(s)**, group (2 or more individuals); **97139-Unlisted therapeutic procedure** (specify) minutes; **97003- occupational therapy evaluation**; **97004- re-evaluation**	Staff Initial
	Add total score here -Maximum Score 40 pt. each form per activity
	See scale below or use own/facilities optional score system

(Score 1-8)=1 (9-16) =2 (17-24) =3 (25-32) =4 (33-40) =5 If w/device add d if wish, ex: 1d, 2d, or If using 1-7 scale: (41-48) =6 (49-56)

Theme Baskets
Physical Goals, Objectives, and Methods

Skill	Goal	Objectives Sample	Method Sample
Fine Motor Skills	Increase fine motor skills, meaningful/fulfilling activities	-will glue, paste, mix, and pour items, will pick up small items, manipulate materials	Staff will encourage residents to pick up and manipulate materials
Gross Motor Skills	Increase large motor skills, meaningful/fulfilling activities	-will lift items using large motor skills, will walk to group (with device or support)	Staff will encourage residents to lift items using gross motor skills
Perceptual Speed and Motor Function	Increase speed and motor ability for function, safety, meaningful/fulfilling activities	-will increase speed of actions by using skills (with Dr. approval)	Staff will encourage residents to do the activity and decrease reaction times by shortening amount of time allotted, or observation of resident ability increasing on own
Hand-Eye Coordination	Increase hand-eye coordination	-will paste items on craft	Staff will encourage residents to place items using hand-eye fine motor abilities, detailed fine motor activities

TABLE 32.2

Recreational Objectives Observational Form
Theme Baskets- Physical Skills

PATIENT	Dependent (Totally dependent)	High Assistance (25+ ability)	Moderate Assist. (50+ ability)	Mild Assistance (75+ability)	Independent (Totally independent)
	1	2	3	4	5
SEE CODES BELOW USE OPTIONAL CODES IF APPROPRIATE	3 cue/ 2-3 physical	2-3 cues/ 2 physical	2-3 cues/ 1 physical	1-2 cues	Encouragement

97530- Therapeutic activities or	SKILL	GOAL	OBJECTIVES ____times per ____	METHOD	OUTCOME DATE			
Therapeutic Activity 97530	FINE MOTOR SKILLS							
97530	EYE-HAND COORDINATION							
97110/ 97530	GROSS MOTOR SKILLS							
97530 If under cognitive code 97532	PERCEPTUAL SPEED/MOTOR FUNCTION							

97530 Therapeutic activities, direct (one on one) patient contact by the provider (use of dynamic activities to improve functional performance),each 15 minutes; **97110 Therapeutic procedure, one or more areas**, each 15 minutes; therapeutic exercises to develop strength and endurance, range of motion and flexibility; ; **97150 Therapeutic procedure(s), group (2 or more individuals**; **97535-Self care/home management training** (e.g., activities of daily living and compensatory training, meal preparation, safety procedures, and instructions in use of adaptive equipment), direct (one-on-one) contact by provider, each 15 minutes; **Physical therapy 97001 evaluation, 97002 Re-evaluation. occupational therapy evaluation 97003, re-evaluation. 97004**	Staff Initials				
	Add total score here Maximum Score 20 pt. each form per activity				
	See scale below or use own/facilities optional score system				

(Score 1-4)=1 (5-8) =2 (9-12) =3 (13-16) =4 (17-20) =5 If w/device add d if wish, ex: 1d, 2d, or If using 1-7 scale: (21-24) =6 (25-28) =7

THEME BASKETS
SOCIO-EMOTIONAL GOALS, OBJECTIVES AND METHODS

Skill	Goal	Objectives Sample	Method Sample
Socialization/Community Integration	Increase social interactions, meaningful/fulfilling activities	-will interact with peers, will engage in community integration experiences (for community adaptation and social skills); will use manners, share, practice social skills	Staff will offer activities that support/encourage residents to socialize through community integration and being w/groups
Team Playing/Sharing	Increase teamwork/sharing, meaningful/fulfilling activities	-will join in on a craft/ activity with others and share, wait turn, support peers _____ time(s) this week.	Staff will encourage residents to create items, share, work as a team, support/use patience, show compassion to other residents
Initiative and Motivation	Increase initiative and motivation/wellness, and quality of life	-will choose if wishes to do craft, will try new crafts, will increase amount of crafts done _____ time(s) a week	Staff will support/encourage the resident to prepare for craft activities in a timely fashion for their own personal gains of attending activity , -Staff will offer new techniques and creative materials to motivate residents to make a creative craft
Emotional Gratification	Increase emotional gratification/wellness, and quality of life	-will state that making crafts is a gratifying experience or will show pleasure by smiling, laughing, deep focus on activities	Staff will ask residents if they enjoyed the activity and what they liked through verbal discussion, group discussions
Sense of Accomplishment	Increase feelings of self-worth, pride, productivity, dignity/wellness, and quality of life	-will use gestures to express pride in self , will show crafts to others	Staff will offer activities as a way to support residents' desire to use creativity and imagination, and produce items
Self-esteem/self-identity	Increase self-esteem, feelings of belonging, dignity, self-worth, integrity, self-identity/wellness, and quality of life	-will state/communicate positive feelings about self, will join craft class to take an active role in maintaining health though arts/crafts, volunteer work, will join the craft class based on own choices	Staff will educate residents on the value of doing crafts/learning talents for brain muscle/stimulant benefits and healing qualities, and will encourage residents to join classes and share crafts
Sensory Integration/Tolerating Stimulation	Increase sensory processing and enhance awareness of sensations and toleration/adaptation of sensory stimulations and demands	-will adjust to the smells, lights, sounds, etc. in environment	-Staff will offer activities and residents will be exposed to sensory stimulating experiences of tactile stimulation, sights, hearing, communication, and possibly smell sensory stimulations -Staff will support residents as they adjust to the stimulus a step at a time
Fostering Appropriate Behaviors	Increase social interaction, social opportunities and adjustment, safety, using appropriate behaviors during an activity for a calm environment/wellness, and quality of life	-will join in on class, share items/tools, listen and follow instructions, use appropriate behavior for the setting; will wait turn, stand in line quietly, will quiet down when asked	Before class begins, staff will discuss the rules, appropriate behaviors, respect of property, safety, and respect of fellow peers/staff

TABLE 32.3

Recreational Objectives Observational Form
Theme Baskets- Socio-emotional Skills

PATIENT	Dependent (Totally dependent)	High Assistance (25+ ability)	Moderate Assist. (50+ ability)	Mild Assistance (75+ability)	Independent (Totally independent.)
SEE CODES BELOW USE OPTIONAL CODES IF APPROPRIATE	1	2	3	4	5
	3 cue/ 2-3 physical	2-3 cues/ 2 physical	2-3 cues/ 1 physical	1-2 cues	Encouragement

97530-Therapeutic activities or	SKILL	GOAL	OBJECTIVES ____times per ____	METHOD	OUTCOME DATE			
97537 Or 97535	SOCIALIZATION/ COMMUNITY INTEGRATION							
97537 Or 97535	TEAM PLAYING /SHARING							
97537 Or 97535	INITIATIVE AND MOTIVATION							
97537 Or 97535	EMOTIONAL GRATIFICATION							
97537 Or 97535	SENSE OF ACCOMPLISHMENT							
97537 Or 97535	SELF-ESTEEM/ SELF-IDENTITY							
97537 Or 97535	FOSTERING APPROPRIATE BEHAVIORS							
97533	SENSORY INTEGRATION/ TOLERATING							

97537-Community/work reintegration training (e.g., shopping, transportation, money management, avocational activities and/or work environment/modification analysis, work task analysis), direct (one-on-one) contact by provider, each 15 minutes; **97535-Self care/home management training** (e.g., activities of daily living and compensatory training, meal preparation, safety procedures, and instructions in use of adaptive equipment), direct (one-on-one) contact by provider, each 15 minutes; **97530-Therapeutic activities, direct (one-on-one)** patient contact by the provider (use of dynamic activities to improve functional performance), each 15 minutes; **97150-Therapeutic procedure(s), group (2 or more individuals); 97533-Sensory integration techniques** to enhance sensory processing and promote adaptive responses to environmental demands, direct (one-on-one) patient contact by the provider, each 15 minutes; **occupational therapy evaluation 97003, re-evaluation . 97004**	Staff Initial			
	Add total score here-Maximum Score 40 pt. each form per activity			
	See scale below or use own/facilities optional score system			

(Score 1-8)=1 (9-16) =2 (17-24) =3 (25-32) =4 (33-40) =5 If w/device add d if wish, ex: 1d, 2d, or If using 1-7 scale: (41-48) =6 (49-56)

Wind Chimes

Objectives and benefits:

Cognitive Challenges: attention, memory, language, orientation, following patterns, following directions, productivity, mastering a task

Physical Needs: fine motor skills, gross motor skills, hand-eye coordination, perceptual speed and motor function, manipulation of materials, dexterity

Socio-emotional Needs: socialization, community integration, initiative and motivation, emotional gratification, sense of accomplishment, fostering appropriate behaviors, nurturing, * Reminiscing Qualities, Healing Qualities

Supplies: Fishing string, hanging ornaments, a cardboard circle. Be sure to have a nice variety of ornaments. You could do this on a theme such as the Fourth of July or spring.

Time: 30 minutes.

Staff/older adult ratio: 1:4

Instructions: Have each resident's supplies set up for them. This should include four strings tied in a knot. Take five strings and tie a knot at the top of the string. This knot should be slightly open so they can hang their chime from it. They should also have a cardboard circle with five holes punched in it to put the strings through. This will help to spread out the ornaments that will hang down. There will be four holes placed roughly at the four directions of a compass as well as one middle hole.

Have them put the strings through the holes, then have them attach chimes to the four compass direction strings, and a stone or ornament to the middle string. Either tie the string to hold the chimes and ornament or, if more security is needed, use a glue gun to secure the items. Then have them hang their wind chime in a windy place and enjoy the relaxing sound.

Research has shown activities that help cognition of sensory/motor and speed processing will be geared towards help in visual and motor memory, discrimination, comparison, and categorizing areas. Reminiscing activities may help improve memory skills. Long-term studies (Arbuckle and others, 1998) have consistently showed that stimulating the brain with activities helps cognitive function in a similar way exercise helps muscle function. Staying productive has been shown to enhance socio-emotional wellness

WIND CHIMES
Cognitive Goals, Objectives, and Methods

Skill	Goal	Objectives Sample	Method Sample
Orientation	Show increased awareness of, time/"timeframe," people, circumstances, and past experiences vs. present experiences, to engage in present-time activities, or for a reminiscing intended question	-will respond with correct answer to two choice questions Or yes/no answer, will state where they are, time of day, present company of people on own and with the correct answer	Staff will ask residents a series of questions to stimulate focus to the present setting (Ex: "What talents are you going to share? Have you made Wind Chimes before?")
Attention	Show increased attention span, task for function, and to engage in meaningful, recreational/fulfilling activities	-will make eye-contact with staff for _____ sec., will verbalize with staff and instructor, will read/listen to rules, say yes/no to show understand or do the action	Staff will address or stand in front of resident, make eye-contact, ask questions, or use others methods to get resident's attention
Memory	Show increased memory skills of recall, recognition, retention of information, working memory	-will repeat/recall how to make project, will remember lesson at next class	Staff will show steps and actions on how to make bookmarks, and residents will repeat the action using short-term memory/recall, working memory
Language	Show increased ability to communicate use of words, phrases, sentence structure, comprehension, interpretation	-will be asked a question and answer yes or no, will be asked what is included in project, will state ingredients, methods, items; will interact with peers, staff; will interpret instructor's request and follow	Staff will ask questions to stimulate a communication (Ex: "What materials are you using to make your bookmarks?") Interpretation/Lang. skills (Ex: "You need to add paste to make it stick well.") and then note resident's actions to show they understood
Cognitive Stimulation (awareness, seeks information in)	Increased stimulus/exposure for visual/ motor memory, cognitive experiences/awareness and brain stimulation to enhance (function, pragmatics, neuron-plasticity)	-will look around the room, will listen/seek cognitive stimulation, will accept challenge of input information and engage/interact in bookmark activity	Staff will set up crafts and put out a wide variety of arts and craft materials to encourage creativity, discrimination, comparison, categorizing, etc.
Perceptual Awareness	Show increased abilities of depth perception, visual-spatial awareness, and acuity (for discrimination, comparison, and categorizing), safety	-will use ingredients/items, will discriminate and compare, will maneuver around work area, will put items away in proper containers associated with proper area (buttons with buttons, glitter with glitter)	Staff will engage residents in an activity that requires use of acuity, discrimination, comparison and categorizing for visual-spatial awareness (Ex: placing items on the bookmark using visual acuity)
Problem-solving (goes beyond thinking/stimulus and initiates thinking process)	Increase problem-solving ability, processing of information, thinking, reasoning, and use of good judgment and decision-making	-will think up a story, use creativity, or comprehend and process the information, will judge appropriate materials	-Staff will engage residents in a creative project and decision-making regarding whom to send the bookmarks to. -Staff will show the resident the step-by-step actions to make a bookmark to stimulate working memory
Complete a Task	Increase ability to complete a task	will recall/retain, sort/gather information, problem-solve, and complete activity	-Staff will support resident's ability to follow through with the project, -Staff will encourage residents, supply adaptive devices/programs if needed, and supply necessary materials and support

TABLE 33.1

Recreational Objectives Observational Form

WIND CHIMES- COGNITIVE SKILLS

PATIENT		Dependent (Totally dependent)	High Assistance (25+ ability)	Moderate Assist. (50+ ability)	Mild Assistance (75+ability)	Independent (Totally independent)			
SEE CODES BELOW USE OPTIONAL CODES IF APPROPRIATE		1	2	3	4	5			
		3 cue/ 2-3 physical	2-3 cues/ 2 physical	2-3 cues/ 1 physical	1-2 cues	Encouragement			
97530- Therapeutic activities or	**SKILL**	**GOAL**	**OBJECTIVES** ____times per ____		**METHOD**	**OUTCOME DATE**			
97532 Cognitive skills	ORIENTATION								
97532 Cognitive skills	ATTENTION								
97532 Cognitive skills	MEMORY								
97532 Cognitive skills	PROBLEM-SOLVING								
97532 Cognitive skills	COMPLETE A TASK								
97139 Speech Therapy 97532 Cognitive skills	LANGUAGE								
97533	SENSORY STIMULATION/ COGNITIVE STIMULATION								
97532	PERCEPTUAL AWARENESS								

97532-Development of cognitive skills to improve attention, memory, problem-solving, includes compensatory training and/or sensory integrative activities, direct (one-on-one) patient contact by the provider, each 15 minutes; **97530-Therapeutic activities**, direct (one-on-one) patient contact by the provider (use of dynamic activities to improve functional performance), each 15 minutes; **97533-Sensory integration techniques** to enhance sensory processing and promote adaptive responses to environmental demands, direct (one-on-one) patient contact by the provider, each 15 minutes; **97150-Therapeutic procedure(s)**, group (2 or more individuals); **97139-Unlisted therapeutic procedure** (specify) minutes; **97003- occupational therapy evaluation**; **97004- re-evaluation**	Staff Initial				
	Add total score here -Maximum Score 40 pt. each form per activity				
	See scale below or use own/facilities optional score system				

(Score 1-8)=1 (9-16) =2 (17-24) =3 (25-32) =4 (33-40) =5 If w/device add d if wish, ex: 1d, 2d, or If using 1-7 scale: (41-48) =6 (49-56)

Wind Chimes

Physical Goals, Objectives, and Methods

Skill	Goal	Objectives Sample	Method Sample
Fine Motor Skills	Increase fine motor skills, meaningful/fulfilling activities	-will glue, paste, mix, pour, items; will pick up small items, manipulate materials	Staff will encourage residents to pick up and manipulate materials
Gross Motor Skills	Increase large motor skills, meaningful/fulfilling activities	-will lift items using large motor skills, will walk to group (with device or support)	Staff will encourage residents to lift items using gross motor skills
Perceptual Speed and Motor Function	Increase speed and motor ability for function, safety, meaningful/fulfilling activities	-will increase speed of actions by using skills (Dr. approval)	Staff will encourage to do the activity and decrease reaction times by shortening amount of time allotted, or observation of resident ability increasing on own
Hand-Eye Coordination	Increase hand-eye coordination	-will paste items on craft	Staff will encourage residents to place items on the craft using hand-eye fine motor abilities and detailed fine motor activities

TABLE 33.2

Recreational Objectives Observational Form

WIND CHIMES- PHYSICAL SKILLS

<table>
<tr><td colspan="2">PATIENT</td><td>Dependent (Totally dependent)</td><td>High Assistance (25+ ability)</td><td>Moderate Assist. (50+ ability)</td><td>Mild Assistance (75+ability)</td><td colspan="4">Independent (Totally independent)</td></tr>
<tr><td colspan="2"></td><td>1</td><td>2</td><td>3</td><td>4</td><td colspan="4">5</td></tr>
<tr><td colspan="2">SEE CODES BELOW
USE OPTIONAL CODES IF APPROPRIATE</td><td>3 cue/
2-3 physical</td><td>2-3 cues/
2 physical</td><td>2-3 cues/
1 physical</td><td>1-2 cues</td><td colspan="4">Encouragement</td></tr>
<tr><td>97530- Therapeutic activities or</td><td>SKILL</td><td>GOAL</td><td colspan="2">OBJECTIVES
____times per ____</td><td>METHOD</td><td colspan="4">OUTCOME DATE</td></tr>
<tr><td>Therapeutic Activity 97530</td><td>FINE MOTOR SKILLS</td><td></td><td colspan="2"></td><td></td><td></td><td></td><td></td><td></td></tr>
<tr><td>97530</td><td>EYE-HAND COORDINATION</td><td></td><td colspan="2"></td><td></td><td></td><td></td><td></td><td></td></tr>
<tr><td>97110/ 97530</td><td>GROSS MOTOR SKILLS</td><td></td><td colspan="2"></td><td></td><td></td><td></td><td></td><td></td></tr>
<tr><td>97530 If under cognitive code 97532</td><td>PERCEPTUAL SPEED/MOTOR FUNCTION</td><td></td><td colspan="2"></td><td></td><td></td><td></td><td></td><td></td></tr>
<tr><td colspan="5" rowspan="3">97530 Therapeutic activities, direct (one on one) patient contact by the provider (use of dynamic activities to improve functional performance),each 15 minutes; 97110 Therapeutic procedure, one or more areas, each 15 minutes; therapeutic exercises to develop strength and endurance, range of motion and flexibility; ; 97150 Therapeutic procedure(s), group (2 or more individuals; 97535-Self care/home management training (e.g., activities of daily living and compensatory training, meal preparation, safety procedures, and instructions in use of adaptive equipment), direct (one-on-one) contact by provider, each 15 minutes; Physical therapy 97001 evaluation, 97002 Re-evaluation. occupational therapy evaluation 97003, re-evaluation. 97004</td><td colspan="5">Staff Initials</td></tr>
<tr><td>Add total score here Maximum Score 20 pt.
each form per activity</td><td></td><td></td><td></td><td></td></tr>
<tr><td>See scale below or use own/facilities optional score system</td><td></td><td></td><td></td><td></td></tr>
</table>

(Score 1-4)=1 (5-8) =2 (9-12) =3 (13-16) =4 (17-20) =5 If w/device add d if wish, ex: 1d, 2d, or If using 1-7 scale: (21-24) =6 (25-28) =7Current Procedural Terminology © 2005 American Medical Association. All rights reserved. Recreational Objectives Observational forms© 2005. All rights reserved. Patent pending.

WIND CHIMES
Socio-emotional Goals, Objectives, and Methods

Skill	Goal	Objectives Sample	Method Sample
Socialization/Community Integration	Increase social interactions, meaningful/fulfilling activities	-will interact with peers, will engage in community integration experiences (for community adaptation and social skills), will use manners, share, practice social skills	Staff will offer activities that support/encourage residents to socialize through community integration and being w/groups
Team Playing/Sharing	Increase teamwork/sharing, meaningful/fulfilling activities	-will join in on a craft/activity with others and share, wait turn, support peers _____ time(s) this week.	Staff will encourage residents to create items, share, work as a team, support/use patience, show compassion to other residents
Initiative and Motivation	Increase initiative and motivation/wellness, and quality of life	-will choose if wishes to do craft, will try new crafts, will increase amount of crafts done _____ time(s) a week	Staff will support/encourage the resident to prepare for craft activities in a timely fashion for their own personal gains of attending activity, -Staff will offer new techniques/creative materials to motivate residents to make a creative craft
Emotional Gratification	Increase emotional gratification/wellness, and quality of life	-will state that making crafts is a gratifying experiences or will show pleasure by smiling, laughing, deep focus on activities	Staff will ask residents if they enjoyed the activity and what they liked through verbal discussion, group discussions
Sense of Accomplishment	Increase feelings of self-worth, pride, productivity, dignity/wellness, and quality of life	-will use gestures to express pride in self, will show crafts to others	Staff will offer activities as a way to support resident's desire to use creativity, imagination, and produce items
Self-esteem/self-identity	Increase self-esteem, feelings of belonging, dignity, self-worth, integrity, self-identity/wellness, and quality of life	-will state/communicate positive feelings about self, will join craft class to take an active role in maintaining health though arts/crafts, volunteer work; will join the craft class based on own choices	Staff will educate residents on the value of doing crafts and learning talents for brain muscle/stimulant benefits and healing qualities -Staff will encourage residents to join classes/share crafts
Sensory Integration/Tolerating Stimulation	Increase social interaction, social opportunities and adjustment, safety, using appropriate behaviors during an activity for a calm environment/wellness, and quality of life	-will adjust to the smells, lights, sounds, etc. in environment	Staff will offer activities and residents will be exposed to sensory stimulating experiences of tactile stimulation, sights, hearing, communication, and possibly smell sensory stimulations -Staff will support residents as they adjust to the stimulus one step at a time
Fostering Appropriate Behaviors	Increase sensory processing and enhance awareness of sensations and toleration/adaptation of sensory stimulations and demands	-will join in on class, share items/tools, listen and follow instructions, use appropriate behavior for the setting; will wait turn, stand in line quietly, will quiet down when asked	Before class begins, staff will discuss the rules, appropriate behaviors, respect of property, safety, and respect of fellow peers and staff

TABLE 33.3

Recreational Objectives Observational Form

WIND CHIMES- SOCIO-EMOTIONAL SKILLS

PATIENT	Dependent (Totally dependent)	High Assistance (25+ ability)	Moderate Assist. (50+ ability)	Mild Assistance (75+ability)	Independent (Totally independent.)
SEE CODES BELOW USE OPTIONAL CODES IF APPROPRIATE	1	2	3	4	5
	3 cue/ 2-3 physical	2-3 cues/ 2 physical	2-3 cues/ 1 physical	1-2 cues	Encouragement

97530-Therapeutic activities or	SKILL	GOAL	OBJECTIVES ____times per ____	METHOD	OUTCOME DATE			
97537 Or 97535	SOCIALIZATION/ COMMUNITY INTEGRATION							
97537 Or 97535	TEAM PLAYING /SHARING							
97537 Or 97535	INITIATIVE AND MOTIVATION							
97537 Or 97535	EMOTIONAL GRATIFICATION							
97537 Or 97535	SENSE OF ACCOMPLISHM ENT							
97537 Or 97535	SELF-ESTEEM/ SELF-IDENTITY							
97537 Or 97535	FOSTERING APPROPRIATE BEHAVIORS							
97533	SENSORY INTEGRATION/ TOLERATING							

97537-Community/work reintegration training (e.g., shopping, transportation, money management, avocational activities and/or work environment/modification analysis, work task analysis), direct (one-on-one) contact by provider, each 15 minutes; **97535-Self care/home management training** (e.g., activities of daily living and compensatory training, meal preparation, safety procedures, and instructions in use of adaptive equipment), direct (one-on-one) contact by provider, each 15 minutes; **97530-Therapeutic activities, direct (one-on-one)** patient contact by the provider (use of dynamic activities to improve functional performance), each 15 minutes; **97150-Therapeutic procedure(s), group (2 or more individuals); 97533-Sensory integration techniques** to enhance sensory processing and promote adaptive responses to environmental demands, direct (one-on-one) patient contact by the provider, each 15 minutes; **occupational therapy evaluation 97003, re-evaluation . 97004**	Staff Initial				
	Add total score here-Maximum Score 40 pt. each form per activity				
	See scale below or use own/facilities optional score system				

(Score 1-8)=1 (9-16) =2 (17-24) =3 (25-32) =4 (33-40) =5 If w/device add d if wish, ex: 1d, 2d, or If using 1-7 scale: (41-48) =6 (49-56)

Relaxation, Self-Nurturing Activity
OR
Sensory Integration Activities

(High Socio-emotional Stimulation) or
(High Cognitive Sensory Stimulus)

Reminiscing activities may help improve memory and sensory skills. Self-Nurturing activities can have positive effects on reducing stress, promoting relaxation, solace and be beneficial to physical well-being.

Aromatherapy

Objectives and benefits:

Cognitive Challenges: attention, memory, language, orientation, following patterns, following directions, productivity, mastering a task

Physical Needs: fine motor skills, gross motor skills, hand-eye coordination, perceptual speed and motor function, manipulation of materials, dexterity

Socio-emotional Needs: socialization, community integration, initiative and motivation, emotional gratification, sense of accomplishment, fostering appropriate behaviors, nurturing, * Reminiscing Qualities, Healing Qualities

Supplies: A variety of aromatherapy materials such as candles, incense, etc.

Time: As long as desired.

Staff/older adult ratio: As assessed per needs of individuals or group.

Instructions: Offer a variety of aromatherapy items/scents. You can generally find information on the qualities and benefits of different aroma scents and supplies. You can also use different smells for different themes. For example: gingerbread for Christmas or apples for autumn. You can also look into information on the healing qualities of incense. There is particular incense that produces relaxation or energy and so on. Generally, you can check at stores that specialize in candles and aromatherapy, or you may find such information through online sites.

Be sure no candles or incense are left unattended. Also, be sure you do not have older adults with allergies to the incense or candles used for any aromatherapy activities. Awareness of all older adults/staff allergies should be known before starting any activities.

Reminiscing activities may help improve memory and sensory skills. Self-Nurturing activities can have positive effects on reducing stress, promoting relaxation, solace and be beneficial to physical well-being.

Aromatherapy
Cognitive Goals, Objectives, and Methods

Skill	Goal	Objectives Sample	Method Sample
Orientation	Show increased awareness of time/ "timeframe," people, circumstances, and past experiences vs. present experiences, to engage in present- time activities or for a reminiscing intended question	-will respond with correct answer to two choice questions; will state where they are, time of day, present company of people on own and with a correct answer	The resident will be asked a series of questions to stimulate focus to the present setting Or past if reminiscing exercise (Ex: "What do these smells remind you of?")
Attention	Show increased attention span, task for function, and to engage in meaningful, recreational/fulfilling activities	-will make eye-contact with staff for _____ sec., will verbalize with staff, instructor	Staff will address or stand in front of resident, make eye-contact, ask questions, or use others methods to get resident's attention
Memory	Show increased memory skills of recall, recognition, retention of information, working memory	-will repeat/recall smells from past experiences	Staff will use aroma-therapy to stimulate recall/memories
Language	Show increased ability to communicate use of words, phases, sentence structure, comprehension, interpretation	-will be asked a question and answer yes or no, will be asked what fragrance is being used, will interact with peers and staff, will engage in a sensory game, will consider smells and try to answer the type of smells	Staff will ask questions to stimulate a mmunication (Ex: what does this smell remind you of?") Interpretation/Lang. skills
Sensory integration/ Cognitive Stimulation (awareness, seeks information in)	Increased stimulus/exposure for visual/motor memory, cognitive experiences/awareness and brain stimulation to enhance (sensory processing function, pragmatics, neuroplasticity)	-will listen/seek cognitive stimulation, accept challenge of input information and engage/interact in aroma-therapy activity	Staff will engage residents in an aroma-therapy project and promote making choices, processing information, engaging in recall/recognition of sensory items
Perceptual Awareness	Show increased awareness of depth perception, visio-spatical, acuity for discrimination, comparison, and categorize safety, meaningful activities	-will sort, discriminate colors of candles, oils, etc.	Staff will use various types of objects to support resident's needs of perceptual discrimination, comparing for function and safety
Problem solving (goes beyond thinking/stimulus and initiates thinking process)	Increase problem-solving ability, processing of information, thinking, reasoning, and use of good judgment and decision-making	-will consider and process smell sensory of previous sensory experiences or knowledge	Staff will engage residents in an aroma-therapy project and promote making choices, processing information, engaging in recall, recognition of sensory items
Healing/ Self-Nurturing	Increase ability to accept/ experience nurturing, healing experiences	-will engage in self nurturing activities, will continue to accept nurturing from others and to nurture self	Staff will engage residents in an aromatherapy project and promote self-nurturing and being nurtured.

TABLE 34.1

Recreational Objectives Observational Form
Aromatherapy- Cognitive skills

PATIENT	Dependent (Totally dependent)	High Assistance (25+ ability)	Moderate Assist. (50+ ability)	Mild Assistance (75+ability)	Independent (Totally independent)
SEE CODES BELOW USE OPTIONAL CODES IF APPROPRIATE	1	2	3	4	5
	3 cue/ 2-3 physical	2-3 cues/ 2 physical	2-3 cues/ 1 physical	1-2 cues	Encouragement

97530- Therapeutic activities or	SKILL	GOAL	OBJECTIVES ____times per ____	METHOD	OUTCOME DATE			
97532 Cognitive skills	ORIENTATION							
97532 Cognitive skills	ATTENTION							
97532 Cognitive skills	MEMORY							
97532 Cognitive skills	PROBLEM-SOLVING							
97532 Cognitive skills	COMPLETE A TASK							
97139 Speech Therapy 97532 Cognitive skills	LANGUAGE							
97533	SENSORY STIMULATION/ COGNITIVE STIMULATION							
97532	PERCEPTUAL AWARENESS							

97532-Development of cognitive skills to improve attention, memory, problem-solving, includes compensatory training and/or sensory integrative activities, direct (one-on-one) patient contact by the provider, each 15 minutes; **97530-Therapeutic activities**, direct (one-on-one) patient contact by the provider (use of dynamic activities to improve functional performance), each 15 minutes; **97533-Sensory integration techniques** to enhance sensory processing and promote adaptive responses to environmental demands, direct (one-on-one) patient contact by the provider, each 15 minutes; **97150-Therapeutic procedure(s)**, group (2 or more individuals); **97139-Unlisted therapeutic procedure** (specify) minutes; **97003- occupational therapy evaluation**; **97004- re-evaluation**	Staff Initial				
	Add total score here -Maximum Score 40 pt. each form per activity				
	See scale below or use own/facilities optional score system				

(Score 1-8)=1 (9-16) =2 (17-24) =3 (25-32) =4 (33-40) =5 If w/device add d if wish, ex: 1d, 2d, or If using 1-7 scale: (41-48) =6 (49-56)

Aromatherapy
Physical Goals, Objectives, and Methods
(if used in conjunction with other activity)

Skill	Goal	Objectives	Method
Fine motor skills	Increase fine motor skills, meaningful /fulfilling activities	-will use fingers, hands, dexterity, etc. when manipulating items or exercising, yoga, etc.	Staff will give resident fine motor sensory stimulating activities, items for smell etc. for stimuli activities and may include baking, yoga exercise etc.
Gross motor skills	Increase large motor skills, meaningful /fulfilling activities	-will bend, stretch, and do movements if required	Staff will give resident gross motor sensory stimulating activities, items for smell, touch, taste, vision, etc. for stimuli activities
Perceptual speed and motor function	Increase speed and motor ability for function, safety, meaningful /fulfilling activities	-will react and do motor movement of activity (if required during activity)	Staff will give resident items that increase perceptual function (Ex: slow dance movements or to help set up items for aroma-therapy class, or baking as part of event
Following step patterns/backwards forward movement	Increase strength, balance, endurance, meaningful /fulfilling activities	ill walk backwards, forwards, etc. If activity requires	Staff will decrease the amount of time waited between actions to do a task
Range of motion	Increase strength, endurance, agility and flexibility	-will lift arms, legs (to capacity-set by Dr./clinician) -will extend and flex (to capacity-set by clinician)	Staff/Clinician will ask resident to lift arms and legs (to capacity-set by Dr./clinician) and to extend and flex (to capacity-set by clinician)
Posture	Increase improve body alignment, flexibility	-will sit in chair and increase posture during activity	Staff/clinician will ask resident to sit in chair and increase/hold posture for 3-5 min. during activity
Balance and Gait	Increase balance and gait	-will stand up without losing balance, will walk a safe pace (approved by Dr. and capacity tests) If approved clinical specialist: ____ ft. ________________________	Staff/clinician will ask resident to stand up without losing balance and walk a safe pace (approved by Dr. and capacity tests) If approved clinical specialist: ____ ft. ________________________
Cardio-vascular workout	Increase circulation, blood flow, stamina	-will play the game/do movements at a safe pace (approved by Dr. and capacity tests) If approved clinical specialist: ________________________	If applicable, staff will engage residents in a game at a safe pace (approved by Dr. and capacity tests) If approved clinical specialist: ________________________

TABLE 34.2

Recreational Objectives Observational Form
Aromatherapy- Physical Skills
(If resident participates and exhibits action/ demand)

PATIENT		Dependent (Totally dependent)	High Assistance (25+ ability)	Moderate Assist. (50+ ability)	Mild Assistance (75+ability)	Independent (Totally independent)
		1	2	3	4	5
SEE CODES BELOW USE OPTIONAL CODES IF APPROPRIATE		3 cue/ 2-3 physical	2-3 cues/ 2 physical	2-3 cues/ 1 physical	1-2 cues	Encouragement
97530- Therapeutic activities or	**SKILL**	**GOAL**	**OBJECTIVES** ____times per ____		**METHOD**	**OUTCOME DATE**
Therapeutic Activity 97530	FINE MOTOR SKILLS					
97530	EYE-HAND COORDINATION					
97110/ 97530	GROSS MOTOR SKILLS					
97530 If under cognitive code 97532	PERCEPTUAL SPEED/MOTOR FUNCTION					

97530 Therapeutic activities, direct (one on one) patient contact by the provider (use of dynamic activities to improve functional performance),each 15 minutes; **97110 Therapeutic procedure, one or more areas**, each 15 minutes; therapeutic exercises to develop strength and endurance, range of motion and flexibility; ; **97150 Therapeutic procedure(s), group (2 or more individuals**; **97535-Self care/home management training** (e.g., activities of daily living and compensatory training, meal preparation, safety procedures, and instructions in use of adaptive equipment), direct (one-on-one) contact by provider, each 15 minutes; **Physical therapy 97001 evaluation, 97002 Re-evaluation. occupational therapy evaluation 97003, re-evaluation. 97004**

Staff Initials				
Add total score here Maximum Score 20 pt. each form per activity				
See scale below or use own/facilities optional score system				

(Score 1-4)=1 (5-8) =2 (9-12) =3 (13-16) =4 (17-20) =5 If w/device add d if wish, ex: 1d, 2d, or If using 1-7 scale: (21-24) =6 (25-28) =7Current Procedural Terminology © 2005 American Medical Association. All rights reserved. Recreational Objectives Observational forms© 2005. All rights reserved. Patent pending.

Aromatherapy
Socio-emotional Goals, Objectives, and Methods

Skill	Goal	Objectives Sample	Method Sample
Socialization/Community Integration	Increase social interactions, meaningful/fulfilling activities	-will respond with correct answer to two choice questions, will state where they are, time of day, present company of people on own and with a correct answer	Staff will offer residents aroma-therapy for memory stimulation and relaxation encourage residents to socialize with others in the group (if group activity)
Team Playing/Sharing	Increase teamwork/sharing, meaningful/fulfilling activities	-will make eye-contact with staff for _____ sec., will verbalize with staff and instructor	Staff will encourage residents to work together to choose aroma-therapy smells, candles, crèmes, oils, etc.
Initiative and Motivation	Increase initiative and motivation/wellness, and quality of life	-will repeat/recall smells from past experiences	Staff will support and encourage the resident to come to activity in a timely fashion, for their own personal gains -Staff will offer new techniques to motivate
Emotional Gratification	Increase emotional gratification/wellness, and quality of life	-will be asked a question and answer (yes/no, will be asked what fragrance is being used, will interact with peers and staff, will engage in a sensory game, will consider smells and try to swer the type of smells	Staff will ask resident if they enjoyed the activity and what they liked through verbal discussion, group discussions
Sense of Accomplishment	Increase feelings of self-worth, pride, productivity, dignity/wellness, and quality of life	-will request/partake in an aroma-therapy activity, will engage in self-nurturing activities, will continue to accept nurturing from others and to nurture self, will request/partake in activities that involve healing qualities	-Staff will provide the availability and opportunity for residents to experience aroma-therapy -Staff will engage residents in experiences to promote self-nurturing and being nurtured, or for healing qualities, smell, recall/reminiscing
Self-esteem/self-identity	Increase self-esteem, feelings of belonging, dignity, self-worth, integrity, self-identity/wellness, and quality of life	-will choose aromas , smells, candles, oils, etc.	Staff will provide educational materials on the value of relaxation exercises, the healing qualities, and encourage residents to continue the activity.
Fostering Appropriate Behaviors	Increase social interaction, social opportunities and adjustment, safety, using appropriate behaviors during an activity for a calm environment/wellness, and quality of life	-will consider and process smell(sensory of previous sensory experiences or knowledge), will relax (Ex: sit calmly) and do activity for up to 15 minutes	-Staff will take residents to the activity, and the residents will be exposed to sensory stimulating experiences of smell, touch (crèmes, oils), residents will be supported as they adjust to the stimulus one step at a time -Staff will provide an orderly, transitional, calm environment area for solace
Sensory Integration/Tolerating Stimulation	Increase sensory processing and enhance awareness of sensations and toleration/adaptation of sensory stimulations and demands	-will recall/retain , sort/gather information, problem-solve, and complete activity	Before activity begins, staff will discus rules, appropriate behaviors, respect of property, safety, and respect of peers

TABLE 34.3

Recreational Objectives Observational Form
Aromatherapy- Socio-emotional Skills

PATIENT	Dependent (Totally dependent)	High Assistance (25+ ability)	Moderate Assist. (50+ ability)	Mild Assistance (75+ability)	Independent (Totally independent.)
SEE CODES BELOW USE OPTIONAL CODES IF APPROPRIATE	1	2	3	4	5
	3 cue/ 2-3 physical	2-3 cues/ 2 physical	2-3 cues/ 1 physical	1-2 cues	Encouragement

97530-Therapeutic activities or	SKILL	GOAL	OBJECTIVES ____times per ____	METHOD	OUTCOME DATE			
97537 Or 97535	SOCIALIZATION/ COMMUNITY INTEGRATION							
97537 Or 97535	TEAM PLAYING /SHARING							
97537 Or 97535	INITIATIVE AND MOTIVATION							
97537 Or 97535	EMOTIONAL GRATIFICATION							
97537 Or 97535	SENSE OF ACCOMPLISHMENT							
97537 Or 97535	SELF-ESTEEM/ SELF-IDENTITY							
97537 Or 97535	FOSTERING APPROPRIATE BEHAVIORS							
97533	SENSORY INTEGRATION/ TOLERATING							

97537-Community/work reintegration training (e.g., shopping, transportation, money management, avocational activities and/or work environment/modification analysis, work task analysis), direct (one-on-one) contact by provider, each 15 minutes; **97535-Self care/home management training** (e.g., activities of daily living and compensatory training, meal preparation, safety procedures, and instructions in use of adaptive equipment), direct (one-on-one) contact by provider, each 15 minutes; **97530-Therapeutic activities, direct (one-on-one)** patient contact by the provider (use of dynamic activities to improve functional performance), each 15 minutes; **97150-Therapeutic procedure(s), group (2 or more individuals); 97533-Sensory integration techniques** to enhance sensory processing and promote adaptive responses to environmental demands, direct (one-on-one) patient contact by the provider, each 15 minutes; **occupational therapy evaluation 97003, re-evaluation . 97004**	Staff Initial				
	Add total score here-Maximum Score 40 pt. each form per activity				
	See scale below or use own/facilities optional score system				

(Score 1-8)=1 (9-16) =2 (17-24) =3 (25-32) =4 (33-40) =5 If w/device add d if wish, ex: 1d, 2d, or If using 1-7 scale: (41-48) =6 (49-56)

Beauty and Hair Care

Objectives and benefits:

Cognitive Challenges: attention, language, orientation, cognitive stimulation, sense stimulation.

Physical Needs: possible fine motor skills (if contributing to activity), possible gross motor skills (if contributing to activity), muscle stimulation.

Socio-emotional Needs: community integration, self-esteem, dignity and pride, self-identity, personal hygiene/grooming, semblance of past routines, relaxation, solace, nurturing, healing.

Supplies: As needed or brought in by hair care personnel

Time: Varied

Staff/older adult ratio: As assessed per needs of individuals or group.

Instructions: Once per week, or as able, have hair care personnel come to your center. Have haircuts done as needed. Have hair shampooed and set as older adults would like. If time allows they can have their nails done also. You can also do complete manicures, facials, and make-up applications. This may be a good time to ask older adults about any personal care needs they would like addressed. This would be a good time to have these issues taken care of in honor and dignity of their needs and feelings. Be sure the person performing manicures on the residents is aware of those who might be diabetic, have skin conditions or other factors that may require special permissions or precautions.

Reminiscing activities may help improve memory and sensory skills. Self-Nurturing activities can have positive effects on reducing stress, promoting relaxation, solace and be beneficial to physical well-being. Having the ability to address beauty and hair care needs can promote positive self -identity dignity and personal choices

Beauty and Hair Care
Cognitive Goals, Objectives, and Methods

Skill	Goal	Objectives Sample	Method Sample
Orientation	Show increased awareness of, time/"timeframe," people, circumstances, and past experiences vs. present experiences, to engage in present time activities or for a reminiscing intended question	-will respond with correct answer to two choice questions (Ex: "Who used to do your hair, Mary or Sara?") Or yes/no answer, will state where they are, time of day, present company of people on own and with a correct answer	Staff will ask resident a series of questions to stimulate focus to the present setting (Ex: "Are you at the beauty parlor you always went to?") Or past if reminiscing exercise (Ex: "Who took you to the beauty parlor when you lived at home?")
Attention	Show increased attention span, task for function and to engage in meaningful, recreational/fulfilling activities	-will make eye-contact with staff for _____ sec., will verbalize with staff and instructor	Staff will address or stand in front of resident, make eye contact, ask questions or use others forms to get resident's attention
Memory	Show increased memory skills of recall, recognition, retention of information, working memory	-will repeat/recall routines of past semblance, past trips to beauty parlor	Staff will tell resident what the haircutter will do, or haircutter will ask resident what hair style they would like
Language	Show increased ability to communicate use of words, phases, sentence structure, comprehension, interpretation	-will be asked a question and answer (yes or no), will be asked what kind of hairstyle he or she likes and reply to two choices, will interact with peers and staff, will engage in a sensory game	Staff will ask questions to stimulate a communication k: "What color is your daughters' ir?") Or make a command to Interpretation/Lang. skills (Ex: "Can you tilt your head back into the sink so we can wash your hair?")
Problem solving (goes beyond thinking/stimulus and initiates thinking process)	Increase problem-solving ability, processing of information, thinking, reasoning, and use of good judgment and decision-making	-will make a decision regarding hairstyle, haircut, manicures, pedicures (w/Dr. permission)	Staff will engage residents in a grooming/beauty activity experience, and promote hygiene, making choices, decision-making, engaging in activities of past, sensory experiences
Sensory integration/ Cognitive Stimulation (awareness, seeks information in)	Increased stimulus/exposure for visual/ motor memory, cognitive experiences/ awareness and brain stimulation to enhance (function, pragmatics, neuro-plasticity)	-will listen/seek cognitive stimulation, will accept challenge of input information and engage in beauty and hair care activity	Staff will engage residents in a grooming/beauty activity experience and promote interactions, stimulating conversations

TABLE 35.1

Recreational Objectives Observational Form
Beauty and Hair Care- Cognitive skills

PATIENT		Dependent (Totally dependent)	High Assistance (25+ ability)	Moderate Assist. (50+ ability)	Mild Assistance (75+ability)	Independent (Totally independent)
SEE CODES BELOW USE OPTIONAL CODES IF APPROPRIATE		1	2	3	4	5
		3 cue/ 2-3 physical	2-3 cues/ 2 physical	2-3 cues/ 1 physical	1-2 cues	Encouragement
97530- Therapeutic activities or	**SKILL**	**GOAL**	**OBJECTIVES** ____times per ____		**METHOD**	**OUTCOME DATE**
97532 Cognitive skills	ORIENTATION					
97532 Cognitive skills	ATTENTION					
97532 Cognitive skills	MEMORY					
97532 Cognitive skills	PROBLEM-SOLVING					
97532 Cognitive skills	COMPLETE A TASK					
97139 Speech Therapy 97532 Cognitive skills	LANGUAGE					
97533	SENSORY STIMULATION/ COGNITIVE STIMULATION					
97532	PERCEPTUAL AWARENESS					

97532-Development of cognitive skills to improve attention, memory, problem-solving, includes compensatory training and/or sensory integrative activities, direct (one-on-one) patient contact by the provider, each 15 minutes; **97530-Therapeutic activities**, direct (one-on-one) patient contact by the provider (use of dynamic activities to improve functional performance), each 15 minutes; **97533-Sensory integration techniques** to enhance sensory processing and promote adaptive responses to environmental demands, direct (one-on-one) patient contact by the provider, each 15 minutes; **97150-Therapeutic procedure(s)**, group (2 or more individuals); **97139-Unlisted therapeutic procedure** (specify) minutes; **97003- occupational therapy evaluation**; **97004- re-evaluation**	Staff Initial				
	Add total score here -Maximum Score 40 pt. each form per activity				
	See scale below or use own/facilities optional score system				

(Score 1-8)=1 (9-16) =2 (17-24) =3 (25-32) =4 (33-40) =5 If w/device add d if wish, ex: 1d, 2d, or If using 1-7 scale: (41-48) =6 (49-56)

Beauty and Hair Care
Physical Goals, Objectives, and Methods

Skill	Goal	Objectives Sample	Method Sample
Fine Motor Skills	Increase fine motor skills, meaningful/fulfilling activities	-will pick up small items, manipulate materials	Staff will encourage residents to pick up and manipulate materials
Gross Motor Skills	Increase large motor skills, meaningful/fulfilling activities	-will lift items using large motor skills, will walk to group (with device or support)	Staff will encourage residents to lift items using gross motor skills
Perceptual Speed and Motor Function	Increase speed and motor ability for function, safety, meaningful/fulfilling activities	-will increase speed of actions by using skills (Dr. approval)	Staff will encourage to do the activity and decrease reaction times by shortening amount of time allotted, or observation of resident ability increasing on own
Hand-Eye Coordination	Increase hand-eye coordination	-will brush hair, wash face, polish nails	Staff will encourage residents to place items on the craft using hand-eye fine motor abilities and detailed fine motor activities

Table 35.2

Recreational Objectives Observational Form
Beauty and Hair Care- Physical Skills
(If resident participates and exhibits action/ demand)

PATIENT		Dependent (Totally dependent)	High Assistance (25+ ability)	Moderate Assist. (50+ ability)	Mild Assistance (75+ability)	Independent (Totally independent)			
		1	2	3	4	5			
SEE CODES BELOW USE OPTIONAL CODES IF APPROPRIATE		3 cue/ 2-3 physical	2-3 cues/ 2 physical	2-3 cues/ 1 physical	1-2 cues	Encouragement			
97530- Therapeutic activities or	**SKILL**	**GOAL**	**OBJECTIVES** ____times per ____		**METHOD**	**OUTCOME DATE**			
Therapeutic Activity 97530	FINE MOTOR SKILLS								
97530	EYE-HAND COORDINATION								
97110/ 97530	GROSS MOTOR SKILLS								
97530 If under cognitive code 97532	PERCEPTUAL SPEED/MOTOR FUNCTION								
97530 Therapeutic activities, direct (one on one) patient contact by the provider (use of dynamic activities to improve functional performance),each 15 minutes; **97110 Therapeutic procedure, one or more areas**, each 15 minutes; therapeutic exercises to develop strength and endurance, range of motion and flexibility; ; **97150 Therapeutic procedure(s), group (2 or more individuals**; **97535-Self care/home management training** (e.g., activities of daily living and compensatory training, meal preparation, safety procedures, and instructions in use of adaptive equipment), direct (one-on-one) contact by provider, each 15 minutes; **Physical therapy 97001 evaluation, 97002 Re-evaluation. occupational therapy evaluation 97003, re-evaluation. 97004**					Staff Initials				
					Add total score here Maximum Score 20 pt. each form per activity				
					See scale below or use own/facilities optional score system				

(Score 1-4)=1 (5-8) =2 (9-12) =3 (13-16) =4 (17-20) =5 If w/device add d if wish, ex: 1d, 2d, or If using 1-7 scale: (21-24) =6 (25-28) =7

Beauty and Hair Care
Socio-emotional Goals, Objectives, and Methods

Skill	Goal	Objectives Sample	Method Sample
Socialization/Community Integration	Increase social interactions, meaningful/fulfilling activities	-will interact with peers, will engage in community integration experiences (for social skills), will use manners and social practices (for community adaptation), will put coin in bus pay slot	Staff will take resident to the beauty parlor/hairdresser's and support/encourage the residents to socialize through community integration with other residents at the beauty shop
Team Playing/Sharing	Increase teamwork/sharing, meaningful/fulfilling activities	-will share, wait turn, support peers	Staff will encourage residents to wait patiently for their turn at hairdressers, and resident's behavior in showing care and support to others.
Initiative and Motivation	Increase initiative and motivation/wellness, and quality of life	-will choose to get hair cut for grooming or religious practices, etc.	Staff will support/encourage the resident to prepare for trip to the hairdresser's in a timely fashion, for their own personal gains of a haircut/having hair styled
Emotional Gratification	Increase emotional gratification/wellness, and quality of life	-will state that they like haircut, show pleasure by smiling, laughing, and gazing in mirror	Staff will ask resident if they like their hair style and/or enjoyed the trip to the hairdresser's
Sense of Accomplishment	Increase feelings of self-worth, pride, productivity, dignity/wellness, and quality of life	-will request/partake in a hairdressing/grooming activity, will engage in self-nurturing activities, will continue to accept nurturing from others and to nurture self, will request/partake in activities that involve healing qualities	-Staff will provide the availability and opportunity for residents to have a haircut/new hairstyle or honor request of resident to be taken for a haircut, manicure, pedicure (if approved by Dr.) -Staff will engage residents in experiences to promote self-nurturing and being nurtured/or for healing qualities, grooming
Self-esteem/self-identity	Increase self-esteem, feelings of belonging, dignity, self-worth, integrity, self-identity/wellness, and quality of life	-will state/communicate positive feelings about self and nice new haircut/style	Staff will support resident in obtaining good grooming, feeling good about cleanliness, and obtaining a nice hairstyle
Sensory Integration/Tolerating Stimulation	Increase sensory processing and enhance awareness of sensations and toleration/adaptation of sensory stimulations and demands	-will adjust to the smell of hair salon _____ time(s) this week, will relax (Ex: sit calmly) and do activity for up to 15 minutes	-Staff will take resident to the hairdressers, and the resident will be exposed to sensory stimulating experiences (touch, smell, etc.) -Staff will support residents as they adjust to the stimulus one step at a time -Staff will provide an orderly, transitional, calm environment for solace
Fostering Appropriate Behaviors	Increase social interaction, social opportunities and adjustment, safety, using appropriate behaviors during an activity for a calm environment/wellness, and quality of life	-will join in trip to hair salon, will use appropriate behavior for the setting, will sit patiently, wait turn, and stand in line quietly, will quiet down when asked	Before trip/activity begins, staff will discuss the rules, appropriate behaviors, respect of property, safety, and respect of fellow residents while getting hair cut

TABLE 35.3

Recreational Objectives Observational Form
Beauty and Hair Care- Socio-emotional Skills

PATIENT	Dependent (Totally dependent)	High Assistance (25+ ability)	Moderate Assist. (50+ ability)	Mild Assistance (75+ability)	Independent (Totally independent.)
SEE CODES BELOW USE OPTIONAL CODES IF APPROPRIATE	1	2	3	4	5
	3 cue/ 2-3 physical	2-3 cues/ 2 physical	2-3 cues/ 1 physical	1-2 cues	Encouragement

97530- Therapeutic activities or	SKILL	GOAL	OBJECTIVES ____times per ____	METHOD	OUTCOME DATE			
97537 Or 97535	SOCIALIZATION/ COMMUNITY INTEGRATION							
97537 Or 97535	TEAM PLAYING /SHARING							
97537 Or 97535	INITIATIVE AND MOTIVATION							
97537 Or 97535	EMOTIONAL GRATIFICATION							
97537 Or 97535	SENSE OF ACCOMPLISHM ENT							
97537 Or 97535	SELF-ESTEEM/ SELF-IDENTITY							
97537 Or 97535	FOSTERING APPROPRIATE BEHAVIORS							
97533	SENSORY INTEGRATION/ TOLERATING							

97537-Community/work reintegration training (e.g., shopping, transportation, money management, avocational activities and/or work environment/modification analysis, work task analysis), direct (one-on-one) contact by provider, each 15 minutes; **97535-Self care/home management training** (e.g., activities of daily living and compensatory training, meal preparation, safety procedures, and instructions in use of adaptive equipment), direct (one-on-one) contact by provider, each 15 minutes; **97530-Therapeutic activities, direct (one-on-one)** patient contact by the provider (use of dynamic activities to improve functional performance), each 15 minutes; **97150-Therapeutic procedure(s), group (2 or more individuals); 97533-Sensory integration techniques** to enhance sensory processing and promote adaptive responses to environmental demands, direct (one-on-one) patient contact by the provider, each 15 minutes; **occupational therapy evaluation 97003, re-evaluation . 97004**

Staff Initial				
Add total score here-Maximum Score 40 pt. each form per activity				
See scale below or use own/facilities optional score system				

(Score 1-8)=1 (9-16) =2 (17-24) =3 (25-32) =4 (33-40) =5 If w/device add d if wish, ex: 1d, 2d, or If using 1-7 scale: (41-48) =6 (49-56)

Community Outings/Visitors

Objectives and benefits:

Cognitive Challenges: attention, memory, language, orientation, cognitive stimulation, education.

Physical Needs: fine motor skills, gross motor skills, possible awareness of touch.

Socio-emotional Needs: socialization, community integration, initiative and motivation, tolerating stimulation, fostering appropriate behaviors.

Supplies: Generally the community visitor will bring their own supplies. This may be a zoo, pet mobile, someone from an art exhibit, or someone from an animal shelter to name a few agencies.

Time: 60 minutes.

Staff/older adult ratio: As assessed per needs of individuals or group.

Instructions: Information about community resources is generally easy to find. Community organizations generally offer vans to travel to the center. There are usually people who will come from the library, or the zoo, etc. Dance schools will often come and share what the students have learned. You could invite Irish or other groups to come and entertain the older adults. It might be good to check with your local senior citizen centers and see if they have any ideas or resources to offer.

Research has shown activities that help cognition of sensory/motor and speed processing will be geared towards help in visual and motor memory, discrimination, comparison, and categorizing areas. Reminiscing activities may help improve memory skills. Long-term studies (Arbuckle and others, 1998) have consistently showed that stimulating the brain with activities helps cognitive function in a similar way exercise helps muscle function. Staying productive, making choices regarding community outings and visitors can enhance feelings of independence and has been shown to enhance socio-emotional wellness.

Community Outings/Visitors
Cognitive Goals, Objectives, and Methods

Skill	Goal	Objectives Sample	Method Sample
Orientation	Show increased awareness of, time/"timeframe," people, circumstances, and past experiences vs. present experiences; to engage in present-time activities or for a reminiscing intended question	-will respond with correct answer to two choice questions Or yes/no answer, will state where they are, time of day, present company of people on own and with a correct answer	Staff will ask resident a series of questions to stimulate focus to the present setting Or past if reminiscing exercise (Ex: "Where are we? Have you been to the museum before? With whom? What type of museum is this?")
Attention	Show increased attention span, task for function and to engage in meaningful, recreational/fulfilling activities	-will make eye-contact with instructor for ______ sec., will verbalize with staff and instructor, will read/listen to rules	Staff will address or stand in front of resident, make eye-contact, ask questions or use others methods to get/gauge resident's attention (Ex: "Please, stand by the door.")
Memory	Show increased memory skills of recall, recognition, retention of information, working memory	-will repeat/recall prior experiences, will remember event at a later time/date and talk about it	Staff or center educators will talk about items at the museum and residents will talk about what they saw/remember about the event during a group discussion
Language	Show increased ability to communicate use of words, phases, sentence structure, comprehension, interpretation	-will be asked a question and talk about it, will interact with peers and staff, will interpret instructors request and follow	Staff will ask questions to stimulate a communication (Ex: "Tell me about your experience at the museum.") Or for interpretation/Lang. skills (Ex: "What is this object used for?")
Sensory integration/ Cognitive Stimulation (awareness, seeks information in)	Increased stimulus/exposure for visual/motor memory, cognitive experiences/awareness and brain stimulation to enhance (function, pragmatics, neuron-plasticity)	-will explore, listen to information, read signs , seek and accept challenge of input information, and interact in community outing	Staff will introduce residents to stimulating educational experiences and introduce residents to various mediums of arts
Perceptual Awareness	Show increased awareness of depth perception, visual-spatial, acuity for discrimination, comparison, and categorize safety, meaningful activities	-will look at art abstract and try to capture/see the visual fields, discriminate, categorize, compare, etc., will also stay within own space and maneuver around area	Staff will introduce art works that challenge, stimulate visual awareness, observations, staff will also observe how well the residents maneuver around the rooms, onto the bus, use vision-abilities to distinguish, compare painters' works and exhibits, compare works support if necessary
Problem solving (goes beyond thinking/stimulus and initiates thinking process)Problem-Solving	Increase problem-solving ability, processing of information, thinking, reasoning, and use of good judgment and decision-making	-will ask questions, interact, talk about exhibits; will understand instructions regarding trip routine and exhibits by verbal cue or imitation of actions	Staff will talk about the exhibits, offer the residents educational materials and stimulating questions to spark thinking, and offer hands-on experiences if possible
Complete a Task	Increase ability to complete a task	-will recall, retain, sort, and gather information, problem-solve, and complete activity; residents will stay with the group (after being given two minutes to look at each exhibit, will follow routine of walking along with the group)	-Staff will explain the procedure/agenda regarding events they will be seeing at the museum and answer questions regarding understanding to support resident's ability to follow procedure -Staff will instruct, encourage, and make use of adaptive devices if needed, and supply necessary materials and support

TABLE 36.1

Recreational Objectives Observational Form
Community Outings/Community Visitors - Cognitive skills

PATIENT		Dependent (Totally dependent)	High Assistance (25+ ability)	Moderate Assist. (50+ ability)	Mild Assistance (75+ability)	Independent (Totally independent)			
SEE CODES BELOW USE OPTIONAL CODES IF APPROPRIATE		1	2	3	4	5			
		3 cue/ 2-3 physical	2-3 cues/ 2 physical	2-3 cues/ 1 physical	1-2 cues	Encouragement			
97530- Therapeutic activities or	**SKILL**	**GOAL**	**OBJECTIVES** ____times per ____		**METHOD**	**OUTCOME DATE**			
97532 Cognitive skills	ORIENTATION								
97532 Cognitive skills	ATTENTION								
97532 Cognitive skills	MEMORY								
97532 Cognitive skills	PROBLEM-SOLVING								
97532 Cognitive skills	COMPLETE A TASK								
97139 Speech Therapy 97532 Cognitive skills	LANGUAGE								
97533	SENSORY STIMULATION/ COGNITIVE STIMULATION								
97532	PERCEPTUAL AWARENESS								
97532-Development of cognitive skills to improve attention, memory, problem-solving, includes compensatory training and/or sensory integrative activities, direct (one-on-one) patient contact by the provider, each 15 minutes; **97530-Therapeutic activities**, direct (one-on-one) patient contact by the provider (use of dynamic activities to improve functional performance), each 15 minutes; **97533-Sensory integration techniques** to enhance sensory processing and promote adaptive responses to environmental demands, direct (one-on-one) patient contact by the provider, each 15 minutes; **97150-Therapeutic procedure(s)**, group (2 or more individuals); **97139-Unlisted therapeutic procedure** (specify) minutes; **97003- occupational therapy evaluation**; **97004- re-evaluation**					Staff Initial				
					Add total score here -Maximum Score 40 pt. each form per activity				
					See scale below or use own/facilities optional score system				

(Score 1-8)=1 (9-16) =2 (17-24) =3 (25-32) =4 (33-40) =5 If w/device add d if wish, ex: 1d, 2d, or If using 1-7 scale: (41-48) =6 (49-56)

Community Outing/Visitors
Physical Goals, Objectives, and Methods

Skill	Goal	Objectives Sample	Method Sample
Fine Motor skills	Increase fine motor skills, meaningful /fulfilling activities	-will pick items (if appropriate) and manipulate	If appropriate, staff will encourage residents to touch and pick up items during a community outing/visitor 1x wk. using fine motor skills
Gross Motor skills	Increase large motor skills, meaningful/fulfilling activities	-will lift, bend, stretch , etc. when appropriate	Staff will lead group in a sub-maximal warm-up before activity and/or walking activity
Perceptual Speed and Motor Function	Increase speed and motor ability for function, safety, meaningful/fulfilling activities	-will react and follow direction of activity with increased ability and speed (Ex: will put money in machine for pet food at zoo with adequate timing.	While on a trip, staff will ask residents to do an activity with increased speed of actions (Ex: walk a bit faster, pay ticket and sit sooner)
Following Step Patterns/Backwards Forward Movement	Increase strength, balance, endurance, meaningful/fulfilling activities	-will walk backwards, forwards, turn all directions while walking	Staff will ask residents to move back/forward during observation at an event or as a natural progression of actions
Range of Motion	Increase strength, endurance, agility, flexibility	-will lift arms and legs (to capacity-set by Dr./clinician)	Staff will lead residents in a sub-maximal warm up before activity that include flexing and extending muscles
Posture	Increase body alignment, flexibility	-will sit in chair and maintain posture, will stand and maintain posture	Staff will show residents proper posture and ask them to hold body in straight alignment/posture
Balance and Gait	Increase balance and gait	-will stand up without losing balance and walk a safe pace (approved by Dr. and capacity tests) If approved clinical specialist: _____ft. ____________________	-Staff will ask residents to walk on the trip -Staff will ask residents to increase balance by strengthening legs, exercise and being asked to hold body in straight alignment/posture
Cardio-vascular Workout	Increase circulation, blood flow, stamina	-will swim at a safe pace (approved by Dr. and capacity tests) If approved clinical specialist: ____________________	Staff will make sure residents are involved in walking, etc. (as approved by Dr.)

TABLE 36.2

Recreational Objectives Observational Form

Community Outings/Community Visitors- Physical Skills

PATIENT	Dependent (Totally dependent)	High Assistance (25+ ability)	Moderate Assist. (50+ ability)	Mild Assistance (75+ability)	Independent (Totally independent.)
SEE CODES BELOW	1	2	3	4	5
USE OPTIONAL CODES IF APPROPRIATE	3 cue/ 2-3 physical	2-3 cues/ 2 physical	2-3 cues/ 1 physical	1-2 cues	Encouragement

97530-Therapeutic activities or	SKILL	GOAL	OBJECTIVES ____times per ____	METHOD	OUTCOME DATE			
97530 Therapeutic Activity	FINE MOTOR SKILLS							
97110/ 97530	GROSS MOTOR SKILLS							
97110/ 97530/ If under cognitive code 97532	PERCEPTUAL SPEED/ MOTOR FUNCTION							
97530 or Gait training 97116-	STEP PATTERNS							
		Licensed/ Clinician	Dr. approved use only	Licensed/ Clinician				
97110	RANGE OF MOTION							
97112	POSTURE AND BALANCE							
97110 Or Gait training 97116-	GAIT (INCLUDES STAIR CLIMBING)							
97110	CARDIO-VASCULAR WORKOUT*							

97110-Therapeutic procedure, one or more areas, each 15 minutes; therapeutic exercises to develop strength and endurance, range of motion, and flexibility; **97112-Neuromuscular reeducation** of movement, balance, coordination, kinesthetic sense, posture, and proprioception; **97113-Aquatic therapy** with therapeutic exercises; **97116-Gait training** (includes stair climbing); **97139-Unlisted therapeutic procedure** (specify); **97150 Therapeutic procedure(s), group** (2 or more individuals); **97750-Physical performance test or measurement** (e.g., musculoskeletal, functional capacity), with written report, each 15 minutes; **97535-Self care/home management training** (e.g., activities of daily living and compensatory training, meal preparation, safety procedures, and instructions in use of adaptive equipment), direct (one-on-one) contact by provider, each 15 minutes **Physical therapy 97001 evaluation, 97002 Re-evaluation. occupational therapy** evaluation **97003, re-evaluation 97004**	Staff Initial			
	Add total score here Maximum Score 40 pt. each form per activity			
	See scale below or use own/facilities optional score system			

Score 1-8) =1 (9-16) =2 (17-24) =3 (25-32) =4 (33-40) =5 If w/device add d if wish, ex: 1d, 2d, or If using 1-7 scale: (41-48) =6 (49-56) Current Procedural Terminology

Community Outing/Visitors
Socio-emotional Goals, Objectives, and Methods

Skill	Goal	Objectives Sample	Method Sample
Socialization/Community Integration	Increase social interactions, meaningful/fulfilling activities	-will interact with peers for pleasure (for social skills), will use manners, social practices (for community adaptation), will put coin in bus pay slot	-Staff will take residents on a community outing or have a visitor, -Staff will support/encourage to socialize through community integration and pairing w/peers
Team Playing/Sharing	Increase teamwork/sharing, meaningful/fulfilling activities	-will join in on an activity with others and share, wait turn, support peers _____ time(s) this week.	During activity, staff will encourage residents to play, share, and form teams, strategize together, show empathy and compassion for peers (Ex: wait, support w/words of encouragement, etc.)
Initiative and Motivation	Increase initiative and motivation/wellness, and quality of life	-will choose if wishes to go on outing , will choose if wishes to join in activity while on outing, will do activity on own (or with assistance)	-Staff will support/encourage the resident to prepare for outing or visitors by being prepared (dressing, getting items ready) in a timely fashion for their own personal gains of activity -Staff will offer new activities to motivate
Emotional Gratification	Increase emotional gratification/wellness, and quality of life	-will state that the activity is a gratifying experience or will show pleasure by smiling, laughing, deep focus on activity	Staff will ask residents if they enjoyed the activity and what they liked through verbal discussion, group discussions
Sense of Accomplishment	Increase feelings of self-worth, pride, productivity, dignity/wellness, and quality of life	-will use gestures to express pride in self, will talk about what they did or experienced on trip	Staff will encourage residents to join in on a discussion about the event about what they learned, how it applies to them, and how they can help out (volunteer, etc.)
Self-esteem/self-identity	Increase self-esteem, feelings of belonging, dignity, self-worth, integrity, self-identity/wellness, and quality of life	-will state/communicate positive feelings about self, will join activity to take an active role in health though experiences, will join the activity based on own choices	-Staff will educate residents on the value of educational experiences -Staff will talk to residents about what the topics/events meant to them
Sensory Integration/Tolerating Stimulation	Increase social interaction, social opportunities and adjustment, safety, using appropriate behaviors during an activity for a calm environment/wellness, and quality of life	-will adjust to the environment, noises, people, etc.; will show adjustment to stimulus by staying in area with increased timing _____ time(s) this week	-Staff will take residents to an activity and will expose them to sensory stimulating experiences -Staff will support residents as they adjust to the stimulus one step at a time
Fostering Appropriate Behaviors	Increase sensory processing and enhance awareness of sensations and toleration/adaptation of sensory stimulations and demands	-will join in on activity, listen and follow instructions, use appropriate behavior for the setting, wait turn, stand in line quietly; will quiet down when asked	Before activity begins, staff will discuss the rules, appropriate behaviors, respect of property, safety, and respect of fellow peers and staff

TABLE 36.3

Recreational Objectives Observational Form
Community Outings/Community Visitors- Socio-emotional Skills

PATIENT	Dependent (Totally dependent)	High Assistance (25+ ability)	Moderate Assist. (50+ ability)	Mild Assistance (75+ability)	Independent (Totally independent.)
SEE CODES BELOW USE OPTIONAL CODES IF APPROPRIATE	1	2	3	4	5
	3 cue/ 2-3 physical	2-3 cues/ 2 physical	2-3 cues/ 1 physical	1-2 cues	Encouragement

97530- Therapeutic activities or	SKILL	GOAL	OBJECTIVES ____times per ____	METHOD	OUTCOME DATE			
97537 Or 97535	SOCIALIZATION/ COMMUNITY INTEGRATION							
97537 Or 97535	TEAM PLAYING /SHARING							
97537 Or 97535	INITIATIVE AND MOTIVATION							
97537 Or 97535	EMOTIONAL GRATIFICATION							
97537 Or 97535	SENSE OF ACCOMPLISHM ENT							
97537 Or 97535	SELF-ESTEEM/ SELF-IDENTITY							
97537 Or 97535	FOSTERING APPROPRIATE BEHAVIORS							
97533	SENSORY INTEGRATION/ TOLERATING							

97537-Community/work reintegration training (e.g., shopping, transportation, money management, avocational activities and/or work environment/modification analysis, work task analysis), direct (one-on-one) contact by provider, each 15 minutes; **97535-Self care/home management training** (e.g., activities of daily living and compensatory training, meal preparation, safety procedures, and instructions in use of adaptive equipment), direct (one-on-one) contact by provider, each 15 minutes; **97530-Therapeutic activities, direct (one-on-one)** patient contact by the provider (use of dynamic activities to improve functional performance), each 15 minutes; **97150-Therapeutic procedure(s), group (2 or more individuals); 97533-Sensory integration techniques** to enhance sensory processing and promote adaptive responses to environmental demands, direct (one-on-one) patient contact by the provider, each 15 minutes; **occupational therapy evaluation 97003, re-evaluation . 97004**	Staff Initial				
	Add total score here-Maximum Score 40 pt. each form per activity				
	See scale below or use own/facilities optional score system				

(Score 1-8)=1 (9-16) =2 (17-24) =3 (25-32) =4 (33-40) =5 If w/device add d if wish, ex: 1d, 2d, or If using 1-7 scale: (41-48) =6 (49-56)

Movies

Objectives and benefits:

Cognitive Challenges: attention, memory, language, orientation, cognitive stimulation, education.

Physical Needs: fine motor skills, gross motor skills, possible awareness of touch.

Socio-emotional Needs: socialization, community integration, initiative and motivation, tolerating stimulation, fostering appropriate behaviors.

Supplies: A movie, DVD player or VCR

Time: As long as desired

Staff/older adult ratio: As assessed per needs of individuals or group

Instructions: Have older adults take turns choosing a special movie they would like to watch. Although they may certainly watch movies on their own throughout the week, make this time special. Offer snacks, juice, etc. Really celebrate as if you were at a movie theater. If possible, visit a real movie theater or show.

> Research has shown activities that help cognition of sensory/motor and speed processing will be geared towards help in visual and motor memory, discrimination, comparison, and categorizing areas. Reminiscing activities may help improve memory skills. Long-term studies (Arbuckle and others, 1998) have consistently showed that stimulating the brain with activities helps cognitive function in a similar way exercise helps muscle function.

Movies
Cognitive Goals, Objectives, and Methods

Skill	Goal	Objectives Sample	Method Sample
Orientation	Show increased awareness of, time/"timeframe," people, circumstances, and past experiences vs. present experiences to engage in present time activities, or for a reminiscing intended question	-will respond with correct answer to two choice questions Or yes/no answer, will state where they are, time of day, present company of people on own and with correct context	Staff will ask resident a series of questions to stimulate focus to the present setting (Ex: "Do you know what movie we are watching?") Or past if a reminiscing exercise (Ex: "What is your favorite movie?")
Attention	Show increased attention span, task for function; to engage in meaningful recreational/fulfilling activities	-will make eye contact with staff and watch movie for _____ sec., will verbalize with staff and instructor	Staff will address or stand in front of resident, make eye contact, ask questions, or use others forms to get resident's attention
Memory	Show increased memory skills of recall, recognition, retention of information, working memory	-will repeat/recall events of the movie	-Staff will engage resident in reminiscing about past movies -Staff will ask residents about the movie and what they remember
Language	Show increased ability to communicate use of words, phases, sentence structure, comprehension, interpretation	-will be asked a question and answer yes or no, will be asked what happened in the movie and state in proper words and sequence -will interact with peers and staff, will interpret instructors request and follow (Ex: "Please walk to the bus.")	Staff will ask questions to stimulate communication (Ex: "Tell me a bit of what happened in the movie from beginning to end."
Sensory integration/ Cognitive Stimulation (awareness, seeks information in)	Increased stimulus/exposure for visual/motor memory, cognitive experiences/awareness and brain stimulation to enhance (function, pragmatics, neuroplasticity)	-will watch a movie and be stimulated by sights, learning (if learning /documentary, etc.), will listen and seek cognitive stimulation, will accept challenge of input information and engage/interact during a movie	Staff will support resident's needs for cognitively stimulating activities by offering the resident a quality movie
Perceptual Awareness	Show increased awareness of depth perception, visio-spatical, acuity for discrimination, comparison, and categorize safety, meaningful activities	-will stay within own space next to others	Staff will encourage perceptual acuity and visual exercises by offering residents movies to watch
Problem solving (goes beyond thinking/stimulus and initiates thinking process)	Increase problem-solving ability, processing of information, thinking, reasoning, and use of good judgment and decision-making	-will answer questions about the movie, will reflect or comment on the movie, will use processing skills to do exercising program (if an exercise video)	-Staff will take residents to a movie and residents will be asked to follow rules and keep up to an adequate pace with others -Staff will ask residents a series of questions about the movie to stimulate episodic memories
Complete a task	Increase ability to complete a task	-will recall, retain, sort, and gather information, will problem-solve and complete activity	Staff will support resident's ability to do the project by following instruction, encouragement, using adaptive devices/programs if needed, and supplying necessary materials and support

TABLE 37.1

Recreational Objectives Observational Form
Movies- Cognitive skills

PATIENT	Dependent (Totally dependent)	High Assistance (25+ ability)	Moderate Assist. (50+ ability)	Mild Assistance (75+ability)	Independent (Totally independent)
SEE CODES BELOW USE OPTIONAL CODES IF APPROPRIATE	1	2	3	4	5
	3 cue/ 2-3 physical	2-3 cues/ 2 physical	2-3 cues/ 1 physical	1-2 cues	Encouragement

97530-Therapeutic activities or	SKILL	GOAL	OBJECTIVES ____times per ____	METHOD	OUTCOME DATE			
97532 Cognitive skills	ORIENTATION							
97532 Cognitive skills	ATTENTION							
97532 Cognitive skills	MEMORY							
97532 Cognitive skills	PROBLEM-SOLVING							
97532 Cognitive skills	COMPLETE A TASK							
97139 Speech Therapy 97532 Cognitive skills	LANGUAGE							
97533	SENSORY STIMULATION/ COGNITIVE STIMULATION							
97532	PERCEPTUAL AWARENESS							

97532-Development of cognitive skills to improve attention, memory, problem-solving, includes compensatory training and/or sensory integrative activities, direct (one-on-one) patient contact by the provider, each 15 minutes; **97530-Therapeutic activities**, direct (one-on-one) patient contact by the provider (use of dynamic activities to improve functional performance), each 15 minutes**; 97533-Sensory integration techniques** to enhance sensory processing and promote adaptive responses to environmental demands, direct (one-on-one) patient contact by the provider, each 15 minutes; **97150-Therapeutic procedure(s)**, group (2 or more individuals); **97139-Unlisted therapeutic procedure** (specify) minutes; **97003- occupational therapy evaluation**; **97004- re-evaluation**	Staff Initial				
	Add total score here -Maximum Score 40 pt. each form per activity				
	See scale below or use own/facilities optional score system				

(Score 1-8)=1 (9-16) =2 (17-24) =3 (25-32) =4 (33-40) =5 If w/device add d if wish, ex: 1d, 2d, or If using 1-7 scale: (41-48) =6 (49-56)

Movies

PHYSICAL GOALS, OBJECTIVES, AND METHODS

Skill	Goal	Objectives Sample	Method Sample
Fine Motor Skills	Increase fine motor skills, meaningful/fulfilling activities	-will pick up small items, manipulate materials	Staff will encourage residents to pick up and manipulate materials
Gross Motor Skills	Increase large motor skills, meaningful/fulfilling activities	-will lift items using large motor skills, will walk to group (with device or support)	Staff will encourage residents to lift items using gross motor skills
Perceptual Speed and Motor Function	Increase speed and motor ability for function, safety, meaningful/fulfilling activities	-will increase speed of actions by using skills (Ex: walking)	Staff will encourage to do the activity and decrease reaction times by shortening amount of time allotted, or observation of resident ability increasing on own
Hand-Eye Coordination	Increase hand-eye coordination	-will pick up drinks, eat during movie using good hand-eye coordination	Staff will encourage residents to Gather snacks for the movie and feed self snacks using hand-eye fine motor abilities and detailed fine motor activities

TABLE 37.2

Recreational Objectives Observational Form
Movies- Physical Skills (if involves walking, exercise, etc)

PATIENT		Dependent (Totally dependent)	High Assistance (25+ ability)	Moderate Assist. (50+ ability)	Mild Assistance (75+ability)	Independent (Totally independent)			
		1	2	3	4	5			
SEE CODES BELOW USE OPTIONAL CODES IF APPROPRIATE		3 cue/ 2-3 physical	2-3 cues/ 2 physical	2-3 cues/ 1 physical	1-2 cues	Encouragement			
97530- Therapeutic activities or	SKILL	GOAL	OBJECTIVES ____times per ____		METHOD	OUTCOME DATE			
Therapeutic Activity 97530	FINE MOTOR SKILLS								
97530	EYE-HAND COORDINATION								
97110/ 97530	GROSS MOTOR SKILLS								
97530 If under cognitive code 97532	PERCEPTUAL SPEED/MOTOR FUNCTION								

97530 Therapeutic activities, direct (one on one) patient contact by the provider (use of dynamic activities to improve functional performance),each 15 minutes; **97110 Therapeutic procedure, one or more areas**, each 15 minutes; therapeutic exercises to develop strength and endurance, range of motion and flexibility; ; **97150 Therapeutic procedure(s), group (2 or more individuals**; **97535-Self care/home management training** (e.g., activities of daily living and compensatory training, meal preparation, safety procedures, and instructions in use of adaptive equipment), direct (one-on-one) contact by provider, each 15 minutes; **Physical therapy 97001 evaluation, 97002 Re-evaluation. occupational therapy evaluation 97003, re-evaluation. 97004**	Staff Initials				
	Add total score here Maximum Score 20 pt. each form per activity				
	See scale below or use own/facilities optional score system				

(Score 1-4)=1 (5-8) =2 (9-12) =3 (13-16) =4 (17-20) =5. If w/device add d if wish, ex: 1d, 2d, or If using 1-7 scale: (21-24) =6 (25-28) =7

Movies
Socio-emotional Goals, Objectives, and Methods

Skill	Goal	Objectives Sample	Method Sample
Socialization/Community Integration	Increase social interactions, meaningful/fulfilling activities	-will interact with peers, will engage in community integration experiences (for social skills), will use manners and social practices (for community adaptation), will put coin in bus pay slot	Staff will take residents to a movie or have residents choose a movie. -Staff may also put on a special movie for a social theme or purpose. -Staff will encourage residents to socialize through community integration and being paired w/ swimmers/group games
Team Playing/Sharing	Increase teamwork/sharing, meaningful/fulfilling activities	-will join in on watching a movie with others, share, wait turn, and support peers _____ time(s) this week.	Staff will encourage residents to work together at choosing a movie, compromise, and share movie choices
Initiative and Motivation	Increase initiative and motivation/wellness, and quality of life	-will choose if wishes to watch movie/watch an exercise tape, will choose if wishes to join in on unit movie time	Staff will encourage the resident to prepare to come to the movie and be ready in a timely fashion for their own personal gain
Emotional Gratification	Increase emotional gratification/wellness, and quality of life	-will state that the movie or exercise program is a gratifying experience or will show pleasure by smiling, laughing , and deep focus on movie	Staff will ask resident if they enjoyed the movie and what they liked through verbal discussion and group discussions
Sense of Accomplishment	Increase feelings of self-worth, pride, productivity, dignity/wellness, and quality of life	-will request/partake in movie, will engage in self-chosen activities, will continue to accept nurturing/respect of choices from others and to respect own choices/wishes ands nurture self, will request/partake in activities that involve healing qualities	-Staff will provide the availability and opportunity for residents to watch special movies or honor request of resident to have special movies and shows available -Staff will engage residents in a movie experience and promote self-nurturing and self-choice activities
Self-esteem/self-identity	Increase self-esteem, feelings of belonging, dignity, self-worth, integrity, self-identity/wellness, and quality of life	-will state/communicate positive feelings about self and ability to engage in workout, will join and take an active role in health though nurturing, funny movies or exercising movies; will join activity based on own choices	Staff will educate residents on the value of joining activities and encourage residents to join the group during a movie
Sensory Integration/Tolerating Stimulation	Increase social interaction, social opportunities and adjustment, safety, using appropriate behaviors during an activity for a calm environment/wellness, and quality of life	-will tolerate environment noises, lights, and peers _____ time(s) this week, will relax (Ex: sit calmly) and do activity for up to 15 minutes	-Staff will take residents to the movie or put on a movie during activity time. ----- Staff will expose residents to sensory stimulating experiences -Staff will support residents as they adjust to the stimulus -Staff will provide an orderly, transitional, calm environment and area for enhancement of solace
Fostering Appropriate Behaviors	Increase sensory processing and enhance awareness of sensations and toleration/adaptation of sensory stimulations and demands	-will join in on movie/movie with exercises, will listen and follows instructions, will use appropriate behavior for the setting, will wait turn and stand in line quietly; will quiet down when asked	Before going to the movie, or turning movie on, staff will discuss the rules, appropriate behaviors, respect of property, and respect of others

TABLE 37.3

Recreational Objectives Observational Form

Movies- Socio-emotional Skills Socio-emotional Skills

PATIENT	Dependent (Totally dependent)	High Assistance (25+ ability)	Moderate Assist. (50+ ability)	Mild Assistance (75+ability)	Independent (Totally independent.)
SEE CODES BELOW USE OPTIONAL CODES IF APPROPRIATE	1	2	3	4	5
	3 cue/ 2-3 physical	2-3 cues/ 2 physical	2-3 cues/ 1 physical	1-2 cues	Encouragement

97530- Therapeutic activities or	SKILL	GOAL	OBJECTIVES ____times per ____	METHOD	OUTCOME DATE			
97537 Or 97535	SOCIALIZATION/ COMMUNITY INTEGRATION							
97537 Or 97535	TEAM PLAYING /SHARING							
97537 Or 97535	INITIATIVE AND MOTIVATION							
97537 Or 97535	EMOTIONAL GRATIFICATION							
97537 Or 97535	SENSE OF ACCOMPLISHMENT							
97537 Or 97535	SELF-ESTEEM/ SELF-IDENTITY							
97537 Or 97535	FOSTERING APPROPRIATE BEHAVIORS							
97533	SENSORY INTEGRATION/ TOLERATING							

97537-Community/work reintegration training (e.g., shopping, transportation, money management, avocational activities and/or work environment/modification analysis, work task analysis), direct (one-on-one) contact by provider, each 15 minutes; **97535-Self care/home management training** (e.g., activities of daily living and compensatory training, meal preparation, safety procedures, and instructions in use of adaptive equipment), direct (one-on-one) contact by provider, each 15 minutes; **97530-Therapeutic activities, direct (one-on-one)** patient contact by the provider (use of dynamic activities to improve functional performance), each 15 minutes; **97150-Therapeutic procedure(s), group (2 or more individuals); 97533-Sensory integration techniques** to enhance sensory processing and promote adaptive responses to environmental demands, direct (one-on-one) patient contact by the provider, each 15 minutes; **occupational therapy evaluation 97003, re-evaluation . 97004**	Staff Initial				
	Add total score here-Maximum Score 40 pt. each form per activity				
	See scale below or use own/facilities optional score system				

(Score 1-8)=1 (9-16) =2 (17-24) =3 (25-32) =4 (33-40) =5 If w/device add d if wish, ex: 1d, 2d, or If using 1-7 scale: (41-48) =6 (49-56)

Sensory Room

Objectives and benefits:

Cognitive Challenges: attention, memory, language, orientation, cognitive stimulation, education.

Physical Needs: fine motor skills, gross motor skills, possible awareness of touch.

Socio-emotional Needs: socialization, community integration, initiative and motivation, tolerating stimulation, fostering appropriate behaviors.

Supplies: Tactile materials, mobiles, computer screen with pictures, musical tapes, sand table or box with different types of materials to manipulate, scent items, a bowl with strong flavored treats. A fish bowl is also wonderful to have in a sensory room.

Time: This activity can be set up in a room and/or available at all times.

Staff/older adult ratio: As assessed per needs of individuals or group

Instructions: Sensory material can be set up in a room or you could bring sensory material into a group setting. Encourage residents to touch, taste, smell, listen, and observe sensory items.

Research has shown activities that help cognition of sensory/motor and speed processing will be geared towards help in visual and motor memory, discrimination, comparison, and categorizing areas. Reminiscing activities may help improve memory and sensory skills. Long-term studies (Arbuckle and others, 1998) have consistently showed that stimulating the brain with activities helps cognitive function in a similar way exercise helps muscle function.

Sensory Room
Cognitive Goals, Objectives, and Methods

Skill	Goal	Objectives Sample	Method Sample
Orientation	Show increased awareness of, time/"timeframe," people, circumstances, past experiences vs. present experiences, to engage in present-time activities, or for a reminiscing intended question	-will respond with correct answer to two choice questions, will answer yes/ no , etc.; will state where they are, time of day, present company of people on own and with correct answer	The resident will be asked a series of questions to stimulate focus to the present setting (Ex: "Did you just have lunch? What did you have for lunch? Soup or pasta?"), Or past if reminiscing exercise (Ex: "Have you used the computer before?")
Attention	Show increased attention span and task for function, and to engage in meaningful, recreational/fulfilling activities	-will make eye contact with staff for ______ sec. -will verbalize with staff and instructor, will be given an item and use it to show they understand	Staff will address or stand in front of resident, make eye contact, ask questions, or use others forms to get resident's attention
Memory	Show increased memory skills of recall, recognition, retention of information, and working memory	-will repeat/recall items and their known use, will repeat /recall how to use item, will remember how to use and recall item at next class/time	Staff will show steps on how to do the activity, etc., Or game: Teach steps of game
Language	Show increased ability to communicate use of words, phases, sentence structure, comprehension, interpretation	-will be asked a question and answer yes or no, will be asked what color or texture an item is and give a reply, will interpret instructors request and follow	Staff will ask questions to stimulate a communication (Ex: "What color float do you like?") Or make a command (Ex: "Can you hand me the float, please?")
Following Patterns/ complete a task	Show increased cognition for thinking, processing information, and ability to complete a task	-will look at the item, shake it, or do action necessary, etc.	-Staff will show the resident the step-by-step actions to do the activity/game -Staff will give instructions
Sensory integration/ Cognitive Stimulation (awareness, seeks information in)	Increased stimulus for visual/motor memory, cognitive experiences/awareness, and brain stimulation to enhance function, pragmatics, neuroplasticity	-will use sight, touch, smell, taste, and ears to item, will seek cognitive stimulation, will accept challenge of input information and engage in sensory activity	Staff will set up game and have residents use critical thinking to complete the task (Ex: find all the pictures that are the same)
Perceptual Awareness	Show increased awareness of depth perception, visio-spatical, acuity for discrimination, comparison, and categorize safety, meaningful activities	-will be able to discriminate and compare items, and place items on the board correctly, fit into spot, etc.	Staff will support resident with activities that stimulate awareness to visio-spatical fields, depth perception, etc. through the use of sensory stimulation activities (Ex: building sculptures with clay)
Problem solving (goes beyond thinking/stimulus and initiates thinking process)	Increase problem-solving ability, processing of information, thinking, reasoning, and use of good judgment, decision-making	-will sort/put beads on paper with background lights for color/tactile stimulation	Staff will engage residents in a sensory activity that includes problem solving strategies, decisions ex: simple or complex beads sorting for picture
Complete a task	Increase ability to complete a task	-will recall, retain, sort, and gather information, problem-solve, and complete activity by being involved in sensory activities	Staff will support resident's ability to engage in sensory experiences by offering sensory activities through use of sensory items, instruction, encouragement, adaptive devices/programs if needed, and supplying necessary materials and support

TABLE 38.1

Recreational Objectives Observational Form
Sensory Room- Cognitive skills

PATIENT		Dependent (Totally dependent)	High Assistance (25+ ability)	Moderate Assist. (50+ ability)	Mild Assistance (75+ability)	Independent (Totally independent)
SEE CODES BELOW USE OPTIONAL CODES IF APPROPRIATE		1	2	3	4	5
		3 cue/ 2-3 physical	2-3 cues/ 2 physical	2-3 cues/ 1 physical	1-2 cues	Encouragement
97530-Therapeutic activities or	**SKILL**	**GOAL**	**OBJECTIVES** ____times per ____		**METHOD**	**OUTCOME DATE**
97532 Cognitive skills	ORIENTATION					
97532 Cognitive skills	ATTENTION					
97532 Cognitive skills	MEMORY					
97532 Cognitive skills	PROBLEM-SOLVING					
97532 Cognitive skills	COMPLETE A TASK					
97139 Speech Therapy 97532 Cognitive skills	LANGUAGE					
97533	SENSORY STIMULATION/ COGNITIVE STIMULATION					
97532	PERCEPTUAL AWARENESS					

97532-Development of cognitive skills to improve attention, memory, problem-solving, includes compensatory training and/or sensory integrative activities, direct (one-on-one) patient contact by the provider, each 15 minutes; **97530-Therapeutic activities**, direct (one-on-one) patient contact by the provider (use of dynamic activities to improve functional performance), each 15 minutes**; 97533-Sensory integration techniques** to enhance sensory processing and promote adaptive responses to environmental demands, direct (one-on-one) patient contact by the provider, each 15 minutes; **97150-Therapeutic procedure(s)**, group (2 or more individuals); **97139-Unlisted therapeutic procedure** (specify) minutes; **97003- occupational therapy evaluation**; **97004- re-evaluation**	Staff Initial	
	Add total score here -Maximum Score 40 pt. each form per activity	
	See scale below or use own/facilities optional score system	

(Score 1-8)=1 (9-16) =2 (17-24) =3 (25-32) =4 (33-40) =5 If w/device add d if wish, ex: 1d, 2d, or If using 1-7 scale: (41-48) =6 (49-56)

Sensory Room
Physical Goals, Objectives, and Methods

Skill	Goal	Objectives	Method
Fine motor skills	Increase fine motor skills, meaningful /fulfilling activities	-will use fingers, hands, dexterity, etc. when manipulating items	Staff will give resident fine motor sensory stimulating activities, items for smell, touch, taste, vision, etc. for stimuli activities
Gross motor skills	Increase large motor skills, meaningful /fulfilling activities	-will bend, stretch, and do movements if required	Staff will give resident gross motor sensory stimulating activities, items for smell, touch, taste, vision, etc. for stimuli activities
Perceptual speed and motor function	Increase speed and motor ability for function, safety, meaningful /fulfilling activities	-will react and do motor movement of activity (Ex: tap light when makes sound, etc.)	Staff will give resident items that increase perceptual function (Ex: computer games, typing, placing pegs on boards, etc.)
Following step patterns/backwards forward movement	Increase strength, balance, endurance, meaningful /fulfilling activities	ill walk backwards, forwards, etc. If activity requires	Staff will decrease the amount of time waited between actions to do a task
Range of motion	Increase strength, endurance, agility and flexibility	-will lift arms, legs (to capacity-set by Dr./clinician) -will extend and flex (to capacity-set by clinician)	Staff/Clinician will ask resident to lift arms and legs (to capacity-set by Dr./clinician) and to extend and flex (to capacity-set by clinician)
Posture	Increase improve body alignment, flexibility	-will sit in chair and increase posture during activity	Staff/clinician will ask resident to sit in chair and increase/hold posture for 3-5 min. during activity
Balance and Gait	Increase balance and gait	-will stand up without losing balance, will walk a safe pace (approved by Dr. and capacity tests) If approved clinical specialist: ____ ft. ______________________	Staff/clinician will ask resident to stand up without losing balance and walk a safe pace (approved by Dr. and capacity tests) If approved clinical specialist: ____ ft. ______________________
Cardio-vascular workout	Increase circulation, blood flow, stamina	-will play the game at a safe pace (approved by Dr. and capacity tests) If approved clinical specialist: ______________________	If applicable, staff will engage residents in a game at a safe pace (approved by Dr. and capacity tests) If approved clinical specialist: ______________________

Table 38.2

Recreational Objectives Observational Form
Sensory Room
Physical Skills (if resident participates and exhibits actions/ demand)

PATIENT		Dependent (Totally dependent)	High Assistance (25+ ability)	Moderate Assist. (50+ ability)	Mild Assistance (75+ability)	Independent (Totally independent.)
SEE CODES BELOW USE OPTIONAL CODES IF APPROPRIATE		1 3 cue/ 2-3 physical	2 2-3 cues/ 2 physical	3 2-3 cues/ 1 physical	4 1-2 cues	5 Encouragement
97530-Therapeutic activities or	**SKILL**	**GOAL**	**OBJECTIVES** ____times per ____		**METHOD**	**OUTCOME DATE**
97530 Therapeutic Activity	FINE MOTOR SKILLS					
97110/ 97530	GROSS MOTOR SKILLS					
97110/ 97530/ If under cognitive code 97532	PERCEPTUAL SPEED/ MOTOR FUNCTION					
97530 or Gait training 97116-	STEP PATTERNS					
		Licensed/ Clinician	Dr. approved use only		Licensed/ Clinician	
97110	RANGE OF MOTION					
97112	POSTURE AND BALANCE					
97110 Or Gait training 97116-	GAIT (INCLUDES STAIR CLIMBING)					
97110	CARDIO-VASCULAR WORKOUT*					

97110-Therapeutic procedure, one or more areas, each 15 minutes; therapeutic exercises to develop strength and endurance, range of motion, and flexibility; **97112-Neuromuscular reeducation** of movement, balance, coordination, kinesthetic sense, posture, and proprioception; **97113-Aquatic therapy** with therapeutic exercises; **97116-Gait training** (includes stair climbing); **97139-Unlisted therapeutic procedure** (specify); **97150 Therapeutic procedure(s), group** (2 or more individuals); **97750-Physical performance test or measurement** (e.g., musculoskeletal, functional capacity), with written report, each 15 minutes; **97535-Self care/home management training** (e.g., activities of daily living and compensatory training, meal preparation, safety procedures, and instructions in use of adaptive equipment), direct (one-on-one) contact by provider, each 15 minutes **Physical therapy 97001 evaluation, 97002 Re-evaluation. occupational therapy** evaluation **97003, re-evaluation 97004**

Staff Initial	
Add total score here Maximum Score 40 pt. each form per activity	
See scale below or use own/facilities optional score system	

Score 1-8) =1 (9-16) =2 (17-24) =3 (25-32) =4 (33-40) =5 If w/device add d if wish, ex: 1d, 2d, or If using 1-7 scale: (41-48) =6 (49-56) Current Procedural Terminology © 2005 American Medical Association. All rights reserved. Recreational Objectives Observational forms © 2005. All rights reserved. Patent pending.

Sensory Room
Socio-emotional Goals, Objectives, and Methods

Skill	Goal	Objectives Sample	Method Sample
Socialization/ Community Integration	Increase social interactions, meaningful/fulfilling activities	-will interact with peers (if group setting), will engage in community integration experiences (for social skills); will use manners, social practices (for community adaptation)	Staff will support/encourage residents to socialize through community integration and being paired w/group if applicable
Team Playing/ Sharing	Increase teamwork/sharing, meaningful/fulfilling activities	-will join in on activity with others and share, wait turn, support peers (if group setting)	Staff will encourage residents to play, share sensory items, form teams, show compassion and patience to residents who need extra time to adjust
Initiative and Motivation	Increase initiative and motivation/wellness, and quality of life	-will choose if wishes to do activity, will choose if wishes to join in on team game using sensory items, will try new sensory techniques, will increase amount of sensory stimulation after stating own goal	-Staff will support/encourage the resident to prepare for activity in a timely fashion for their own personal gains of sensory stimulation - Staff will offer new techniques to motivate
Emotional Gratification	Increase emotional gratification/wellness, and quality of life	-will state that the sensory experience is gratifying or will show pleasure by smiling, laughing, having deep focus on activity	Staff will be asked if they enjoyed the activities and what they liked through verbal discussion and group discussions
Sense of Accomplishment	Increase feelings of self-worth, pride, productivity, dignity/wellness, and quality of life	-will use gestures to express pride in self, or will talk about their accomplishments of tolerating stimulation/experience, will continue to accept nurturing/ respect of choices from others and to respect own choices and wishes, and nurture self; will partake in and accept healing qualities	-Staff will reinforce pride and recognition of resident's ability to tolerate stimulus by offering praise, listening to the resident about accomplishments -Staff will engage residents in a project and promote self-nurturing/self-choice activities and being nurtured -Staff will provide the availability and opportunity for residents to use meaningful objects or honor request of resident to have special objects/sensory stimulation.
Self-esteem/self-identity	Increase self-esteem, feelings of belonging, dignity, self-worth, integrity, self-identity/wellness, and quality of life	-will state positive feelings about self and ability, will take an active role in maintaining health though exploring sensory activities	Staff will educate residents on the benefits of stimuli and exercise and encourage them to continue to engage in stimulating sensory activities
Fostering Appropriate Behaviors	Increase social interaction, social opportunities and adjustment, safety, using appropriate behaviors during an activity for a calm environment/wellness, and quality of life	-will adjust to the smell, taste, touch, sound, and sight, and stay at activity for ___ minutes, etc. ____ time(s) this week. -will relax (Ex: sit calmly) and do activity for up to 15 minutes	-Staff will be involved in a sensory activity and will expose residents to sensory stimulating experiences -Staff will support residents as they adjust to the stimulus one step at a time -Staff will provide an orderly, transitional, and calm environment -Staff will provide an area for enhancement of solace (along w/targeted sensory activity focus)
Sensory Integration/Tolerating Stimulation	Increase sensory processing and enhance awareness of sensations and toleration/adaptation of sensory stimulations and demands	-will join in on activity, will listen and follow instructions, will use appropriate behavior for the setting, will wait turn, stand, sit quietly; will quiet down when asked	Before activity begins, staff will discuss the rules, appropriate behaviors, respect of property, safety, and respect of fellow peers

TABLE 38.3

Recreational Objectives Observational Form
Sensory Room- Socio-emotional Skills

PATIENT	Dependent (Totally dependent)	High Assistance (25+ ability)	Moderate Assist. (50+ ability)	Mild Assistance (75+ability)	Independent (Totally independent.)
SEE CODES BELOW USE OPTIONAL CODES IF APPROPRIATE	1	2	3	4	5
	3 cue/ 2-3 physical	2-3 cues/ 2 physical	2-3 cues/ 1 physical	1-2 cues	Encouragement

97530- Therapeutic activities or	**SKILL**	**GOAL**	**OBJECTIVES** ____times per ____	**METHOD**	**OUTCOME DATE**			
97537 Or 97535	SOCIALIZATION/ COMMUNITY INTEGRATION							
97537 Or 97535	TEAM PLAYING /SHARING							
97537 Or 97535	INITIATIVE AND MOTIVATION							
97537 Or 97535	EMOTIONAL GRATIFICATION							
97537 Or 97535	SENSE OF ACCOMPLISHM ENT							
97537 Or 97535	SELF-ESTEEM/ SELF-IDENTITY							
97537 Or 97535	FOSTERING APPROPRIATE BEHAVIORS							
97533	SENSORY INTEGRATION/ TOLERATING							

97537-Community/work reintegration training (e.g., shopping, transportation, money management, avocational activities and/or work environment/modification analysis, work task analysis), direct (one-on-one) contact by provider, each 15 minutes; **97535-Self care/home management training** (e.g., activities of daily living and compensatory training, meal preparation, safety procedures, and instructions in use of adaptive equipment), direct (one-on-one) contact by provider, each 15 minutes; **97530-Therapeutic activities, direct (one-on-one)** patient contact by the provider (use of dynamic activities to improve functional performance), each 15 minutes; **97150-Therapeutic procedure(s), group (2 or more individuals); 97533-Sensory integration techniques** to enhance sensory processing and promote adaptive responses to environmental demands, direct (one-on-one) patient contact by the provider, each 15 minutes; **occupational therapy evaluation 97003, re-evaluation . 97004**

Staff Initial				
Add total score here-Maximum Score 40 pt. each form per activity				
See scale below or use own/facilities optional score system				

(Score 1-8)=1 (9-16) =2 (17-24) =3 (25-32) =4 (33-40) =5 If w/device add d if wish, ex: 1d, 2d, or If using 1-7 scale: (41-48) =6 (49-56)

Special Consideration Activities

The following activities will require additional considerations and special safety features. These activities have been separated due to the nature of higher cautionary needs, the necessities to implement the activity beyond general barriers and the need for certified or licensed professionals.

The tremendous benefit of these activities warrants considerations to include these activities for older adults whenever possible.

Studies respectively point to the high value of aerobics for cognitive function. While the first section of this book does include exercise and weight lifting, the use of more intense exercises such as aerobic and formal weight training are included in this section. Today many older adults take pride in not only exercising but more formalized aerobic workouts, weight training programs, Pilates and the use of massage therapy.

Whenever possible a rehabilitation program can benefit from the inclusion of personal trainers to support those living in specialty housing or those joining a fitness program in the community. Personal training, Pilate's instructors and the availability of massage therapists are all of great value to the older adult. All of these activities should be taught and supervised by qualified certified or licensed personal trainers, instructors and therapists.

Fishing is a pastime many older adults lose access to when placed in a nursing home setting or in a community setting due to limited support/supervision and or the family's inability to take them fishing.

Programs inclusive of necessary aquatic therapists/licensed swim instructors and one on one staffing can allow the older adult to continue to benefit from this highly therapeutic activity. The need for high safety has often made fishing a huge challenge, and perhaps at times unobtainable. Depending on individual circumstances the activity may indeed be too risky, unsafe, and unadvisable. You will need to consider all safety issue.

Aerobics, Exercise and Weight Training

Objectives and benefits:

Cognitive Challenges: attention, memory, language, orientation, following patterns, keeping rhythm, perceptual awareness

Physical Needs: fine motor skills, gross motor skills, range of motion, posture, balance, gait, following step patterns, cardio-vascular workout

Socio-emotional Needs: socialization, community integration, initiative and motivation, emotional gratification, self-esteem, tolerating stimulation, fostering appropriate behaviors

Supplies: Weights for weight lifting, exercise tapes, a room with floor mats or carpet

Time: 10–30 minutes as capable and prescribed as a suitable workout time

Staff/older adult ratio: 1:1 or as assessed per needs of individuals or group

Instructions: Have older adults join together for aerobics, an exercise class or formal weight training. Have them warm up for exercising by leading them in them in a sub maximal active warm-up first. This will gradually increase their body temperature, blood flow to the muscles, and synovial fluid to the joints. Then you may lead them in a three to five minute stretching exercise. Have a staff member show the older adults the exercise moves. Have them repeat and follow the exercise routine. You can use weights or to enhance exercise or introduce a formal weight training program. You can also introduce weight lifting as the next level of strengthening in a progressive exercise program.

The CDC recommends that older adults participate in moderate-intensity aerobic activity 3-5 days a week for at least 30 minutes. This will help older adults to increase endurance, strength, and balance. It is also recommended that older adults engage in activities that include stretching everyday and strength training activities 2-3 days per week. (CDC, NCCDPHP. Special focus: healthy aging. Chronic Disease Notes and Reports 1999; 12(3): 10-11. Insert CDC recommendations obtained from aoa.hhs.gov 2005

Aerobics, Exercise and Weight Training
Cognitive Goals, Objectives, and Methods

Skill	Goal	Objectives Sample	Method Sample
Orientation	Show increased awareness of, time/"timeframe," people, circumstances, and past experiences vs. present experiences, to engage in present-time activities, or for a reminiscing intended question	-will respond with correct answer to two choice questions Or yes/no answer, will state where they are, time of day, present company of people on own and with the correct answer	Staff will ask resident a series of questions to stimulate focus to the present setting Or past if reminiscing exercise (Ex: "Where are you in the exercise room, the YWCA or at home?")
Attention	Show increased attention span, task for function, and to engage in meaningful, recreational/fulfilling activities	-will make eye-contact with instructor for _____ sec(s), will verbalize with staff and instructor, will read/listen to exercise room rules, will say yes/no to show understand	Staff will address, instruct, or stand in front of resident, make eye-contact, ask questions or use others forms to get resident's attention/gauge attention
Memory	Show increased memory skills of recall, recognition, retention of information, working memory	-will repeat/recall how to do push ups, will repeat/recall how to do side kicks, will remember lesson at next class	Staff will show steps on how to do the exercise, and ask residents to repeat the actions after an increased amount of time
Language	Show increased ability to communicate use of words, phrases, sentence structure, comprehension, interpretation	-will be asked a question and answer yes/no, will be asked what favorite exercise is and reply on own or with two choice method, will interact with peers and staff; will interpret instructor's request and follow	Staff will ask questions to stimulate communication (Ex: "What kinds of exercise did you do?") Or for Interpretation/Lang. skills (Ex: "Let me see you do a side kick, etc.")
Cognitive Stimulation (awareness, seeks information in)	Increased stimulus/exposure for visual/ motor memory, cognitive experiences/awareness and brain stimulation to enhance (function, pragmatics, neuroplasticity)	-will look around the room, will interact with peers while doing an exercise workout, will listen/seek cognitive stimulation, will accept challenge of input information and engage/interact in dancing	Staff will offer exercises to stimulate motor memory functions
Perceptual Awareness	Show increased abilities of depth perception, visio-spatical awareness, and acuity (for discrimination, comparison, and categorizing), safety	-will stay within own space next to others, will maneuver around room, will put items away in proper containers in associated area, will play basketball and hit the target	-Staff will instruct the residents on where they need to stay in their area of exercise mat -Staff may use equipment (if safe ability) -Staff may use punching bags to help with vision concerns
Problem-solving (goes beyond thinking/stimulus and initiates thinking process)	Increase problem-solving ability, processing of information, thinking, reasoning, and use of good judgment and decision-making	-will follow rhythm of workout, will do synchronized workouts, will repeat the rhythm movements when asked to, will stretch, bend, and move arms, legs, etc.; will use light weights and do a set as instructed	Staff will direct the residents in an exercise using a series (Ex: arm lifts and saying 1,2,3 lift, for following rhythms of exercise workout and timing)
Complete a Task	Increase ability to complete a task	will recall/retain and sort/gather information, problem-solve, and complete activity	Staff will show the resident the step-by-step actions of the exercise, and ask resident to repeat the steps until all the steps have been done

Table 39.1
Recreational Objectives Observation Form
Aerobics, Exercise and Weight Training - Cognitive skills

Patient		Dependent (Totally dependent)	High Assistance (25+ ability)	Moderate Assist. (50+ ability)	Mild Assistance (75+ability)	Independent (Totally independent)
SEE CODES BELOW USE OPTIONAL CODES IF APPROPRIATE		1	2	3	4	5
		3 cue/ 2-3 physical	2-3 cues/ 2 physical	2-3 cues/ 1 physical	1-2 cues	Encouragement
97530-Therapeutic activities or	**Skill**	**Goal**	**Objectives** ____times per ____		**Method**	**Outcome Date**
97532 Cognitive skills	Orientation					
97532 Cognitive skills	Attention					
97532 Cognitive skills	Memory					
97532 Cognitive skills	Problem-Solving					
97532 Cognitive skills	Complete a Task					
97139 Speech Therapy 97532 Cognitive skills	Language					
97533	Sensory Stimulation/ Cognitive Stimulation					
97532	Perceptual Awareness					

97532-Development of cognitive skills to improve attention, memory, problem-solving, includes compensatory training and/or sensory integrative activities, direct (one-on-one) patient contact by the provider, each 15 minutes; **97530-Therapeutic activities**, direct (one-on-one) patient contact by the provider (use of dynamic activities to improve functional performance), each 15 minutes; **97533-Sensory integration techniques** to enhance sensory processing and promote adaptive responses to environmental demands, direct (one-on-one) patient contact by the provider, each 15 minutes; **97150-Therapeutic procedure(s)**, group (2 or more individuals); **97139-Unlisted therapeutic procedure** (specify) minutes; **97003- occupational therapy evaluation**; **97004- re-evaluation**

Staff Initial	
Add total score here -Maximum Score 40 pt. each form per activity	
See scale below or use own/facilities optional score system	

(Score 1-8)=1 (9-16) =2 (17-24) =3 (25-32) =4 (33-40) =5 If w/device add d if wish, ex: 1d, 2d, or If using 1-7 scale: (41-48) =6 (49-56)

Aerobics, Exercise and Weight Training
Physical Goals, Objectives, and Methods

Skill	Goal	Objectives Sample	Method Sample
Fine motor skills	Increase fine motor skills, including: using fingers, toes, hand-eye coordination, and dexterity	-will use hands, fingers, toes in extension/flexion, will pick up small weights	Staff will give residents instructions, and residents will be involved in an exercise workout which includes small motor skills (lifting fingers, hands)
Gross motor skills	Increase large motor skills	-will bend, stretch, and do movements during workout, involving large motor skills (legs, arms, trunk)	Staff will give residents instructions, and residents will be involved in an exercise workout, which includes large motor skills (lifting legs, arms, etc.) (Ex: do 10 sidekicks)
Perceptual speed and motor function	Increase speed and motor ability for function, safety, meaningful/fulfilling activities	-will do movement 3-5 min., will do movement 5-10 min., etc.; will increase own time, will join in on a race game (with Dr. approval)	-Staff will direct residents in an exercise workout involving movement and reaction time -Staff will increase the exercise speed as resident's ability allows (dry approved or safe) (Ex: touch nose 10 x by bending elbow and touching nose)
Following step patterns/backwards forward movement	Increase strength, balance, endurance, meaningful/fulfilling activities	-will walk forward, will turn, will walk backwards, will walk backwards and forwards, will walk backwards, forwards, and turn all directions	Staff will ask residents to walk forwards/ backwards and turn during (support device if needed) exercise routine
For clinician/Dr. approved use only	For clinician/Dr. approved use only	-will lift arms, legs (to capacity - set by Dr./clinician), will extend and flex (to capacity - set by clinician)	Staff will instruct resident to do exercises that include flexing, extending muscles (with Dr. approval)
Balance and Posture (approved by Dr. and capacity tests)	Increase balance and improve body alignment and flexibility	-will sit in chair and maintain posture, will stand using adequate posture	Staff will show residents proper posture and how to hold body in straight alignment/posture
Gait/Following Step patterns/ Backwards/Forward movement	Increase strength, balance, endurance, meaningful/fulfilling activities	-will stand up without losing balance and walk a safe pace (approved by Dr. and capacity tests) If approved clinical specialist: ______ ft. ______________________________	Staff will show residents proper stance/alignment to increase balance by standing still, building strength in lower legs (Dr./clinician approved) (support if needed)
Cardio-vascular Workout*	Increase circulation, blood flow, stamina	-will exercise at a safe pace (approved by Dr. and capacity tests), If approved clinical specialist: ________________ ___________________________	Staff will offer residents an exercise class/workout according to ability and Dr./clinician approved amount of exercise

TABLE 39.2

Recreational Objectives Observation Form
Aerobics, Exercise and Weight Training - Physical Skills

PATIENT	Dependent (Totally dependent)	High Assistance (25+ ability)	Moderate Assist. (50+ ability)	Mild Assistance (75+ability)	Independent (Totally independent.)
SEE CODES BELOW	1	2	3	4	5
USE OPTIONAL CODES IF APPROPRIATE	3 cue/ 2-3 physical	2-3 cues/ 2 physical	2-3 cues/ 1 physical	1-2 cues	Encouragement

97530- Therapeutic activities or	SKILL	GOAL	OBJECTIVES ____times per ____	METHOD	OUTCOME DATE
97530 Therapeutic Activity	FINE MOTOR SKILLS				
97110/ 97530	GROSS MOTOR SKILLS				
97110/ 97530/ If under cognitive code 97532	PERCEPTUAL SPEED/ MOTOR FUNCTION				
97530 or Gait training 97116-	STEP PATTERNS				
		Licensed/ Clinician	Dr. approved use only	Licensed/ Clinician	
97110	RANGE OF MOTION				
97112	POSTURE AND BALANCE				
97110 Or Gait training 97116-	GAIT (INCLUDES STAIR CLIMBING)				
97110	CARDIO-VASCULAR WORKOUT*				

97110-Therapeutic procedure, one or more areas, each 15 minutes; therapeutic exercises to develop strength and endurance, range of motion, and flexibility; 97112-Neuromuscular reeducation of movement, balance, coordination, kinesthetic sense, posture, and proprioception; **97113-Aquatic therapy** with therapeutic exercises; **97116-Gait training** (includes stair climbing); **97139-Unlisted therapeutic procedure** (specify); **97150 Therapeutic procedure(s)**, group (2 or more individuals); **97750-Physical performance test or measurement** (e.g., musculoskeletal, functional capacity), with written report, each 15 minutes; **97535-Self care/home management training** (e.g., activities of daily living and compensatory training, meal preparation, safety procedures, and instructions in use of adaptive equipment), direct (one-on-one) contact by provider, each 15 minutes; **Physical therapy 97001 evaluation, 97002 Re-evaluation. occupational therapy evaluation 97003, re-evaluation. 97004; Athlete training 97005; re-evaluation 97006**

Staff Initial	
Add total score here Maximum Score 40 pt. each form per activity	
See scale below or use own/facilities optional score system	

Score 1-8) =1 (9-16) =2 (17-24) =3 (25-32) =4 (33-40) =5 If w/device add d if wish, ex: 1d, 2d, or If using 1-7 scale: (41-48) =6 (49-56)

Aerobics, Exercise and Weight Training
Socio-emotional Goals, Objectives, and Methods

Skill	Goal	Objectives Sample	Method Sample
Socialization/Community Integration	Increase social interactions, meaningful/fulfilling activities	-will interact with peers, will engage in community integration experiences (for social skills), will use manners, social practices (for community adaptation), will attend the "YMCA", etc.	Staff will take residents to a center or implement an exercise routine to support and encourage socialization through community integration and being paired w/partners and teams
Team Playing/Sharing	Increase teamwork/sharing, meaningful/fulfilling activities	-will join in on a sport game, or exercise with others and share, wait turn, support peers	Staff will encourage residents to share equipment, strategize, work as a team, include all members
Initiative and Motivation	Increase initiative and motivation/wellness, and quality of life	-will choose if they wish to exercise, will choose if they wish to join in on team game/workout, will try a new technique, game; will do all moves on own (or with assistance), but own imitative; will increase amount of exercise after stating goal	Staff will support and encourage the resident to prepare to exercise by changing or putting on sneakers. etc. in a timely fashion for their own personal gains of exercising -Staff will offer new exercise routines to motivate
Emotional Gratification	Increase emotional gratification/wellness, and quality of life	-will state that the class is a gratifying experience, or will show pleasure by smiling, laughing, deep focus on exercise workout	Staff will ask resident if they enjoyed the exercise class to stimulate communication of emotional well-being
Sense of Accomplishment	Increase feelings of self-worth, pride, productivity, dignity/wellness, and quality of life	-will use gestures to express pride in self, will talk about their accomplishments of exercise, amount of weights they can lift, pace, etc. during lunch time	Staff will place a chart on the unit wall or hand out a paper to the residents that reflects "steps to success exercise program" and residents' accomplishments
Self-esteem/self-identity	Increase self-esteem, feelings of belonging, dignity, self-worth, integrity, self-identity/wellness, and quality of life	-will state/communicate positive feelings about self and ability to do exercises, will join class to take an active role in health though exercising, will join the swim class based on own choices	Staff will educate residents on the value of exercise and will encourage them to exercise -Staff will design a wall chart showing swimmers names and personal swim time and endurance
Fostering Appropriate Behaviors	Increase social interaction, social opportunities and adjustment, safety, using appropriate behaviors during an activity for a calm environment/wellness, and quality of life	-will adjust to noises (sounds of equipment, peers), and vibration of machines	-Staff will have residents join in on exercises and be exposed to sensory experiences -Staff will support residents as they adjust to the stimulus one step at a time
Sensory Integration/Tolerating Stimulation	Increase sensory processing and enhance awareness of sensations and toleration/adaptation of sensory stimulations and demands	-will join in on exercise class, listen, and follow instructions, use appropriate behavior for the setting; will wait turn, stand in line quietly; will quiet down when asked	Before exercise class, staff will discuss the gym rules, appropriate behaviors, respect of property, safety, and respect of peers and staff

TABLE 39.3

Recreational Objectives Observation Form
Aerobics, Exercise and Weight Training Socio-emotional Skills

PATIENT		Dependent (Totally dependent)	High Assistance (25+ ability)	Moderate Assist. (50+ ability)	Mild Assistance (75+ability)	Independent (Totally independent.)
SEE CODES BELOW USE OPTIONAL CODES IF APPROPRIATE		1	2	3	4	5
		3 cue/ 2-3 physical	2-3 cues/ 2 physical	2-3 cues/ 1 physical	1-2 cues	Encouragement
97530- Therapeutic activities or	**SKILL**	**GOAL**	**OBJECTIVES** ____times per ____		**METHOD**	**OUTCOME DATE**
97537 Or 97535	SOCIALIZATION/ COMMUNITY INTEGRATION					
97537 Or 97535	TEAM PLAYING /SHARING					
97537 Or 97535	INITIATIVE AND MOTIVATION					
97537 Or 97535	EMOTIONAL GRATIFICATION					
97537 Or 97535	SENSE OF ACCOMPLISHMENT					
97537 Or 97535	SELF-ESTEEM/ SELF-IDENTITY					
97537 Or 97535	FOSTERING APPROPRIATE BEHAVIORS					
97533	SENSORY INTEGRATION/ TOLERATING					

97537-Community/work reintegration training (e.g., shopping, transportation, money management, avocational activities and/or work environment/modification analysis, work task analysis), direct (one-on-one) contact by provider, each 15 minutes; **97535-Self care/home management training** (e.g., activities of daily living and compensatory training, meal preparation, safety procedures, and instructions in use of adaptive equipment), direct (one-on-one) contact by provider, each 15 minutes; **97530-Therapeutic activities, direct (one-on-one)** patient contact by the provider (use of dynamic activities to improve functional performance), each 15 minutes; **97150-Therapeutic procedure(s), group (2 or more individuals); 97533-Sensory integration techniques** to enhance sensory processing and promote adaptive responses to environmental demands, direct (one-on-one) patient contact by the provider, each 15 minutes; **occupational therapy evaluation 97003, re-evaluation . 97004**	Staff Initial
	Add total score here-Maximum Score 40 pt. each form per activity
	See scale below or use own/facilities optional score system

(Score 1-8)=1 (9-16) =2 (17-24) =3 (25-32) =4 (33-40) =5 If w/device add d if wish, ex: 1d, 2d, or If using 1-7 scale: (41-48) =6 (49-56)

Massage Therapy

Objectives and benefits:

Cognitive Challenges: attention, memory, language, orientation, following patterns, keeping rhythm, perceptual awareness

Physical Needs: Relaxes tight muscles, revitalizes skin, exfoliates skin, stimulates lymphatic system, stimulates circulation, helps misaligned bones, detoxes the body, improves sleep patterns

Socio-emotional Needs: socialization, community integration, initiative and motivation, emotional gratification, self-esteem, tolerating stimulation, fostering appropriate behaviors, relaxation, solace, nurturing, healing qualities

Supplies/ professional: Massage therapist or knowledgeable staffs, lotions, massage oils

Time: 20–30 minutes

Staff/older adult ratio: 1:1

Instructions: Talk to them in a soothing voice and gently massage their muscles. Encourage them to communicate. This is a good opportunity to talk to clients about the benefits of drinking water, stretching, and other actions they can do to take charge of their personal well being.

Massage therapy can enhance physical well-being as well as promote healing qualities of socializing, relaxation and solace for positive emotional /psycho-social benefits

Massage Therapy
Cognitive Goals, Objectives, and Methods

Skill	Goal	Objectives Sample	Method Sample
Orientation	Show increased awareness of, time/"timeframe," people, circumstances, and past experiences vs. present experiences; to engage in present time activities, or for a reminiscing intended question	-will respond with correct answer to two choice questions (Ex: "Are you at the mall or at the activity center?") Or yes/no answer; will state where they are, time of day, present company of people on own with a correct answer	Staff will ask the resident a series of questions to stimulate focus to the present setting (Ex: "Is this your first massage?") Or past if reminiscing exercise (Ex: "When was your last massage?")
Attention	Show increased attention span, task for function, and to engage in meaningful, recreational/fulfilling activities	-will make eye contact with masseuse instructor for _____ sec., will verbalize with staff and instructor, will listen and do an action to show they understand	Staff will address or stand in front of resident, make eye contact, ask questions, or use others methods to get resident's attention
Memory	Show increased memory skills of recall, recognition, retention of information, working memory	-will repeat/recall information of past events, current events while talking to masseur, will recognize the masseur at next visit	Staff/masseuse will engage resident in reminiscing about past events if the resident wishes to talk during the massage (Ex: "Have you had a massage before? What activities do you do to nurture yourself?")
Language	Show increased ability to communicate use of words, phrases, sentence structure, comprehension, interpretation	-will be asked a question and answer yes /no, will be asked (Ex: "What is your favorite relaxing music?") and will give a reply, will interact with peers and staff, will interpret instructor's questions and words	Staff will ask questions to stimulate mmunication (Ex: "How many children grandchildren do you ve?") Or resident will listen to soothing music
Sensory integration/ Cognitive Stimulation (awareness, seeks information in)	Increased stimulus/exposure for visual/ motor memory, cognitive experiences/awareness and brain stimulation to enhance (function, pragmatics, neuroplasticity)	-listens and seeks cognitive stimulation, accepts challenge of input information, and engages/interacts in massage	Staff will engage residents in a visit with a masseuse to promote awareness of healthy activities and relaxation techniques

TABLE 40.1

Recreational Objectives Observational Form
Massage Therapy- Cognitive skills

PATIENT	Dependent (Totally dependent)	High Assistance (25+ ability)	Moderate Assist. (50+ ability)	Mild Assistance (75+ability)	Independent (Totally independent)
SEE CODES BELOW USE OPTIONAL CODES IF APPROPRIATE	1	2	3	4	5
	3 cue/ 2-3 physical	2-3 cues/ 2 physical	2-3 cues/ 1 physical	1-2 cues	Encouragement

97530-Therapeutic activities or	SKILL	GOAL	OBJECTIVES ____times per ____	METHOD	OUTCOME DATE			
97532 Cognitive skills	ORIENTATION							
97532 Cognitive skills	ATTENTION							
97532 Cognitive skills	MEMORY							
97532 Cognitive skills	PROBLEM-SOLVING							
97532 Cognitive skills	COMPLETE A TASK							
97139 Speech Therapy 97532 Cognitive skills	LANGUAGE							
97533	SENSORY STIMULATION/ COGNITIVE STIMULATION							
97532	PERCEPTUAL AWARENESS							
97532-Development of cognitive skills to improve attention, memory, problem-solving, includes compensatory training and/or sensory integrative activities, direct (one-on-one) patient contact by the provider, each 15 minutes; **97530-Therapeutic activities**, direct (one-on-one) patient contact by the provider (use of dynamic activities to improve functional performance), each 15 minutes; **97533-Sensory integration techniques** to enhance sensory processing and promote adaptive responses to environmental demands, direct (one-on-one) patient contact by the provider, each 15 minutes; **97150-Therapeutic procedure(s)**, group (2 or more individuals); **97139-Unlisted therapeutic procedure** (specify) minutes; **97003-occupational therapy evaluation**; **97004- re-evaluation**					Staff Initial			
					Add total score here -Maximum Score 40 pt. each form per activity			
					See scale below or use own/facilities optional score system			

(Score 1-8)=1 (9-16) =2 (17-24) =3 (25-32) =4 (33-40) =5 If w/device add d if wish, ex: 1d, 2d, or If using 1-7 scale: (41-48) =6 (49-56)

Massage Therapy
Physical Goals and Methods

****************	Goal	Objectives	***************
Licensed massage therapist only	Increase or support ability to relax tight muscles	-will improve/ relaxation of tight muscles	Licensed massage therapist only
Licensed massage therapist only	Increase lymphatic system function	-will improve lymphatic system function	Licensed massage therapist only
Licensed massage therapist only	Increase Stimulation to the nervous system	-will improve nervous system	Licensed massage therapist only
Licensed massage therapist only	Increase circulation	-will improve circulation	Licensed massage therapist only
Licensed massage therapist only	Improve proper alignment of body/ bones	-will aligned bones	Licensed massage therapist only
Licensed massage therapist only	boost detoxification methods to improve health and well-being	-will support Detoxification of the body	Licensed massage therapist only
Licensed massage therapist only	Improve sleep patterns	-will Improve sleep patterns	Licensed massage therapist only

TABLE **40.2**

Recreational Objectives Observational Form
Massage Therapy- Physical Skills
(If resident participates and exhibits actions/ demand)

PATIENT		Dependent (Totally dependent)	High Assistance (25+ ability)	Moderate Assist. (50+ ability)	Mild Assistance (75+ability)	Independent (Totally independent.)
SEE CODES BELOW USE OPTIONAL CODES IF APPROPRIATE		1	2	3	4	5
		3 cue/ 2-3 physical	2-3 cues/ 2 physical	2-3 cues/ 1 physical	1-2 cues	Encouragement

97530- Therapeutic activities or	**SKILL**	**GOAL**	**OBJECTIVES** ____times per ____	**METHOD**	**OUTCOME DATE**
97530 Therapeutic Activity	FINE MOTOR SKILLS				
97110/ 97530	GROSS MOTOR SKILLS				
97110/ 97530/ If under cognitive code 97532	PERCEPTUAL SPEED/ MOTOR FUNCTION				
97530 or Gait training 97116-	STEP PATTERNS				
		Licensed/ Clinician	Dr. approved use only	Licensed/ Clinician	
97110	RANGE OF MOTION				
97112	POSTURE AND BALANCE				
97110 Or Gait training 97116-	GAIT (INCLUDES STAIR CLIMBING)				
97110	CARDIO-VASCULAR WORKOUT*				

97110-Therapeutic procedure, one or more areas, each 15 minutes; therapeutic exercises to develop strength and endurance, range of motion, and flexibility; **97112-Neuromuscular reeducation** of movement, balance, coordination, kinesthetic sense, posture, and proprioception; **97113-Aquatic therapy** with therapeutic exercises; **97116-Gait training** (includes stair climbing); **97139-Unlisted therapeutic procedure** (specify); **97150 Therapeutic procedure(s), group** (2 or more individuals); **97750-Physical performance test or measurement** (e.g., musculoskeletal, functional capacity), with written report, each 15 minutes; **97535-Self care/home management training** (e.g., activities of daily living and compensatory training, meal preparation, safety procedures, and instructions in use of adaptive equipment), direct (one-on-one) contact by provider, each 15 minutes **Physical therapy 97001 evaluation, 97002 Re-evaluation. occupational therapy** evaluation **97003, re-evaluation 97004**	Staff Initial Add total score here Maximum Score 40 pt. each form per activity See scale below or use own/facilities optional score system

Score 1-8) =1 (9-16) =2 (17-24) =3 (25-32) =4 (33-40) =5 If w/device add d if wish, ex: 1d, 2d, or If using 1-7 scale: (41-48) =6 (49-56)

Massage Therapy
Socio-emotional Goals, Objectives, and Methods

Skill	Goal	Objectives Sample	Method Sample
Socialization /Community Integration	Increase social interactions, meaningful/fulfilling activities	-will interact with peers, will engage in community integration experiences (for social skills), will use manners and social practices (for community adaptation), will put coin in bus pay slot	Staff will take resident to the massage center
Team Playing/Sharing	Increase teamwork/sharing, meaningful/fulfilling activities	-will be given massage, wait turn, support peers _____ time(s) this week.	Staff will encourage residents to wait patiently for their turn
Initiative and Motivation	Increase initiative and motivation/wellness, and quality of life	-will choose if wishes to have a massage, will try a new technique	-Staff will support/encourage the resident to prepare to go to massage center in a timely fashion, for their own personal gains of having a massage -Staff will offer new techniques to motivate
Emotional Gratification	Increase emotional gratification/wellness, and quality of life	-will state that the massage is a gratifying experiences or will show pleasure by smiling, laughing, and/or deep relaxation of muscles	Staff will ask residents if they enjoyed the massage and what they liked through verbal discussion
Sense of Accomplishment	Increase feelings of self-worth, pride, productivity, dignity/wellness, and quality of life	-will request/partake in a massage, will engage in self-nurturing activities, will continue to accept nurturing from others and to nurture self, will request/partake in activities that involve healing qualities	-Staff will provide the availability and opportunity for residents to have a massage or honor request of resident to be taken for a massage -Staff will engage residents in an aroma-therapy experience/project and promote self-nurturing and being nurtured or for healing qualities
Self-esteem/self-identity	Increase self-esteem, feelings of belonging, dignity, self-worth, integrity, self-identity/wellness, and quality of life	-will state/communicate positive feelings about self and increasing health though massage, will join the massage based on own choices	Staff will listen to resident's request to have a massage and will ensure the resident is given the opportunity to have a massage
Fostering Appropriate Behaviors	Increase social interaction, social opportunities and adjustment, safety, using appropriate behaviors during an activity for a calm environment/wellness, and quality of life	-will adjust to the smell and temperatures of massage oils and crèmes _____ time(s) this week -will relax (Ex: sit calmly) and do activity for up to 15 minutes	-Staff will set up the resident to have a massage and for the resident to be exposed to sensory stimulating experiences -Staff will support the resident as they adjust to the stimulus one step at a time -Staff will provide an orderly, transitional, and calm environment, and enhancement of solace
Sensory Integration/Tolerating Stimulation	Increase sensory processing and enhance awareness of sensations and toleration/adaptation of sensory stimulations and demands	-will listen and follow instructions, use appropriate behavior for the setting, will quiet down when/if asked	Before going to the massage center, staff will discuss the rules, appropriate behaviors, respect of property, safety, and respect of peers

TABLE 40.3

Recreational Objectives Observational Form Massage therapy- Socio-emotional Skills

PATIENT			Dependent (Totally dependent)	High Assistance (25+ ability)	Moderate Assist. (50+ ability)	Mild Assistance (75+ability)	Independent (Totally independent.)			
SEE CODES BELOW USE OPTIONAL CODES IF APPROPRIATE			1	2	3	4	5			
			3 cue/ 2-3 physical	2-3 cues/ 2 physical	2-3 cues/ 1 physical	1-2 cues	Encouragement			
97530- Therapeutic activities or	SKILL	GOAL	OBJECTIVES ____times per ____			METHOD	OUTCOME DATE			
97537 Or 97535	SOCIALIZATION/ COMMUNITY INTEGRATION									
97537 Or 97535	TEAM PLAYING /SHARING									
97537 Or 97535	INITIATIVE AND MOTIVATION									
97537 Or 97535	EMOTIONAL GRATIFICATION									
97537 Or 97535	SENSE OF ACCOMPLISHM ENT									
97537 Or 97535	SELF-ESTEEM/ SELF-IDENTITY									
97537 Or 97535	FOSTERING APPROPRIATE BEHAVIORS									
97533	SENSORY INTEGRATION/ TOLERATING									
97537-Community/work reintegration training (e.g., shopping, transportation, money management, avocational activities and/or work environment/modification analysis, work task analysis), direct (one-on-one) contact by provider, each 15 minutes; **97535-Self care/home management training** (e.g., activities of daily living and compensatory training, meal preparation, safety procedures, and instructions in use of adaptive equipment), direct (one-on-one) contact by provider, each 15 minutes; **97530-Therapeutic activities, direct (one-on-one)** patient contact by the provider (use of dynamic activities to improve functional performance), each 15 minutes; **97150-Therapeutic procedure(s), group (2 or more individuals); 97533-Sensory integration techniques** to enhance sensory processing and promote adaptive responses to environmental demands, direct (one-on-one) patient contact by the provider, each 15 minutes; **occupational therapy evaluation 97003, re-evaluation . 97004**						Staff Initial				
						Add total score here-Maximum Score 40 pt. each form per activity				
						See scale below or use own/facilities optional score system				

(Score 1-8)=1 (9-16) =2 (17-24) =3 (25-32) =4 (33-40) =5 If w/device add d if wish, ex: 1d, 2d, or If using 1-7 scale: (41-48) =6 (49-56) Current Procedural Terminology © 2005 American Medical Association. All rights reserved. Recreational Objectives Observational form© 2005. All rights reserved. Patent pending.

Pilates

Objectives and benefits:

Cognitive Challenges: attention, memory, language, orientation, following patterns, keeping rhythm, perceptual awareness

Physical Needs: fine motor skills, gross motor skills, range of motion, posture, balance, gait, following step patterns, cardio-vascular workout

Socio-emotional Needs: socialization, community integration, initiative and motivation, emotional gratification, self-esteem, tolerating stimulation, fostering appropriate behaviors

Supplies: Pilate's equipment includes special machines which uses spring-loaded items to create taut/ resistance. This equipment is used with pulleys, handles and a stationary bike. Special boards may be used to increase balance, and strength. Other items may include large balls, a room with floor mats or carpet, etc. The Pilates workout includes pushing or pulling against resistance while lying, sitting or kneeling.

Time: 10–30 minutes as capable and prescribed as a suitable workout time

Staff/older adult ratio: 1:1, Pilates is done by a certified instructor. As Pilates has become more popular group classes have become more prevalent. However Pilates should be done with a certified instructor at all times.

Instructions: Have older adults join together for aerobics, an exercise class or formal weight training. Have them warm up for exercising by leading them in them in a sub maximal active warm-up first. This will gradually increase their body temperature, blood flow to the muscles, and synovial fluid to the joints. Then you may lead them in a three to five minute stretching exercise. Have a staff member show the older adults the exercise moves. Have them repeat and follow the exercise routine. A certified instructor should only do the actual Pilates workout.

The CDC recommends that older adults participate in moderate-intensity aerobic activity 3-5 days a week for at least 30 minutes. This will help older adults to increase endurance, strength, and balance. It is also recommended that older adults engage in activities that include stretching everyday and strength training activities 2-3 days per week. (CDC, NCCDPHP. Special focus: healthy aging. Chronic Disease Notes and Reports 1999; 12(3): 10-11. Insert CDC recommendations obtained from aoa.hhs.gov 2005

Pilates
Cognitive Goals, Objectives, and Methods

Skill	Goal	Objectives Sample	Method Sample
Orientation	Show increased awareness of, time/"timeframe," people, circumstances, and past experiences vs. present experiences, to engage in present-time activities, or for a reminiscing intended question	-will respond with correct answer to two choice questions Or yes/no answer, will state where they are, time of day, present company of people on own and with the correct answer	Staff will ask resident a series of questions to stimulate focus to the present setting Or past if reminiscing exercise (Ex: "Where are you in the exercise room, the YWCA or at home?")
Attention	Show increased attention span, task for function, and to engage in meaningful, recreational/fulfilling activities	-will make eye-contact with instructor for ______ sec(s), will verbalize with staff and instructor, will read/listen to exercise room rules, will say yes/no to show understand	Staff will address, instruct, or stand in front of resident, make eye-contact, ask questions or use others forms to get resident's attention/gauge attention
Memory	Show increased memory skills of recall, recognition, retention of information, working memory	-will repeat/recall how to do push ups, will repeat/recall how to do Pilate moves, will remember lesson at next class	Staff will show steps on how to do the exercise, and ask residents to repeat the actions after an increased amount of time
Language	Show increased ability to communicate use of words, phrases, sentence structure, comprehension, interpretation	-will be asked a question and answer yes/no, will be asked what favorite exercise is and reply on own or with two choice method, will interact with peers and staff; will interpret instructor's request and follow	Staff will ask questions to stimulate communication (Ex: "What kinds of exercise did you do?") Or for Interpretation/Lang. skills (Ex: "Let me see you pull on the handles, etc.")
Cognitive Stimulation (awareness, seeks information in)	Increased stimulus/exposure for visual/ motor memory, cognitive experiences/awareness and brain stimulation to enhance (function, pragmatics, neuroplasticity)	-will look around the room, will interact with peers while doing an exercise workout, will listen/seek cognitive stimulation, will accept challenge of input information and engage/interact in dancing	Staff will offer exercises to stimulate motor memory functions
Perceptual Awareness	Show increased abilities of depth perception, visio-spatical awareness, and acuity (for discrimination, comparison, and categorizing), safety	-will stay within own space next to others, will maneuver around room, will put items away in proper containers in associated area	-Staff will instruct the residents on where they need to stay in their area of exercise mat -Staff may use equipment (if safe ability)
Problem-solving (goes beyond thinking/stimulus and initiates thinking process)	Increase problem-solving ability, processing of information, thinking, reasoning, and use of good judgment and decision-making	-will follow rhythm of workout, will do synchronized workouts, will repeat the rhythm movements when asked to, will stretch, bend, and move arms, legs, etc.; will use equipment and do a set as instructed	Staff will direct the residents in an exercise using a series (Ex: arm lifts and saying 1,2,3 lift, for following rhythms of exercise workout and timing)
Complete a Task	Increase ability to complete a task	will recall/retain and sort/gather information, problem-solve, and complete activity	Staff will show the resident the step-by-step actions of the exercise, and ask resident to repeat the steps until all the steps have been done

TABLE 41.1

Recreational Objectives Observation Form
Pilates - Cognitive skills

PATIENT		Dependent (Totally dependent)	High Assistance (25+ ability)	Moderate Assist. (50+ ability)	Mild Assistance (75+ability)	Independent (Totally independent)
SEE CODES BELOW USE OPTIONAL CODES IF APPROPRIATE		1	2	3	4	5
		3 cue/ 2-3 physical	2-3 cues/ 2 physical	2-3 cues/ 1 physical	1-2 cues	Encouragement
97530-Therapeutic activities or	SKILL	GOAL	OBJECTIVES ____times per ____		METHOD	OUTCOME DATE
97532 Cognitive skills	ORIENTATION					
97532 Cognitive skills	ATTENTION					
97532 Cognitive skills	MEMORY					
97532 Cognitive skills	PROBLEM-SOLVING					
97532 Cognitive skills	COMPLETE A TASK					
97139 Speech Therapy 97532 Cognitive skills	LANGUAGE					
97533	SENSORY STIMULATION/ COGNITIVE STIMULATION					
97532	PERCEPTUAL AWARENESS					

97532-Development of cognitive skills to improve attention, memory, problem-solving, includes compensatory training and/or sensory integrative activities, direct (one-on-one) patient contact by the provider, each 15 minutes; **97530-Therapeutic activities**, direct (one-on-one) patient contact by the provider (use of dynamic activities to improve functional performance), each 15 minutes; **97533-Sensory integration techniques** to enhance sensory processing and promote adaptive responses to environmental demands, direct (one-on-one) patient contact by the provider, each 15 minutes; **97150-Therapeutic procedure(s)**, group (2 or more individuals); **97139-Unlisted therapeutic procedure** (specify) minutes; **97003- occupational therapy evaluation**; **97004- re-evaluation**	Staff Initial	
	Add total score here -Maximum Score 40 pt. each form per activity	
	See scale below or use own/facilities optional score system	

(Score 1-8)=1 (9-16) =2 (17-24) =3 (25-32) =4 (33-40) =5 If w/device add d if wish, ex: 1d, 2d, or If using 1-7 scale: (41-48) =6 (49-56)

Pilates
Physical Goals, Objectives, and Methods

Skill	Goal	Objectives Sample	Method Sample
Fine motor skills	Increase fine motor skills, including: using fingers, toes, hand-eye coordination, and dexterity	-will use hands, fingers, toes in extension/flexion, will pick up small weights	Staff will give residents instructions, and residents will be involved in an exercise workout which includes small motor skills (hands, wrists, feet, toes)
Gross motor skills	Increase large motor skills	-will bend, stretch, and do movements during workout, involving large motor skills (legs, arms, trunk)	Staff will give residents instructions, and residents will be involved in an exercise workout, which includes large motor skills (lifting legs, arms, etc.)
Perceptual speed and motor function	Increase speed and motor ability for function, safety, meaningful/fulfilling activities	-will do movement 3-5 min., will do movement 5-10 min., etc.; will increase own time, will join in on a race game (with Dr. approval)	-Staff will direct residents in an exercise workout involving movement and reaction time -Staff will increase the exercise speed as resident's ability allows (dr approved or safe) (Ex: touch nose 10 x by bending elbow and touching nose)
Following step patterns/backwards forward movement	Increase strength, balance, endurance, meaningful/fulfilling activities	-will walk forward, will turn, will walk backwards, will walk backwards and forwards, will walk backwards, forwards, and turn all directions	Staff will ask residents to walk forwards/ backwards and turn during (support device if needed) exercise routine
For clinician/Dr. approved use only	For clinician/Dr. approved use only	-will lift arms, legs (to capacity - set by Dr./clinician), will extend and flex (to capacity - set by clinician)	Staff will instruct resident to do exercises that include flexing, extending muscles (with Dr. approval)
Balance and Posture (approved by Dr. and capacity tests)	Increase balance and improve body alignment and flexibility	-will sit in chair and maintain posture, will stand using adequate posture	Staff will show residents proper posture and how to hold body in straight alignment/posture
Gait/Following Step patterns/ Backwards/Forward movement	Increase strength, balance, endurance, meaningful/fulfilling activities	-will stand up without losing balance and walk a safe pace (approved by Dr. and capacity tests) If approved clinical specialist: _____ ft. ______________________________	Staff will show residents proper stance/alignment to increase balance by standing still, building strength in lower legs (Dr./clinician approved) (support if needed)
Cardio-vascular Workout*	Increase circulation, blood flow, stamina	-will exercise at a safe pace (approved by Dr. and capacity tests), If approved clinical specialist: ________________ ______________________________	Staff will offer residents an exercise class/workout according to ability and Dr./clinician approved amount of exercise

TABLE 41.2

Recreational Objectives Observation Form
Pilates - Physical Skills

PATIENT	Dependent (Totally dependent)	High Assistance (25+ ability)	Moderate Assist. (50+ ability)	Mild Assistance (75+ability)	Independent (Totally independent.)
SEE CODES BELOW	1	2	3	4	5
USE OPTIONAL CODES IF APPROPRIATE	3 cue/ 2-3 physical	2-3 cues/ 2 physical	2-3 cues/ 1 physical	1-2 cues	Encouragement

97530- Therapeutic activities or	SKILL	GOAL	OBJECTIVES ____times per ____	METHOD	OUTCOME DATE			
97530 Therapeutic Activity	FINE MOTOR SKILLS							
97110/ 97530	GROSS MOTOR SKILLS							
97110/ 97530/ If under cognitive code 97532	PERCEPTUAL SPEED/ MOTOR FUNCTION							
97530 or Gait training 97116-	STEP PATTERNS							
		Licensed/ Clinician	Dr. approved use only	Licensed/ Clinician				
97110	RANGE OF MOTION							
97112	POSTURE AND BALANCE							
97110 Or Gait training 97116-	GAIT (INCLUDES STAIR CLIMBING)							
97110	CARDIO-VASCULAR WORKOUT*							

97110-Therapeutic procedure, one or more areas, each 15 minutes; therapeutic exercises to develop strength and endurance, range of motion, and flexibility; 97112-Neuromuscular reeducation of movement, balance, coordination, kinesthetic sense, posture, and proprioception**; 97113-Aquatic therapy** with therapeutic exercises; **97116-Gait training** (includes stair climbing); **97139-Unlisted therapeutic procedure** (specify); **97150 Therapeutic procedure(s)**, group (2 or more individuals); **97750-Physical performance test or measurement** (e.g., musculoskeletal, functional capacity), with written report, each 15 minutes; **97535-Self care/home management training** (e.g., activities of daily living and compensatory training, meal preparation, safety procedures, and instructions in use of adaptive equipment), direct (one-on-one) contact by provider, each 15 minutes; **Physical therapy 97001 evaluation, 97002 Re-evaluation. occupational therapy evaluation 97003, re-evaluation. 97004; Athlete training 97005; re-evaluation 97006**	Staff Initial				
	Add total score here Maximum Score 40 pt. each form per activity				
	See scale below or use own/facilities optional score system				

Score 1-8) =1 (9-16) =2 (17-24) =3 (25-32) =4 (33-40) =5 If w/device add d if wish, ex: 1d, 2d, or If using 1-7 scale: (41-48) =6 (49-56)

Pilates
Socio-emotional Goals, Objectives, and Methods

Skill	Goal	Objectives Sample	Method Sample
Socialization/Community Integration	Increase social interactions, meaningful/fulfilling activities	-will interact with peers, will engage in community integration experiences (for social skills), will use manners, social practices (for community adaptation), will attend the "YMCA", etc.	Staff will take residents to a center or implement an exercise routine to support and encourage socialization through community integration and being paired w/partners and teams
Team Playing/Sharing	Increase teamwork/sharing, meaningful/fulfilling activities	-will join in on a sport game, or exercise with others and share, wait turn, support peers	Staff will encourage residents to share equipment, strategize, work as a team, include all members
Initiative and Motivation	Increase initiative and motivation/wellness, and quality of life	-will choose if they wish to exercise, will choose if they wish to join in on team game/workout, will try a new technique, game; will do all moves on own (or with assistance), but own imitative; will increase amount of exercise after stating goal	Staff will support and encourage the resident to prepare to exercise by changing or putting on sneakers. etc. in a timely fashion for their own personal gains of exercising -Staff will offer new exercise routines to motivate
Emotional Gratification	Increase emotional gratification/wellness, and quality of life	-will state that the class is a gratifying experience, or will show pleasure by smiling, laughing, deep focus on exercise workout	Staff will ask resident if they enjoyed the exercise class to stimulate communication of emotional well-being
Sense of Accomplishment	Increase feelings of self-worth, pride, productivity, dignity/wellness, and quality of life	-will use gestures to express pride in self, will talk about their accomplishments of exercise during lunch time	Staff will place a chart on the unit wall or hand out a paper to the residents that reflects "steps to success exercise program" and residents' accomplishments
Self-esteem/self-identity	Increase self-esteem, feelings of belonging, dignity, self-worth, integrity, self-identity/wellness, and quality of life	-will state/communicate positive feelings about self and ability to do exercises, will join class to take an active role in health though exercising, will join the swim class based on own choices	Staff will educate residents on the value of exercise and will encourage them to exercise -Staff will design a wall chart showing endurance
Fostering Appropriate Behaviors	Increase social interaction, social opportunities and adjustment, safety, using appropriate behaviors during an activity for a calm environment/wellness, and quality of life	-will adjust to noises (sounds of equipment, peers), and vibration of machines	-Staff will have residents join in on exercises and be exposed to sensory experiences -Staff will support residents as they adjust to the stimulus one step at a time
Sensory Integration/Tolerating Stimulation	Increase sensory processing and enhance awareness of sensations and toleration/adaptation of sensory stimulations and demands	-will join in on exercise class, listen, and follow instructions, use appropriate behavior for the setting; will wait turn, stand in line quietly; will quiet down when asked	Before exercise class, staff will discuss the gym rules, appropriate behaviors, respect of property, safety, and respect of peers and staff

TABLE 41.3

Recreational Objectives Observation Form
Pilates -Socio-emotional Skills

PATIENT	Dependent (Totally dependent)	High Assistance (25+ ability)	Moderate Assist. (50+ ability)	Mild Assistance (75+ability)	Independent (Totally independent.)
SEE CODES BELOW USE OPTIONAL CODES IF APPROPRIATE	1	2	3	4	5
	3 cue/ 2-3 physical	2-3 cues/ 2 physical	2-3 cues/ 1 physical	1-2 cues	Encouragement

97530-Therapeutic activities or	SKILL	GOAL	OBJECTIVES ____times per ____	METHOD	OUTCOME DATE			
97537 Or 97535	SOCIALIZATION/ COMMUNITY INTEGRATION							
97537 Or 97535	TEAM PLAYING /SHARING							
97537 Or 97535	INITIATIVE AND MOTIVATION							
97537 Or 97535	EMOTIONAL GRATIFICATION							
97537 Or 97535	SENSE OF ACCOMPLISHM ENT							
97537 Or 97535	SELF-ESTEEM/ SELF-IDENTITY							
97537 Or 97535	FOSTERING APPROPRIATE BEHAVIORS							
97533	SENSORY INTEGRATION/ TOLERATING							

97537-Community/work reintegration training (e.g., shopping, transportation, money management, avocational activities and/or work environment/modification analysis, work task analysis), direct (one-on-one) contact by provider, each 15 minutes; **97535-Self care/home management training** (e.g., activities of daily living and compensatory training, meal preparation, safety procedures, and instructions in use of adaptive equipment), direct (one-on-one) contact by provider, each 15 minutes; **97530-Therapeutic activities, direct (one-on-one)** patient contact by the provider (use of dynamic activities to improve functional performance), each 15 minutes; **97150-Therapeutic procedure(s), group (2 or more individuals); 97533-Sensory integration techniques** to enhance sensory processing and promote adaptive responses to environmental demands, direct (one-on-one) patient contact by the provider, each 15 minutes; **occupational therapy evaluation 97003, re-evaluation . 97004**

Staff Initial				
Add total score here-Maximum Score 40 pt. each form per activity				
See scale below or use own/facilities optional score system				

(Score 1-8)=1 (9-16) =2 (17-24) =3 (25-32) =4 (33-40) =5 If w/device add d if wish, ex: 1d, 2d, or If using 1-7 scale: (41-48) =6 (49-56)

Pet Therapy

Objectives and benefits:

Cognitive Challenges: attention, memory, language, orientation, following patterns, keeping rhythm, perceptual awareness

Physical Needs: fine motor skills, gross motor skills, range of motion, posture, balance, gait, following step patterns, cardio-vascular workout

Socio-emotional Needs: socialization, community integration, initiative and motivation, emotional gratification, self-esteem, tolerating stimulation, fostering appropriate behaviors

Supplies: having a unit pet or visits from pets in the community/zoo pets.

Time: This activity can be set up in a room and/or available at all times.

Staff/older adult ratio: As assessed per needs of individuals or group

Instructions: Check with the facility on the acceptability of pets on the unit. Be sure you are aware of all residents' allergies or feelings regarding a visit or placement of a pet on a unit.

If a pet will reside at your location remember to have the supplies the pet will need. This will include being sure the pet has well-check up and is updated for vaccinations.

Allowing the residents to help make arrangements on the pets' needs, can be very therapeutic to the residents. It allows them to feel they can make decisions and offer care to the pet.

Pet therapy has shown to be of high therapeutic value to those in the nursing home setting or within the home environment. Due to concerns for allergies, germs, potential of aggressive behavior (even innocent or accidental) considerations regarding the allowance of pets on a unit do warrants special precautions.

Despite the need to implement additional precautions the value of introducing pets to the nursing home/setting can be of great joy for older adults.

Pet therapy has been found to be beneficial to physical well-being associated with relaxation, solace and positive healing/ health benefits

Pet Therapy
Cognitive Goals, Objectives, and Methods

Skill	Goal	Objectives Sample	Method Sample
Orientation	Show increased awareness of, time/"timeframe," people, circumstances, past experiences vs. present experiences, to engage in present-time activities, or for a reminiscing intended question	-will respond with correct answer to two choice questions, will answer yes/ no , etc.; will state where they are, time of day, present company of people on own and with correct answer	The resident will be asked a series of questions to stimulate focus to the present setting (Ex: "are we on the unit or at a pet shop? Did you just have lunch?" Or past if reminiscing exercise (Ex: "Have you ever owned a pet?")
Attention	Show increased attention span and task for function, and to engage in meaningful, recreational/fulfilling activities	-will make eye contact with staff for _____ sec. -will verbalize with staff and instructor, will be given an item and use it to show they understand	Staff will address or stand in front of resident, make eye contact, ask questions, or use others forms to get resident's attention
Memory	Show increased memory skills of recall, recognition, retention of information, and working memory	-will repeat/recall items and their known use, will repeat /recall how to pet, care for a pet, will remember recall pet at next visit /time	Staff will show steps on how to do the activity, etc., Or game: Teach steps of game
Language	Show increased ability to communicate use of words, phases, sentence structure, comprehension, interpretation	-will be asked a question and answer yes or no, will be asked what kind of imal this is and give a reply, will interpret instructors request and follow	Staff will ask questions to stimulate a communication (Ex: "What kinds of animals do you like do you like?") Or make a command (Ex: "Can you tell me is that a rabbit or a cat?")
Following Patterns/ complete a task	Show increased cognition for thinking, processing information, and ability to complete a task	-will look at the item, shake it, or do action necessary, etc.	-Staff will show the resident the step-by-step actions to do hold the animal -Staff will give instructions
Sensory integration/ Cognitive Stimulation (awareness, seeks information in)	Increased stimulus for visual/motor memory, cognitive experiences/awareness, and brain stimulation to enhance function, pragmatics, neuroplasticity	-will use sight, touch, smell, taste, and ears to item, will seek cognitive stimulation, will accept challenge of input information and engage in sensory activity	Staff will set up animal visit and have residents use critical thinking to discuss where the pet can visit, what supplies the pet will need while on visit
Perceptual Awareness	Show increased awareness of depth perception, visio-spatical, acuity for discrimination, comparison, and categorize safety, meaningful activities	-will be able to discriminate and compare items, and place items on the board correctly, fit into spot, etc.	Staff will support resident with activities that stimulate awareness to visio-spatical fields, depth perception, etc. through the use of sensory stimulation activities
Problem solving (goes beyond thinking/stimulus and initiates thinking process)	Increase problem-solving ability, processing of information, thinking, reasoning, and use of good judgment, decision-making	-will sort/put beads on paper with background lights for color/tactile stimulation	Staff will engage residents in a sensory activity that includes problem solving strategies, decisions ex: simple or complex decisions on animal visit ex: where visit will take place, kind of animal
Complete a task	Increase ability to complete a task	-will recall, retain, sort, and gather information, problem-solve, and complete activity by being involved in sensory activities	Staff will support resident's ability to engage in sensory experiences by offering sensory activities through use of pet visits or a unit pet

TABLE 42.1

Recreational Objectives Observational Form
Pet Therapy - Cognitive skills

PATIENT		Dependent (Totally dependent)	High Assistance (25+ ability)	Moderate Assist. (50+ ability)	Mild Assistance (75+ability)	Independent (Totally independent)			
SEE CODES BELOW USE OPTIONAL CODES IF APPROPRIATE		1	2	3	4	5			
		3 cue/ 2-3 physical	2-3 cues/ 2 physical	2-3 cues/ 1 physical	1-2 cues	Encouragement			
97530- Therapeutic activities or	**SKILL**	**GOAL**	**OBJECTIVES** ____times per ____		**METHOD**	**OUTCOME DATE**			
97532 Cognitive skills	ORIENTATION								
97532 Cognitive skills	ATTENTION								
97532 Cognitive skills	MEMORY								
97532 Cognitive skills	PROBLEM-SOLVING								
97532 Cognitive skills	COMPLETE A TASK								
97139 Speech Therapy 97532 Cognitive skills	LANGUAGE								
97533	SENSORY STIMULATION/ COGNITIVE STIMULATION								
97532	PERCEPTUAL AWARENESS								

97532-Development of cognitive skills to improve attention, memory, problem-solving, includes compensatory training and/or sensory integrative activities, direct (one-on-one) patient contact by the provider, each 15 minutes; **97530-Therapeutic activities**, direct (one-on-one) patient contact by the provider (use of dynamic activities to improve functional performance), each 15 minutes; **97533-Sensory integration techniques** to enhance sensory processing and promote adaptive responses to environmental demands, direct (one-on-one) patient contact by the provider, each 15 minutes; **97150-Therapeutic procedure(s)**, group (2 or more individuals); **97139-Unlisted therapeutic procedure** (specify) minutes; **97003- occupational therapy evaluation**; **97004- re-evaluation**	Staff Initial				
	Add total score here -Maximum Score 40 pt. each form per activity				
	See scale below or use own/facilities optional score system				

(Score 1-8)=1 (9-16) =2 (17-24) =3 (25-32) =4 (33-40) =5 If w/device add d if wish, ex: 1d, 2d, or If using 1-7 scale: (41-48) =6 (49-56)

Pet Therapy
Physical Goals, Objectives, and Methods

Skill	Goal	Objectives	Method
Fine motor skills	Increase fine motor skills, meaningful /fulfilling activities	-will pet animals, possible use items to feed pet.	Staff will give resident fine motor sensory stimulating activities including pet visits and handling of pets.
Gross motor skills	Increase large motor skills, meaningful /fulfilling activities	-will bend, stretch, lift pet	Staff will give resident gross motor sensory stimulating activities, items for smell, touch, taste, vision, etc. for stimuli activities
Perceptual speed and motor function	Increase speed and motor ability for function, safety, meaningful /fulfilling activities	-will react and do motor movement of activity (Ex: lift pet)	Staff will give resident items that increase perceptual function (Ex: computer games, typing, placing pegs on boards, etc.)
Following step patterns/backwards forward movement	Increase strength, balance, endurance, meaningful /fulfilling activities	ill walk backwards, forward If activity requires	Staff will decrease the amount of time waited between actions to do a task
Range of motion	Increase strength, endurance, agility and flexibility	-will lift arms, legs (to capacity-set by Dr./clinician) -will extend and flex (to capacity-set by clinician)	Staff/Clinician will ask resident to lift arms and legs (to capacity-set by Dr./clinician) and to extend and flex (to capacity-set by clinician)
Posture	Increase improve body alignment, flexibility	-will sit in chair and increase posture during activity	Staff/clinician will ask resident to sit in chair and increase/hold posture for 3-5 min. during activity
Balance and Gait	Increase balance and gait	-will stand up without losing balance, will walk a safe pace (approved by Dr. and capacity tests) If approved clinical specialist: ____ ft. ______________________	Staff/clinician will ask resident to stand up without losing balance and walk a safe pace (approved by Dr. and capacity tests) If approved clinical specialist: ____ ft. ______________________
Cardio-vascular workout	Increase circulation, blood flow, stamina	-will play the game at a safe pace (approved by Dr. and capacity tests) If approved clinical specialist: ______________________	If applicable, staff will engage residents in a game at a safe pace (approved by Dr. and capacity tests) If approved clinical specialist: ______________________

TABLE 42.2

Recreational Objectives Observational Form
Pet Therapy

PHYSICAL SKILLS (IF RESIDENT PARTICIPATES AND EXHIBITS ACTIONS/ DEMAND)

PATIENT		Dependent (Totally dependent)	High Assistance (25+ ability)	Moderate Assist. (50+ ability)	Mild Assistance (75+ability)	Independent (Totally independent)			
		1	2	3	4	5			
SEE CODES BELOW USE OPTIONAL CODES IF APPROPRIATE		3 cue/ 2-3 physical	2-3 cues/ 2 physical	2-3 cues/ 1 physical	1-2 cues	Encouragement			
97530- Therapeutic activities or	SKILL	GOAL	OBJECTIVES ____times per ____		METHOD	OUTCOME DATE			
Therapeutic Activity 97530	FINE MOTOR SKILLS								
97530	EYE-HAND COORDINATION								
97110/ 97530	GROSS MOTOR SKILLS								
97530 If under cognitive code 97532	PERCEPTUAL SPEED/MOTOR FUNCTION								

97530 Therapeutic activities, direct (one on one) patient contact by the provider (use of dynamic activities to improve functional performance),each 15 minutes; **97110 Therapeutic procedure, one or more areas**, each 15 minutes; therapeutic exercises to develop strength and endurance, range of motion and flexibility; ; **97150 Therapeutic procedure(s), group (2 or more individuals**; **97535-Self care/home management training** (e.g., activities of daily living and compensatory training, meal preparation, safety procedures, and instructions in use of adaptive equipment), direct (one-on-one) contact by provider, each 15 minutes; **Physical therapy 97001 evaluation, 97002 Re-evaluation. occupational therapy evaluation 97003, re-evaluation. 97004**	Staff Initials				
	Add total score here Maximum Score 20 pt. each form per activity				
	See scale below or use own/facilities optional score system				

(Score 1-4)=1 (5-8) =2 (9-12) =3 (13-16) =4 (17-20) =5 If w/device add d if wish, ex: 1d, 2d, or If using 1-7 scale: (21-24) =6 (25-28) =7Current Procedural Terminology © 2005 American Medical Association. All rights reserved. Recreational Objectives Observational forms© 2005. All rights reserved. Patent pending.

Pet Therapy
Socio-emotional Goals, Objectives, and Methods

Skill	Goal	Objectives Sample	Method Sample
Socialization/Community Integration	Increase social interactions, meaningful/fulfilling activities	-will interact with peers (if group setting), will engage in community integration experiences (for social skills); will use manners, social practices (for community adaptation)	Staff will support/encourage residents to socialize through community integration and being paired w/group if applicable. -Staff will invite residents to stroke, pet, engage in activity w pets
Team Playing/Sharing	Increase teamwork/sharing, meaningful/fulfilling activities	-will join in on activity with others and share, wait turn, support peers (if group setting)	Staff will encourage residents to share pets, show compassion and patience to residents who need extra time to adjust to pet visit
Initiative and Motivation	Increase initiative and motivation/wellness, and quality of life	-will choose if wishes to do activity, will choose if wishes to join in on team game using sensory items, will try new sensory techniques, will increase amount of sensory stimulation after stating own goal	-Staff will support/encourage the resident to prepare for activity in a timely fashion for their own personal gains of sensory stimulation - Staff will offer new techniques to motivate
Emotional Gratification	Increase emotional gratification/wellness, and quality of life	-will state that the sensory experience is gratifying or will show pleasure by smiling, laughing, having deep focus on activity	Staff will be asked if they enjoyed the activities and what they liked through verbal discussion and group discussions
Sense of Accomplishment	Increase feelings of self-worth, pride, productivity, dignity/wellness, and quality of life	-will use gestures to express pride in self, or will talk about their accomplishments of tolerating stimulation/experience, will continue to accept nurturing/ respect of choices from others and to respect own choices and wishes, and nurture self; will partake in and accept healing qualities	-Staff will reinforce pride and recognition of resident's ability to tolerate stimulus by offering praise, listening to the resident about accomplishments -Staff will engage residents in a pet therapeutic experience and promote self-nurturing/self-choice activities and being nurtured -Staff will provide the availability and opportunity for residents to spend time with pets or honor request of resident to have special time with pets.
Self-esteem/self-identity	Increase self-esteem, feelings of belonging, dignity, self-worth, integrity, self-identity/wellness, and quality of life	-will state positive feelings about self and ability, will take an active role in maintaining health though exploring sensory activities	Staff will educate residents on the benefits of stimuli and encourage them to continue to engage in stimulating sensory activities
Fostering Appropriate Behaviors	Increase social interaction, social opportunities and adjustment, safety, using appropriate behaviors during an activity for a calm environment/wellness, and quality of life	-will adjust to the smell, taste, touch, sound, and sight, and stay at activity for ___ minutes, etc. ____ time(s) this week. -will relax (Ex: sit calmly) and do activity for up to 15 minutes	-Staff will be involved in a sensory activity and will expose residents to sensory stimulating experiences -Staff will support residents as they adjust to the stimulus one step at a time -Staff will provide an orderly, transitional, and calm environment -Staff will provide an area for enhancement of solace (along w/targeted sensory activity focus)
Sensory Integration/Tolerating Stimulation	Increase sensory processing and enhance awareness of sensations and toleration/adaptation of sensory stimulations and demands	-will join in on activity, will listen and follow instructions, will use appropriate behavior for the setting, will wait turn, stand, sit quietly; will quiet down when asked	Before activity begins, staff will discuss the rules, appropriate behaviors, respect of property, safety, and respect of fellow peers and pets

TABLE 42.3

Recreational Objectives Observational Form
Pet Therapy - Socio-emotional Skills

PATIENT	Dependent (Totally dependent)	High Assistance (25+ ability)	Moderate Assist. (50+ ability)	Mild Assistance (75+ability)	Independent (Totally independent.)
SEE CODES BELOW USE OPTIONAL CODES IF APPROPRIATE	1	2	3	4	5
	3 cue/ 2-3 physical	2-3 cues/ 2 physical	2-3 cues/ 1 physical	1-2 cues	Encouragement

97530-Therapeutic activities or	SKILL	GOAL	OBJECTIVES ____times per ____	METHOD	OUTCOME DATE			
97537 Or 97535	SOCIALIZATION/ COMMUNITY INTEGRATION							
97537 Or 97535	TEAM PLAYING /SHARING							
97537 Or 97535	INITIATIVE AND MOTIVATION							
97537 Or 97535	EMOTIONAL GRATIFICATION							
97537 Or 97535	SENSE OF ACCOMPLISHM ENT							
97537 Or 97535	SELF-ESTEEM/ SELF-IDENTITY							
97537 Or 97535	FOSTERING APPROPRIATE BEHAVIORS							
97533	SENSORY INTEGRATION/ TOLERATING							

97537-Community/work reintegration training (e.g., shopping, transportation, money management, avocational activities and/or work environment/modification analysis, work task analysis), direct (one-on-one) contact by provider, each 15 minutes; **97535-Self care/home management training** (e.g., activities of daily living and compensatory training, meal preparation, safety procedures, and instructions in use of adaptive equipment), direct (one-on-one) contact by provider, each 15 minutes; **97530-Therapeutic activities, direct (one-on-one)** patient contact by the provider (use of dynamic activities to improve functional performance), each 15 minutes; **97150-Therapeutic procedure(s), group (2 or more individuals); 97533-Sensory integration techniques** to enhance sensory processing and promote adaptive responses to environmental demands, direct (one-on-one) patient contact by the provider, each 15 minutes; **occupational therapy evaluation 97003, re-evaluation . 97004**	Staff Initial			
	Add total score here-Maximum Score 40 pt. each form per activity			
	See scale below or use own/facilities optional score system			

(Score 1-8)=1 (9-16) =2 (17-24) =3 (25-32) =4 (33-40) =5 If w/device add d if wish, ex: 1d, 2d, or If using 1-7 scale: (41-48) =6 (49-56)

Fishing

Objectives and benefits:

Cognitive Challenges: attention, memory, language, orientation, following patterns, keeping rhythm, perceptual awareness

Physical Needs: fine motor skills, gross motor skills, range of motion, posture, balance, gait, following step patterns, cardio-vascular workout

Socio-emotional Needs: socialization, community integration, initiative and motivation, emotional gratification, self-esteem, tolerating stimulation, fostering appropriate behaviors

Supplies: Certified swim instructors with all protocol and guidelines of established licensing for swim courses. Availability of small pond. First aid supplies, swim vest, good sneakers, and weather-suitable outfit. If you will be fishing for an extended time period, remember to bring drinks, snacks, necessary safety equipment and supplies. Be responsible, plan ahead and always use "defensive safety strategies" to ensure the older adults safety.

Time: 20–30 minutes

Staff/older adult ratio: This activity requires full supervision of a certified swim instructor at all times. It is very important to pay close attention to the whereabouts and safety of the residents while fishing. They could fall in the water or wander off.

Depending on residents/older adult's abilities, you may need to only fish within a safe circumstances/environment.

Also, be careful of weather changes while on the fishing trip. Keep in mind the different strengths of the residents. It is best to use caution and maintain a one on one staff ratio at all times. This activity could be a special activity planned as a special get away for one resident at a time or a limited number of residents at a time with a ratio of one patient and one staff. Staff must also educate residents on safety practices when casting the line, using caution regarding hooks on the end of the fishing line, distance to others when tossing the line. Caution will also be required regarding the placement of fishing bait onto the line. This may need to be done by the staff. Any injury even a possible nick by a hook should be cleaned and treated with safe antibacterial crème. Depending on protocol and regulations, you may not be able to bring the fish back to the "center". You need to be aware of the guidelines of your particular site/state, etc.

Time: 20–30 minutes or as needed

Instructions: Have them warm up for activity by leading them in a sub maximal active warm-up first. This will gradually increase their body temperature, blood flow to the muscles, and synovial fluid to the joints. You may then lead them in a three to five minute stretching exercise. The activity could be done as a freestyle activity that allows older adults to fish at their own pace, with peers for with the help of instructor.

Due to medications, or falling potential, older adults should be supervised very carefully. Older adults with restrictions may be able to use special equipment available for the use of the physically challenged. Some of these items may include one-hand fishing rods, special wheelchairs to help the resident gain access to a pond area. Please read the adaptive equipment section for suggestions.

Many elders may be "fishing experts" and can offer much help and advice to fellow fishing buddies. In many states fishing licenses are discounted for seniors and disabled adults. Facilities may qualify for facility fishing permits. Please check in your state for particular information. You may find this information by looking up parks and recreation centers in your state.

Research has shown activities that help cognition of sensory/motor and speed processing will be geared towards help in visual and motor memory, discrimination, comparison, and categorizing areas. Reminiscing activities may help improve memory skills and be beneficial to physical well-being (relaxation, solace etc.)

Fishing
Cognitive Goals, Objectives, and Methods

Skill	Goal	Objectives Sample	Method Sample
Orientation	Show increased awareness of, time/"timeframe," people, circumstances, and past experiences vs. present experiences, to engage in present-time activities, or for a reminiscing intended question	-will respond with correct answer to two choice questions (Ex: "Are you at the mall or at the sports center?") Or yes/no answer, will state where they are, time of day, present company of people on own and with the correct answer	Staff will ask residents a series of questions to stimulate focus to the present setting, Or past if reminiscing exercise (Ex: "When have you gone fishing before? Where are we?")
Attention	Show increased attention span, task for function, and to engage in meaningful, recreational/fulfilling activities	-will make eye-contact with instructor for _____ sec(s), will verbalize with staff, will read/listen to rules, will say yes/no to show understand	Staff will address or stand in front of resident, make eye-contact, ask questions, or use others methods to get resident's attention/gauge attention
Memory	Show increased memory skills of recall, recognition, retention of information, working memory	-will repeat/recall and retain rules, will repeat /recall how to cast the line , will remember lesson at next class	Staff will show steps on how to play the game and ask residents to repeat the actions
Language	Show increased ability to communicate use of words, phrases, sentence structure, comprehension, interpretation	-will be asked a question and answer yes/no to a two choice question; will interact with peers and staff, will interpret instructor's request and follow directions	Staff will ask questions to stimulate a communication (Ex: "Do you like to fish?",, what your favorite part of fishing?) Or for Interpretation/Lang. skills (Ex: "Hand me the net please ,,)
Cognitive Stimulation (awareness, seeks information in)	Increased stimulus/exposure for visual/ motor memory, cognitive experiences/awareness and brain stimulation to enhance (function, pragmatics, neuron-plasticity)	-will listen/seek cognitive stimulation, will accept challenge of input information and engage/interact in game	Staff will provide equipment to fish and introduce residents to stimulation experiences
Perceptual Awareness	Show increased abilities of depth perception, visual-spatial awareness, and acuity (for discrimination, comparison, and categorizing), safety	-will gauge distance to cast line). will stay within own space next to others, will maneuver around peers, net	-Staff will instruct the residents on where they need to stay in their area -Staff will use the game to help residents understand/practice/ increase depth perception skills -Staff will talk about safety factors regarding fishing hooks and safety to others.
Problem-solving (goes beyond thinking/stimulus and initiates thinking process)	Increase problem-solving ability, processing of information, thinking, reasoning, and use of good judgment and decision-making	-will use good judgment of speed and motor coordination, movement or strength and distance to hit club/ to hole; will consider dimensions, force of arm strength to aim/swing; will consider strategies to hit the ball	-Staff will direct the residents on using a series of techniques for golf -Staff will answer questions regarding understanding of steps and offer the residents challenging strategies for processing info, step judgments -Staff will have residents attempt to hit the ball, considering dimensions, strategies
Complete a Task	Increase ability to complete a task		

TABLE 43.1

Recreational Objectives Observation Form
Fishing- Cognitive skills

PATIENT		Dependent (Totally dependent)	High Assistance (25+ ability)	Moderate Assist. (50+ ability)	Mild Assistance (75+ability)	Independent (Totally independent)			
SEE CODES BELOW USE OPTIONAL CODES IF APPROPRIATE		1	2	3	4	5			
		3 cue/ 2-3 physical	2-3 cues/ 2 physical	2-3 cues/ 1 physical	1-2 cues	Encouragement			
97530- Therapeutic activities or	**SKILL**	**GOAL**	**OBJECTIVES** ____times per ____		**METHOD**	**OUTCOME DATE**			
97532 Cognitive skills	ORIENTATION								
97532 Cognitive skills	ATTENTION								
97532 Cognitive skills	MEMORY								
97532 Cognitive skills	PROBLEM-SOLVING								
97532 Cognitive skills	COMPLETE A TASK								
97139 Speech Therapy 97532 Cognitive skills	LANGUAGE								
97533	SENSORY STIMULATION/ COGNITIVE STIMULATION								
97532	PERCEPTUAL AWARENESS								

97532-Development of cognitive skills to improve attention, memory, problem-solving, includes compensatory training and/or sensory integrative activities, direct (one-on-one) patient contact by the provider, each 15 minutes; **97530-Therapeutic activities**, direct (one-on-one) patient contact by the provider (use of dynamic activities to improve functional performance), each 15 minutes; **97533-Sensory integration techniques** to enhance sensory processing and promote adaptive responses to environmental demands, direct (one-on-one) patient contact by the provider, each 15 minutes; **97150-Therapeutic procedure(s)**, group (2 or more individuals); **97139-Unlisted therapeutic procedure** (specify) minutes; **97003- occupational therapy evaluation**; **97004- re-evaluation**	Staff Initial				
	Add total score here -Maximum Score 40 pt. each form per activity				
	See scale below or use own/facilities optional score system				

(Score 1-8)=1 (9-16) =2 (17-24) =3 (25-32) =4 (33-40) =5 If w/device add d if wish, ex: 1d, 2d, or If using 1-7 scale: (41-48) =6 (49-56)

Fishing
Physical Goals, Objectives, and Methods

Skill	Goal	Objectives Sample	Method Sample
Fine motor skills	Increase fine motor skills, including: using fingers, toes, hand-eye coordination, and dexterity	-will use club/hands to hit the ball, will pick up ball	Staff will give instructions, and residents will be involved in a game that requires small motor skills
Gross motor skills	Increase large motor skills	-will bend, stretch, jump, hit the ball (may also do from chair)	Staff will give instructions, and residents will be involved in a fishing adventure that requires large motor skills
Perceptual speed and motor function	Increase speed and motor ability for function, safety, meaningful/fulfilling activities	-will increase acuity and hit the ball faster (with Dr. approval)	-Staff will give residents instructions on how to fish -Staff will use varied types of game equipment to support resident's ability to fish
Following step patterns/backwards forward movement	Increase strength, balance, endurance, meaningful/fulfilling activities	-will stand/sit and swing b to make contact with the ball	Staff will ask residents to walk to the fishing area.(support device if needed), or can be done sitting in a chair
For clinician/Dr. approved use only	For clinician/Dr. approved use only	-will lift arms, legs, bend, reach (to capacity - set by Dr./clinician), will extend and flex (to capacity - set by clinician)	Staff/clinician will instruct residents to do exercises that include flexing, extending muscles
Balance and Posture (approved by Dr. and capacity tests)	Increase balance and improve body alignment and flexibility	-will maintain posture, will stand and maintain posture	Staff will remind residents of proper posture and ask residents to hold body in straight alignment/ posture
Gait/Following Step patterns/ Backwards/Forward movement	Increase strength, balance, endurance, meaningful/fulfilling activities	-will stand up without losing balance and walk a safe pace (approved by Dr. and capacity tests), If approved clinical specialist: ____ ft. ____________________ __________	Staff will call residents to the activity and have them walk to activity (w/device if needed) to work on leg strength (if approved by clinician etc.)
Cardio-vascular Workout*	Increase circulation, blood flow, stamina	-will play the game at a safe pace (approved by Dr. and capacity tests), If approved clinical specialist: ____________________ __________	Staff/clinician will have residents join a fishing excursion (according to doctor approved ability and approved amount of exercise)

TABLE 43.2

Recreational Objectives Observation Form
Fishing-Physical Skills

PATIENT	Dependent (Totally dependent)	High Assistance (25+ ability)	Moderate Assist. (50+ ability)	Mild Assistance (75+ability)	Independent (Totally independent.)
SEE CODES BELOW USE OPTIONAL CODES IF APPROPRIATE	1	2	3	4	5
	3 cue/ 2-3 physical	2-3 cues/ 2 physical	2-3 cues/ 1 physical	1-2 cues	Encouragement

97530- Therapeutic activities or	SKILL	GOAL	OBJECTIVES ____times per ____	METHOD	OUTCOME DATE			
97530 Therapeutic Activity	FINE MOTOR SKILLS							
97110/ 97530	GROSS MOTOR SKILLS							
97110/ 97530/ If under cognitive code 97532	PERCEPTUAL SPEED/ MOTOR FUNCTION							
97530 or Gait training 97116-	STEP PATTERNS							
		Licensed/ Clinician	Dr. approved use only	Licensed/ Clinician				
97110	RANGE OF MOTION							
97112	POSTURE AND BALANCE							
97110 Or Gait training 97116-	GAIT (INCLUDES STAIR CLIMBING)							
97110	CARDIO-VASCULAR WORKOUT*							

97110-Therapeutic procedure, one or more areas, each 15 minutes; therapeutic exercises to develop strength and endurance, range of motion, and flexibility; **97112-Neuromuscular reeducation** of movement, balance, coordination, kinesthetic sense, posture, and proprioception; **97113-Aquatic therapy** with therapeutic exercises; **97116-Gait training** (includes stair climbing); **97139-Unlisted therapeutic procedure** (specify); **97150 Therapeutic procedure(s), group** (2 or more individuals); **97750-Physical performance test or measurement** (e.g., musculoskeletal, functional capacity), with written report, each 15 minutes; **97535-Self care/home management training** (e.g., activities of daily living and compensatory training, meal preparation, safety procedures, and instructions in use of adaptive equipment), direct (one-on-one) contact by provider, each 15 minutes **Physical therapy 97001 evaluation, 97002 Re-evaluation. occupational therapy** evaluation **97003, re-evaluation 97004**	Staff Initial				
	Add total score here Maximum Score 40 pt. each form per activity				
	See scale below or use own/facilities optional score system				

Score 1-8) =1 (9-16) =2 (17-24) =3 (25-32) =4 (33-40) =5 If w/device add d if wish, ex: 1d, 2d, or If using 1-7 scale: (41-48) =6 (49-56) Current Procedural Terminology © 2005 American Medical Association. All rights reserved. Recreational Objectives Observational forms © 2005. All rights reserved. Patent pending.

Fishing
Socio-emotional Goals, Objectives and Methods

Skill	Goal	Objectives Sample	Method Sample
Socialization/Community Integration	Increase social interactions, meaningful/fulfilling activities	-will interact with peers, will engage in community integration experiences (for social skills), will use manners, social practices	Staff will engage residents in a sport and support/encourage residents to socialize through community integration and being paired w/group for games
Team Playing/Sharing	Increase teamwork/sharing, meaningful/fulfilling activities	-will join in on the game with others and share, wait turn, support peers	Staff will encourage residents to play, form teams, strategize together, include all members in play
Initiative and Motivation	Increase initiative and motivation/wellness, and quality of life	-will choose if they wish to play or not, will try a new technique, will initiate playing on own (or with assistance), will increase amount of practice after stating own goal	-Staff will support and encourage the residents to prepare/join activities for their own personal gains -Staff will offer new techniques to motivate resident's interests and desires
Emotional Gratification	Increase emotional gratification/wellness, and quality of life	-will state that the game was a gratifying experience or will show pleasure by smiling, laughing, deep focus, and involvement during the game	Staff will ask residents if they enjoyed fishing and what they liked through the use of verbal discussion, group discussions or as observed
Sense of Accomplishment	Increase feelings of self-worth, pride, productivity, dignity/wellness, and quality of life	-will use gestures to express pride in self , will talk about their accomplishments while playing he game	Staff will place a chart on the unit wall or hand a paper to the residents that reflect the fish caught on a charts/paper etc. will be available for residents to see
Self-esteem/self-identity	Increase self-esteem, feelings of belonging, dignity, self-worth, integrity, self-identity/wellness, and quality of life	-will state/communicate positive feelings about self and ability to fish, will join fishing excursion to take an active role in health though exercising, will join the trip based on own choices	Staff will educate residents on the value of exercise and will encourage residents to join sports/outdoor activities
Fostering Appropriate Behaviors	Increase social interaction, social opportunities and adjustment, safety, using appropriate behaviors during an activity for a calm environment/wellness, and quality of life	-will adjust to the noises, other's movements, surroundings, etc.	-Staff will engage residents in sports to expose residents to sensory stimulating experiences -Staff will support residents as they adjust to the stimulus one step at a time
Sensory Integration/Tolerating Stimulation	Increase sensory processing and enhance awareness of sensations and toleration/adaptation of sensory stimulations and demands	-will join in on golf lesson, listen and follow instructions, use appropriate behavior for the setting; will wait turn; will quiet down when asked	Before class begins, staff will discuss the rules, appropriate behaviors, respect of property, safety, and respect of fellow team players

Table 43.3

Recreational Objectives Observation Form
Fishing - Socio-emotional Skills

PATIENT	Dependent (Totally dependent)	High Assistance (25+ ability)	Moderate Assist. (50+ ability)	Mild Assistance (75+ability)	Independent (Totally independent.)
SEE CODES BELOW USE OPTIONAL CODES IF APPROPRIATE	1	2	3	4	5
	3 cue/ 2-3 physical	2-3 cues/ 2 physical	2-3 cues/ 1 physical	1-2 cues	Encouragement

97530- Therapeutic activities or	SKILL	GOAL	OBJECTIVES ____times per ____	METHOD	OUTCOME DATE			
97537 Or 97535	SOCIALIZATION/ COMMUNITY INTEGRATION							
97537 Or 97535	TEAM PLAYING /SHARING							
97537 Or 97535	INITIATIVE AND MOTIVATION							
97537 Or 97535	EMOTIONAL GRATIFICATION							
97537 Or 97535	SENSE OF ACCOMPLISHM ENT							
97537 Or 97535	SELF-ESTEEM/ SELF-IDENTITY							
97537 Or 97535	FOSTERING APPROPRIATE BEHAVIORS							
97533	SENSORY INTEGRATION/ TOLERATING							

97537-Community/work reintegration training (e.g., shopping, transportation, money management, avocational activities and/or work environment/modification analysis, work task analysis), direct (one-on-one) contact by provider, each 15 minutes; **97535-Self care/home management training** (e.g., activities of daily living and compensatory training, meal preparation, safety procedures, and instructions in use of adaptive equipment), direct (one-on-one) contact by provider, each 15 minutes; **97530-Therapeutic activities, direct (one-on-one)** patient contact by the provider (use of dynamic activities to improve functional performance), each 15 minutes; **97150-Therapeutic procedure(s), group (2 or more individuals); 97533-Sensory integration techniques** to enhance sensory processing and promote adaptive responses to environmental demands, direct (one-on-one) patient contact by the provider, each 15 minutes; **occupational therapy evaluation 97003, re-evaluation . 97004**	Staff Initial				
	Add total score here-Maximum Score 40 pt. each form per activity				
	See scale below or use own/facilities optional score system				

(Score 1-8)=1 (9-16) =2 (17-24) =3 (25-32) =4 (33-40) =5 If w/device add d if wish, ex: 1d, 2d, or If using 1-7 scale: (41-48) =6 (49-56)

Monthly Recreational Supply and Cost List

Month of: ____________________

Supplies	Cost (approx. or actual)
__________________	__________
__________________	__________
__________________	__________
__________________	__________
__________________	__________
__________________	__________
__________________	__________
__________________	__________
__________________	__________
__________________	__________
__________________	__________

Cost ________

Initialed _____

Supply List/Inventory

Reorder

Physical Activity Helps Seniors Age Successfully

Being physically active can prevent and help treat many of the most common chronic medical conditions associated with old age. Physical activity is one of the most important steps older adults can take to maintain physical and mental health and quality of life. Scientists have proven that being active can help reduce the risk of obesity, high blood pressure, diabetes, osteoporosis, stroke, depression, colon cancer, and premature death. Yet today, more than 60% of older adults are inactive. Older adults face the same obstacles to being more physically active as younger adults but also have special concerns.

The Challenge to Get Moving

Getting older adults to be active is a challenge. The average American lives a long time, but many are sedentary, physically unfit, and experience disability from chronic medical conditions as they age. Physicians and exercise experts hear many reasons from older adults as to why they are not active: It doesn't feel good. It makes my arthritic joints hurt. It takes too much time. It's boring. However, older adults need physical activity like everyone else, at least as much as younger adults. In fact, the loss of strength and stamina often attributed to aging is in part caused by reduced physical activity.

Walking groups and physical activity programs especially designed for older adults can help seniors become—and remain active. For example, senior swim clubs and water aerobic classes are excellent activities for people with arthritis.

The Need for Strength

Strength training is recommended for all adults, but it is a vital link to health for older adults. The reason is that strength training prevents sarcopenia, the muscle deterioration that comes with aging, and also helps maintain bone mass. "Stronger people have better health Outcomes," noted Dr. David Buchner, Chief of CDC's Physical Activity and Health Branch and renowned Gerontologist. However, some elderly people avoid physical activity and become sedentary out of fear of falling and fracturing a bone. Dr. Buchner added that emerging data indicate that physical activity can prevent falls by improving strength, balance, and endurance.

Keeping Young at Heart

Aerobic activity (also known as cardiorespiratory or cardiovascular endurance activity) is also important. It keeps the heart strong, lowers blood pressure, and relieves anxiety and depression. Older adults can obtain significant health benefits with moderate physical activity, such as walking or gardening. „We need to make physical activity part of the daily routine for older adults," said Dr. Buchner. Health clubs also provide older adults with a variety of opportunities to improve their aerobic fitness, muscular strength, and flexibility. Dr. Buchner adds, „Traditionally health and fitness facilities have marketed mainly to body-conscious younger adults, who focus on the cosmetic effects. It's great to see that health clubs have developed more programs for older adults, and we hope this trend continues. CDC, NCCDPHP". Special focus: healthy aging. Chronic Disease Notes and Reports 1999; 12(3):10-11. (Insert obtained from aoa.hhs.gov 2005.)

CDC Recommendations

The CDC/ACSM recommends that all adults should accumulate at least 30 minutes of moderate-intensity physical activity on five or more days of the week. Cardio respiratory (aerobic) endurance, strength, balance, and flexibility exercises should all be part of a physical activity program for older adults. No one type of activity will bring about all the benefits of physical activity. It is important to include all of them. Older adults can meet the physical activity recommendation with a combination of these activities using the following sample schedule:

- Cardio respiratory: Participate in moderate-intensity aerobic activity 3-5 days a week for at least 30 minutes each session.

- Flexibility*: Stretch every day.

- Strength training: Do strength-building activities 2-3 days per week.

*Flexibility refers to how fully one's joints or limbs are able to move. Being flexible allows for easier movements and reduced pain in joints so that it is also easier to perform daily activities of independent living. By adding stretching to your daily physical activity plan, you can help keep your joints flexible which will help you move with more freedom and comfort.

Participating in these types of activities can help you more easily perform many of your day-to-day tasks. For example, being more flexible will help you more easily do things like reaching in your cupboard and tying your shoes. Being stronger and having more balance will help you lift and carry items like sacks of groceries and will make it easier to get in and out of chairs and the bathtub. Improving your cardio respiratory endurance will allow you to do things like climbing stairs, dancing, or playing with grandchildren without getting out of breath. The chart below provides ideas of activities in the areas of cardio respiratory endurance, strength, and flexibility. Many of these activities will also help improve your balance. Most importantly, choose activities that you enjoy. This will make it more likely that you'll keep doing them!

CDC, NCCDPHP. Special focus: healthy aging. Chronic Disease Notes and Reports 1999; 12(3):10-11. Insert obtained from aoa.hhs.gov 2005

FIGURE 8.0
CDC Recommendations

Cardio respiratory
Strength
Flexibility

Walking
Chair exercises
Stretching

Swimming
Lifting weights or cans
Yoga

Dancing
Carrying laundry or groceries
Tai chi

Skating
Working in the yard

Hiking
Washing the car

Rolling your wheelchair
Scrubbing the floor

FIGURE 9.0
Promoting Active Lifestyles Among Older Adults

Promoting Active Lifestyles Among Older Adults

"No one is too old to enjoy the benefits of regular physical activity." — *U.S. Surgeon General, 1996*[1]

Successful aging is largely determined by individual lifestyle choices and not by genetic inheritance. Few factors contribute as much to successful aging as having a physically active lifestyle. Regular physical activity is important for the primary and secondary prevention of many chronic diseases (e.g., coronary heart disease, non-insulin dependent diabetes mellitus, obesity), disabling conditions (e.g., osteoporosis, arthritis), and chronic disease risk factors (e.g., high blood pressure, high cholesterol).

- Regular physical activity substantially delays the onset of functional limitations and loss of independence. It has been reported that inactive, nonsmoking women at age 65 have 12.7 years of active life expectancy, compared with 18.4 years for highly active, nonsmoking women.[2]
- The U.S. Prevention Task Force recommends counseling older adults on strategies to reduce falls; these include balance exercise[3]. One study reported a 58% reduction in falls among older women who began an exercise program.[4]
- The American Academy of Rheumatologists recommends physical activity in arthritis management. One study reported that regular walking reduced pain and improved function among people with arthritis in the knees.[5]
- Evidence suggests regular physical activity can improve the quality of sleep among older adults.[6]
- Physical activity often reduces symptoms of depression. One study found strength training as effective as medication in reducing depressive symptoms among older adults.[7]
- A recent study suggests that physical activity may help older adults reduce the amount of cognitive decline they experience as they age.[8]

Substantial health benefits occur with regular physical activity (e.g., 30 minutes of brisk walking, 5 or more days of the week). Additional health benefits can be gained through greater amounts of physical activity, but even small amounts of activity are healthier than a sedentary lifestyle.[1] Yet, few older adults achieve the minimum recommended 30 minutes of moderate intensity activity on most, preferably all, days of the week.

- CDC surveillance data show that about 16.7% of adults aged 45–64, 23.1% of adults aged 65–74, and 35.9% of adults aged 75 or older are inactive, meaning they engage in no leisure-time, household, or transportation physical activity. (Figure 1).

Figure 1
Prevalence of Inactivity in US Older Adults
BRFSS, 2001

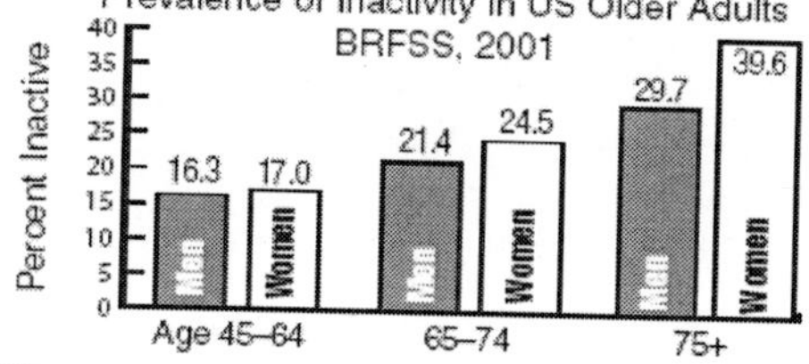

- Reduction in medical costs associated with physical activity increases with age, especially for women (Figure 2).[9]

Figure 2
Annual Medical Costs of Active and Inactive Women Age 45 or Older Without Physical Limitations[9]

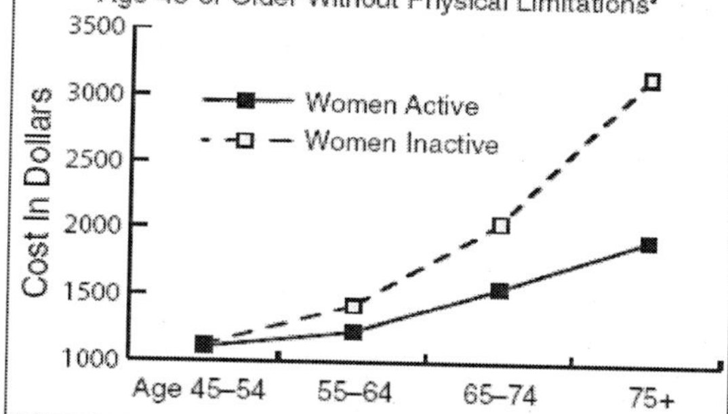

- NHIS data show that only 11% of older adults meet strength training recommendations[10]. The vast majority of older adults are missing opportunities to improve their health through strength training. (Figure 3).

Figure 3
Percentage of US Adults 65 and Older Meeting Strength Training Recommendations, NHIS 2001

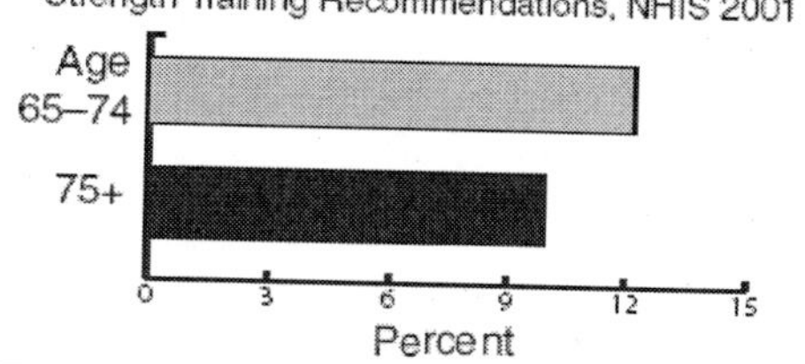

US DEPARTMENT OF HEALTH AND HUMAN SERVICES
CENTERS FOR DISEASE CONTROL AND PREVENTION

CDC
SAFER · HEALTHIER · PEOPLE™

My Pyramid

The 2005 Dietary Guidelines for Americans
and consumer brochure are available at:
www.healthierus.gov/dietaryguidelines

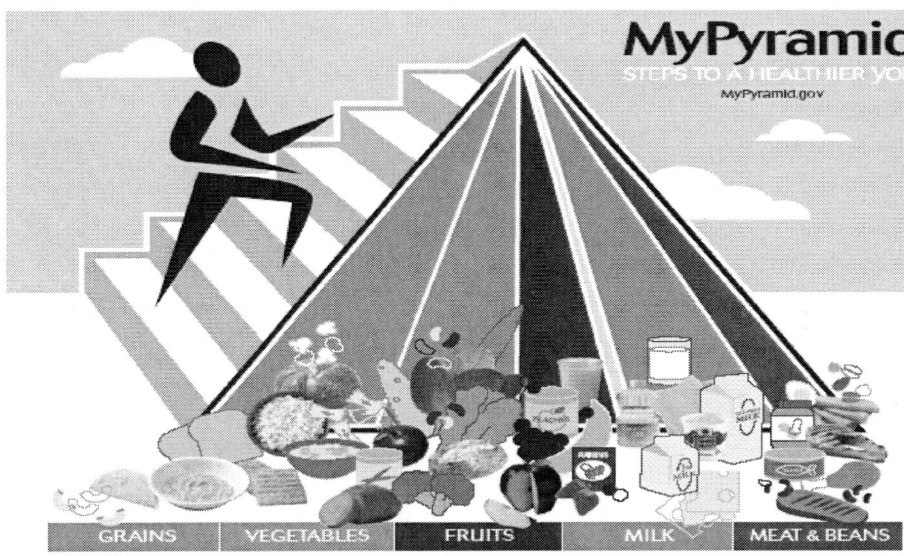

GRAINS Make half your grains whole	VEGETABLES Vary your veggies	FRUITS Focus on fruits	MILK Get your calcium-rich foods	MEAT & BEANS Go lean with protein
Eat at least 3 oz. of whole-grain cereals, breads, crackers, rice, or pasta every day 1 oz. is about 1 slice of bread, about 1 cup of breakfast cereal, or ½ cup of cooked rice, cereal, or pasta	Eat more dark-green veggies like broccoli, spinach, and other dark leafy greens Eat more orange vegetables like carrots and sweetpotatoes Eat more dry beans and peas like pinto beans, kidney beans, and lentils	Eat a variety of fruit Choose fresh, frozen, canned, or dried fruit Go easy on fruit juices	Go low-fat or fat-free when you choose milk, yogurt, and other milk products If you don't or can't consume milk, choose lactose-free products or other calcium sources such as fortified foods and beverages	Choose low-fat or lean meats and poultry Bake it, broil it, or grill it Vary your protein routine — choose more fish, beans, peas, nuts, and seeds
For a 2,000-calorie diet, you need the amounts below from each food group. To find the amounts that are right for you, go to MyPyramid.gov.				
Eat 6 oz. every day	Eat 2½ cups every day	Eat 2 cups every day	Get 3 cups every day; for kids aged 2 to 8, it's 2	Eat 5½ oz. every day

Find your balance between food and physical activity

- Be sure to stay within your daily calorie needs.
- Be physically active for at least 30 minutes most days of the week.
- About 60 minutes a day of physical activity may be needed to prevent weight gain.
- For sustaining weight loss, at least 60 to 90 minutes a day of physical activity may be required.
- Children and teenagers should be physically active for 60 minutes every day, or most days.

Know the limits on fats, sugars, and salt (sodium)

- Make most of your fat sources from fish, nuts, and vegetable oils.
- Limit solid fats like butter, stick margarine, shortening, and lard, as well as foods that contain these.
- Check the Nutrition Facts label to keep saturated fats, *trans* fats, and sodium low.
- Choose food and beverages low in added sugars. Added sugars contribute calories with few, if any, nutrients.

MyPyramid.gov
STEPS TO A HEALTHIER YOU

U.S. Department of Agriculture
Center for Nutrition Policy and Promotion
April 2005
CNPP-15

FIGURE 10.0 USDA Food Pyramid

Functional Assessment Exams and Resources

The Geriatric Observable Activities for Longevity program was formulated and developed using a variety of resources. It consists of professional experiences, as well as input from those working in the field of geriatrics. It includes and utilizes research data derived from clinical tests and studies available regarding older adult care to present a well-rounded knowledge base of test experiences and resources. The primary focus was to build a recreational program specific to assessment areas of cognitive, physical, and socio-emotional needs and abilities. The booklet contains research regarding standardized tests and information used within various types of clinical and home care settings.

Recognizing the importance of testing for dementia, depression, psychological disorders, and other additional issues, this type of testing must be done by a certified doctor. Respectfully, there is no intent to diagnosis patients or to test in clinical areas meant for specialty fields of physicians and clinicians outside of the recreational expertise. The goal was to include research on testing and professional experiences of clinicians in order to appreciate the relevant information that constitutes and encompasses wellness for the older adult. To utilize above testing programs, a diagnosis must be given by an appropriate clinician. This information is then used to decipher where a resident would fall within the range of ability to take part in an activity and gain therapeutic value in recreation. The final step is to integrate clinical diagnosis with activity skill levels to build an inclusive activities program.

In order to determine a value of skill level necessary to obtain goals and benefits of activities, researching standardized tests that are in place would evaluate older adults' needs in cognitive, physical and social development. The Katz Index of Daily Living and the Instrumental Activities of Daily Living were considered to appreciate the needs and abilities addressed for activities of daily living.

When researching the physical needs and abilities of the older adult, the Katz Activities of Daily Living (ADL) and Instrumental Activities of Daily Living (IADL) were considered for their relevance to physical needs. The Modified Barthel Index was also used to gauge physical skills sought. Gerontology research measuring physical needs were also appreciated. These physical needs included small motor skills/dexterity and manipulation of materials, hand-eye coordination, large motor skills, range of motion, tactile stimulation, perceptual speed and motor function, coordination, gait, posture, flexibility, cardio-vascular well-being, and balance.

The Folstein Mini-Mental State Examination and gerontology research measuring cognitive needs and abilities were appreciated when considering the various cognitive elements involving components of memory, recall, recognition, attention, abstract thinking, concrete thinking, orientation, attention, language and communication, perceptual awareness, problem solving, following patterns, and cognitive stimulation. All of these skills were acknowledged to appreciate the needs and abilities of patients in regard to cognitive skill levels.

When assessing socio-emotional skills, it is difficult to pinpoint one standardized exam that encompasses the spectrum of social issues. Therefore, the Folstein Mini-Mental Status Test, Katz ADL and IADL, Modified Barthel Index Performance Assessment and Function, Revised Memory and Behavior Checklist, Norbeck, and a Spiritual Assessments test and gerontology research were considered. It is felt that the Revised Memory and Behavior checklist is helpful for the behavioral aspect of engaging in the activities. When looking at the socio-emotional area, the primary concern is the effects of socio-emotional issues in terms of mood and behavior and its regards to the ability to function. Certainly, mood and behavior are main goal is to look at the effect of ability to function during activities in and of the social aspect. Therefore, mood and behavior are included under socio-emotional skills. Also, social conditions such as living arrangements, cultural and ethnic background, and spiritual needs are included here. Personal activity and the noted meaning of activity theories are important factors when applying the social aspect of any activities program. The goal of including all of these factors in the socio-emotional area is to see how these changes affect the older adult so we can help them adjust to these changes and lead a fulfilled life.

Indeed, in my research, many cognitive, physical, and socio-emotional areas are intertwined. Cognitive, physical, and psychological ability all effect social belonging, feelings of self, and life longevity. The level of cognitive ability to engage in social activities might be completely normal, or social activities could present a challenge due to the presence of dementia. Physical and cognitive developments have a major impact on the elderly person's opportunities to tend to tasks in mind, body, and social atmospheres. Therefore, matching the areas to specific concerns when addressed, goals and activities of any said area is done based on the area most likely consistent to function within the activity.

Keeping in mind that there could be other variables as a result of background, medication, etc., makes it important to not only gauge each individual's ability to do tasks but also their unique factors on testing and ability. At this point, the benefit of this assessment becomes apparent. Rather than assessing generalized impairments and scoring, which fluctuate within cognitive, physical, and socio-emotional scores, each form focuses primarily on each domain. The Recreational Objectives Observation Form allows the documentation of individual skills, goals, objectives and methods to accounts for subtle and distinct circumstances for each resident.

By using resources available, it is hoped that this program can be incorporated along with existing testing by a professional, and become an additional tool in assessing older adults cognitive, physical, and socio-emotional skills. affected and scored by cognitive ability, but the Once assessed, using the activities and forms in this book can help keep track of all progress and decline in these areas, allowing the health care provider to look out for and increase the quality of life for each older adult.

PROGRAM PILOT STUDY

A small-scale pilot study was done to investigate the validity and reliability of the Recreational Observational Objectives Form for use as an observation/ assessment tool. The clientele targeted for this assessment were older adults in a nursing home facility. The primary purpose of the program was to implement activities, assess benefits of older adults engaging in activities and further, documenting individual patients' information for treatment plan goals. The primary purpose of the study was also to validate the use of the program in a nursing home setting and to show validity and reliability of the assessment tool.

Test scores were done using three testing periods. The scale rating was a one to five. Test measures for each scale rate showed measurable rate abilities/distinctions and established appropriate norms. Inter-rater reliability was done and statistical findings are to be submitted on to the Geriatric Society. Content validity was validated through research and standardized tests measuring the skills also mentioned within this assessment tool. The content was also reviewed by a variety of medical, psychological and educational experts in their respected fields.

Construct validity was obtained in appreciation of behaviors and constructs contributing to the abilities to do activities and ADL skills, these constructs where also found in research and standardized tests indicating correlation's, hypothesis and associations.

METHOD

The initial program was administered at a long -term care nursing facility. The nursing home was given the entire book/program including: educative materials, activities and the recreational objectives observational form. The activity director was responsible for overseeing the implementation of the base activities concurrent with the use of the observational /assessment form. There were 15-20 older adults engaging in each of the activities. 5 clients where chosen for observations per activity, additional testing was completed at a later date by two additional raters to increase the number of residents and validate test-retest validity. The recreational observation objectives form targeted, documented and "fine tuned" the area of concern in physical, cognitive, and socio-emotional assessments.

The activity director was certified and qualified to assess and document skill levels. The average time to fill out the individual patient's forms took 10 minutes. The activity director was able to assess and document skill levels based on training and use of the measurable rating scale.

RESULTS

This study was done in a nursing home setting with older adults. As was expected, evaluation of scores showing progression or regression, showed no changes or slight changes at 3 months .Due to the specific clientele studied, this program would/might require longer-term evaluations for these clients to show clear cut observable changes.

However, regarding use of the tool for assessment purposes, it was noted that in even the initial use of forms, the tool was sensitive enough to show a clear picture of specific deficits for patient's present abilities within subsets of particular domains. The staff administering the program commented "that when there has been a slight change during groups with a resident's cognition level, this tool helped to show exactly where these changes were occurring for the residents.

This was validated by analysis of the observation forms .The finding by staff were consistent with score ratings observed within the subset of each domain and patient scoring.

The ability to clue in immediately on specific subsets within domains was helpful in making staff aware of concentrated needs of observation and therefore enhancing the treatment plans and quality programming.

Glossary

Abstract thinking is a cognitive process requiring the ability to consider multi-facet/"far reaching" ideas/ or considering a problem without the benefit of visual targeting and direct mean--ing. This is the opposite of perhaps concrete thinking which is more direct, simple and understandable without complex choices or considerations. Alzheimer's patients do much better with concrete thinking, questions, or without complex need of action. Offer simple directions, facial cues or other hints to help them to understand what you are saying or doing.

Active Assistive Range of Motion- A range of motion exercise that is done with a therapist's assistance, when the patient may be limited to doing the exercises without assistance. It is used to promote stretching and strengthening.

Alzheimer's disease- A neurological brain disorder which causes deterioration to areas of the brain involving memory, thought, language skills, and physical function.

Attention- Reactive focus to a task or information by a stimulus. The goal is to stay focused to the task at hand rather then "taking in" other stimulus. Further this information can then be processed. .

Cognitive functions- The physical aspects of cognitive functions involve the brain as it has developed continues to develop, under develop, and/or declines as a result of physical conditions. It affects speed and ability to process information for sensory functions, motor functions, and perception based on physical abilities. The knowledge aspect of cognitive functions includes thought and reasoning, problem solving, memory, and comprehension of written and spoken language.

Cognitive thinking involves thought, reasoning and the abilities to gather and sort incoming information.

Cognitive stimulation involves stimulating a physical or intellectual process for cognition. An example might be offering a resident a music box (preferably one with music from their time era) the music will be good to stimulate hearing, nurturing qualities of music, and it may also bring up memories.

Cataracts- Opaque colored debris that interferes with light getting to the lens of the eye, making vision difficult.

Community integration- to be integrated or brought together for a group activity with the expressed goal of interaction and adaptation to people, places, and experiences.

Culture is described as the shared values, traditions, norms, customs, arts, history, and folklore and institution of a group of people. Understanding culture helps us to understand how others interpret, perceive, and function. Culture shapes the individuals and the group attitudes, ideals, goals and values.

Disorientation may be the result of many factors, such as dementia, delusional episodes and delirium. An example of being disoriented might be a patient suffering from Alzheimer's disease that has progressed to a point where he or she cannot remember earlier details of the day, such as having had lunch, not recognizing this, and asking for it at four o' clock. They may not even recognize it is four o'clock, or what day or year it is, or even their location. A temporary disorientation might be someone who is depressed and becomes unaware of external happenings in the world, and therefore may be unaware of what day or time it is.

Following patterns is the ability to maintain attention, understand and follow a set course for problem solving. After you make the plans, need to be able to remember where you are going and stay focused on your direction and follow the plan though. Hand-eye coordination - The goal and ability to successfully coordinate perceptual input and fine motor skills to complete a task

Episodic memory- A long-term memory process in which one is able to recall events and time periods that have happened during one's life.

Explicit memory- The conscious ability to recall what is and has taken place. An example of this is when driving to a destination having the ability to remember where you are going and why you are going there, and being able to recount details of the trip.

Fine motor skills- The skills needed for movement and control of the extremities. Mastering of these movements facilitates dexterity, flexibility, and manipulative skills of the hands and fingers.

Gross motor skills- The skills needed for movement and control of the proximal muscles. Mastering of these movements facilitates agility, flexibility, and control of the whole body as well as legs and arms.

Glaucoma- An eye disorder in which there is a build-up of pressure within the eye. It can lead to blindness.

Implicit memory- The unconscious ability to perform a task without the need of deep thought or instruction. The task becomes "automatic," such as driving a car.

Long-term memory- Information permanently embedded within the memory banks of the brain over long periods of time.

Language and communication is the ability to recognize letters, words and understand their meaning, or as in the example of the older adult with hearing problem, the ability to distinguish sounds. To communicate means to be able to give a response in such a way that others can interpret/ comprehend what you are trying to state or the ability to interpret/ comprehend what others are trying to state to you.

Hand-eye motor coordination- coordination of both hand and eye movement to perform a task, controlled by muscles.

Multi-infract- A brain condition that causes obstruction or blockage of blood flow in the cerebral arteries and, as a result, cause mini strokes. These mini strokes eventually lead to loss of intellectual skills and neurological deficits.

Orientation- The cognitive ability to understand the surroundings, time frame, and circumstances within the moment and setting.

Passive Range of Motion-This range of motion exercise is completely done by the therapist, when the patient is completely unable to do the exercise. This involves patients who have paralysis of the body part or other issues of immobility.

Perceptual awareness - The cognitive skills necessary to categorize, discriminate, compare, and gauge depth perception.

Perceptual speed- The cognitive ability to perceive and react to a stimulus. For example, seeing a red light and stepping on the car brakes.

Perceptual and motor development- The level of development whereby perceptual and motor development are coordinated to complete a task.

Parkinson's disease- A progressive brain disease that causes muscle tremors, lack of muscle control, slowed movement, and some facial paralysis.

Problem solving-An example might be making a list to take to the grocery store. You need to be able to consider what you need, write it down, figure out how much it might cost, and how you will get to the store. All of these thoughts must be solved in order to go about the action desired. Problem solving requires comprehension, memory and processing information.

Range of motion is the ability to have full range and movement of the extremities and the proximal muscles. There are various types of range of motion therapies.

Retention is the ability to store and retain information for a short or long time

Recall is the ability to repeat information stored to memory using short or long term memory. Without the ability to recall information, we can not process information or follow through adequately on a task.

Recognition is the ability to perceive and mentally respond/register a situation, person, place, or thing as known and stored in memory

Semantic memory- Knowledge we have learned through books, school, job training, or personal experiences such as learning how to crochet or play chess.

Short-term memory- A stage in the processing of memory in which a person retains information for fifteen to thirty seconds.

Stretching exercises are used to lengthen the muscles/connective tissue to help loosen tight muscles/spasms. The exercises can increase range of motion and lessen pain or spasms.

Tactile stimulation requires the use of a material, human touch, and machine to cause a sensation and promote neurological, muscular, and physical response/awareness. Some types of tactile stimulation include lights, vibration, sounds, smells (like aromatherapy), special foods, and varied texture items.

Working memory- A process of the brain that includes gathering and sorting information, comprehending written or spoken language, solving a problem, and completing a task.

Socio-emotional needs- A term used for meeting the needs of personal well-being in conjunction with changes in life conditions such as the loss of a spouse, a change in living arrangements, the loss of work, or problems with finances.

Self-esteem- How one feels about one's own abilities, goals, worth, and desirability.

Self-identity- A reflection of how we view ourselves in terms of who we are and what we have to offer as an individual within the world. It is based on such issues as interests, views, values, and passions

References

Bonder, Bette R. and Marilyn B. Wagner. Functional Performance in Older Adults. 2nd Ed. Philadelphia: F.A. David Company 2001.

Battiati, L. Francis with Suzanne Meredith, Checchino: A Father & Son Journey Towards Dusk. Battisti Network, 2005.

Brhel, Susan Increasing the Quality of Life for the Older Adult, New York. Brundage Publishing, 2005

Cohen, Elizabeth. House on Beartown Road. Random House, 2000

Flower, Ruth. As We Grow Old. Valley Forge: Judson Press, 1998.

Fuller, Jill and Jennifer Schaller. Health Assessment, A Nursing Approach. Philadelphia: Lippincott, Williams, & Wilkins, 2000.

Finch, C.E. Seeman, T.E. (1999). Stress theories of aging. In V.L. Bengtson, & K.W. Schaie(EDs). Handbook of theories of aging, New York, Springer.

Hauck, S.J., & Bartke, A. (2001) Free radical defenses in the liver and kidney of human growth hormone transgenic mice. Journal of Gerontology, 56A No4, B153-B162

Gallo, Joseph J., Terry Fulmer, Gregory J. Paveza, Cilliam Reichel. Handbook of Geriatric Assessment. 3rd ed. Gaithersburg: Aspen Publishers Inc., 2000.

Hogstel, Mildred O. and Rhonda Keen-Payne. Practical Guide to Health Assessment Through Lifespan. Philadelphia: F.A. Davis Company, 1996.

Kramer, Judy. Changing Place. New York: Riverhead Books, 2000.

Loverde, Joy. The Complete Eldercare Planner. CITY: Silvercare Productions, 1997.

Santrock, John W. Life Span Development. New York: McGraw-Hill, 2002.

Works Cited

Burke, G.L., Arnold, A. M. .,Bild ,D., Cushman, M. ,Fried, O .,Newman, A.,& Robbins, C.(2001).Factors associated with healthy aging. Journal of the American Geriatric Society, 49,254-262.

Evans, W. (2000).Exercise strategies should be designed to increase muscle power. Journal of Gerontology: Medical Sciences, 55A, M309-M310.

Kabitsis, C., Matsouka, O., Harahousou, Y., & Trigonis, I. (1999, November) the effects of a physical activity program on functional ability among elderly women. Paper presented at the meeting of the Gerontology Association of America, San Francisco.

Prohaska, T., & Peters, K., (1999, November) Walking exercise behavior in younger and older adults: An evaluation of a mall walking program. Paper presented at the Gerontology Association of America, San Francisco.

Wang, H., Bashore, T.R. ., & Friedman, E. (1995) Exercise reduces age dependent decrease in platelet protein kinas C activity and translocation. Journal of Gerontology, 50A, M12-M16.

Educational experiences are positively correlated with scores on intelligence tests and information processing tasks, such as memory (Verhaeghen, P., Marcoen, A., & Goossens,L.,(1995).Facts and fiction about memory aging: A quantitative integration of research findings. Journal of Gerontology, 48, P157-P171.

Rodin, J., & Langer, E.J. (1977). Long-term effects of a control-relevant intervention with the institutionalized aged. Studies have shown having a sense of control over decision-making and other choices can increase the older adult's quality of living and satisfaction. Journal of personality and social psychology, 35,397-402.

Define the Biologic and Environmental Factors That Maximize Cognitive, Sensory, and Physical Functions, Identify Social, Psychological, and Lifestyle Factors That Promote Health, well-being, and Longevity, Disassociate Changes of Normal or Usual Aging From Those of Diseases and Disorders. National Institute on Health and aging Subgoal 1: Unlock the Secrets of Aging, Health, and Longevity(2006)

Amber Stary., (2002, February). Aging and Hearing Loss, Stephen F. Austin State University.
Helfer, K.S., (1998). Auditory and auditory-visual recognition of clear and conversational speech by older adults. Journal of the American Academy of Audiology, 9.

National Center for Elder Abuse (NCEA). (2003). www.elderabusecenter.org.
Administration on Aging, Department of Health and Human Services (DHHS, 2003).
The National Elder Abuse Incidence Study, Final Report, http://www.aoa.gov/.

Fire Safety, Department of Health and Human Services (DHHS, 2003). Fire safety (NIOSH 2003)-http://www.cdc.gov/niosh/2003.

http://www.jcaho.org/accreditedorganizations/patientsafety

CDC, NCCDPHP. Special focus: healthy aging. Chronic Disease Notes and Reports 1999; 12(3):10-11.

(Earles, J.L., & Salthouse, T.A. (1995). Interrelations of age, health, and speed. Journal of Gerontology: psychological Sciences 50B, P33-P41

Salthouse, T.A. (1996). General and specific speed mediation of adult age differences in memory. Journal of Gerontology 51A, P30-P42. (2000). Adulthood and aging: Cognitive processes and development .In A.Kazdin(ED), Encyclopedia of psychology. Washington, D.C.7& New York: American Psychological Association and Oxford University press.

Silwinski, M., & Buschke, H. (1999).Cross-sectional and longitudinal relationships among age, cognition, and speed processing. Psychology and Aging, P14, P18-33

Retraining the brain to cope with Illness, Injury, and CBSnews.com (2006) CBS broadcasting Inc.

Riegel, K.F., & Riegel, R.M. (1972) Development, drop, and death. Developmental Psychology, 6,306-319

Baltes, P.B. (1993). The aging mind: Potentials and limits. Gerontologist, 33, 580-594.

Baltes, P.B. (1996, August). On the complete architecture of human ontogenesis. Invited award address presented at the meeting of the American Psychological association, Toronto.

Baltes, P.B., (2000). Life-span developmental theory. In A. Kazdin (ED.), Encyclopedia of psychology. Washington, D.C., & New York: American Psychological Association and Oxford University Press.

Baltes, P.B.., & Baltes, M.M.Baltes (1990) Psychological perspectives on successful aging: The model of selective optimization with compensation.

P.B. Baltes & M.M. Baltes (Eds), Successful aging: Prospectives from behavioral sciences. New York: Cambridge University Press.

Baltes & Baltes, 1990: Mariske & others, 1995) People nominated as wise: A comparison study of wisdom-related knowledge. Psychology and Aging, 10,155-166.

Singh, Clements, & Fiatarone, 1997). A randomized controlled trail of progressive resistance training in depressed elders. Journal of Gerontology, 2A, M27-M35.

In another study, researchers have found that aerobic exercise is related to improved memory and reasoning (Clarkson-Smith & Harley, 1989). Relationships between physical exercise and cognitive abilities in older adults. Psychology and Aging, 4, 183-189.

Observing development of the Young children, Second edition,(1990) Macmillian Publishing Company, New York

The scientific basis for psychotherapeutic interventions with older adults: An overview Knight, B.G. (1999). Journal of Clinical Psychology, 55(8), 927-934.

Psychosocial intervention for individuals with dementia: An integration of theory, therapy, and a clinical understanding of dementia

Coyle, C.P., Kinney, W.B. Riley, B., & Shank, J.W. (Eds.) (1991). Benefits of Therapeutic Recreation: A Consensus View, Ravensdale: Idyll Arbor, Inc.

Functional Fitness Assessment for Adults over 60 years, second edition: Adults over 60; 107 Rehabilitation checklist: 206

Retirement Activities Card Sort Planning Kit, Author -Richard L. Knowdell Rehabilitation checklist J Douglas Salmon jr.Am J Psychiatry. 1982 Sep: 139(9): 1136-9

Family Practice, Family Therapy: A Collaboration of Dialogue **Joan D. Atwood, Ph.D**
Estelle Weinstein, Ph.D,(2005)

The Global Deterioration Scale for assessment of primary degenerative dementia. Reisberg B, Ferris SH, de Leon MJ, Crook

Kasl-Godley, J., & Gatz, M. (2000). Clinical Psychology Review, 20(6), 755-782 Dementia and alz. Patients

G. Cohen, The Myth of the Midlife Crisis (2005) Newsweek, p 82-86: article adapted from The Mature Mind: The Positive Power of the Brain: New York, Basic Books, (2005)

The Global Deterioration Scale for assessment of primary degenerative dementia. Reisberg B, Ferris SH, de Leon MJ, Crook T.

Successful Aging: What does the "good life" look like? Concepts in Gerontology, Lucille B. Bearon, Ph.D., Vol. 1, No. 3, Summer 1996

Resources and Contacts

The American Geriatrics Society,
The Empire State Building,
350 Fifth Avenue, Suite 801,
New York, NY 10118,
info.amger@americangeriatrics.org.

Centers for Medicare & Medicaid Services
7500Security Boulevard, Baltimore MD
21244-1850
http://ppsmds@cms.hhs.gov

http://www.governmentguide.com/govsite.O
SHHA www.osha.gov
Occupational Safety & Health
Administration 200 Constitution
Avenue, NW Washington, DC
20210

The U.S. Department of Health and Human
Services200

Independence Avenue, SW
Washington, D.C. 20201
Telephone: (202) 619-0257
Toll Free: 1 (877) 696-6775

http://www.hhs.gov/ContactUs.html
(202) 690-7850-public domain
3.Information Provided by: The National Institute of Neurological Disorders and Stroke National Institutes of Health Bethesda, MD 20892.
http://www.ninds.nih.gov/health_and_medical/disorders/alzheimersdisease_doc.htm
http://www.healthfinder.gov/orgs/HR0046.htm

Alzheimer's Association. (www.alz.org, http://www.alz.org).
U.S .Department of Health and Human Services

Substance Abuse and Mental Health Services Administration
Substance abuse among older adults
Center for substance abuse Treatment www.samhsa.gov

http://www.hhs.gov/ocr/hipaa/privacy.html

http://www.medicinenet.com/alzheimers_disease/article.htm

http://www.parkinsonsdisease.com/pcp/pcp.htm

The American Academy of Orthopedic Surgeons. permission granted.

http://www.aaos.org/wordhtml/sitemap.htm

- AmericanTherapeuticRecreationAssociation
  1414 Prince St.,
  Suite 204Alexandria, Virginia 22314-2853

- NationalTherapeuticRecreationSociety
  22377 Belmont Ridge Road Ashburn, Virginia 20148-4501

- NationalCouncilforTherapeuticRecreationCertification
  7 Elmwood Drive New City, New York10956

Conclusion

It is my greatest hope that this book will help meet the needs of the older population and better their quality of life. I hope the information in this book helps all health care providers, whether professional clinicians or family caregivers, understand the changes that occur as one ages. I hope this book teaches caregivers how to help older adults cope with some of these changes through the use of recreational activities. May this book bring many hours of fun and satisfaction to all older adults. May this book help provide the older adults with an environment full of creative, supportive, and fulfilling life experiences.

Susan Brhel

A Bio-psychosocial Approach to Therapeutic Activities and Successful Aging is Susan Brhel's second book on Older Adults care and recreational activities. Susan Brhel is also author of the book: Increasing the Quality of life for Older Adults (Geriatric Observable Activities for Longevity Program. It is her hope that education on the benefits of "activities" as an inclusive aspect in the bio-psychosocial framework of human development will promote wellness oriented environments and experience satisfying and fulfilling for our aging population.

Index

A

B

C

D

E

F

G

H

I

K

L

M

N

O

P

T

U

V

W